The Pharmacist's Pocket Guide for Diabetes and Obesity

AF213346

Jennifer Clements
Editor

The Pharmacist's Pocket Guide for Diabetes and Obesity

Practical Strategies, Tips, and Considerations

Springer

Editor
Jennifer Clements
Department of Clinical Pharmacy and Outcomes Sciences
University of South Carolina College of Pharmacy
Greenville, SC, USA

Editorial Contact: Jessica Chio

ISBN 978-3-031-88834-2 ISBN 978-3-031-88835-9 (eBook)
https://doi.org/10.1007/978-3-031-88835-9

© The Editor(s) (if applicable) and The Author(s), under exclusive license to Springer Nature Switzerland AG 2025

This work is subject to copyright. All rights are solely and exclusively licensed by the Publisher, whether the whole or part of the material is concerned, specifically the rights of translation, reprinting, reuse of illustrations, recitation, broadcasting, reproduction on microfilms or in any other physical way, and transmission or information storage and retrieval, electronic adaptation, computer software, or by similar or dissimilar methodology now known or hereafter developed.
The use of general descriptive names, registered names, trademarks, service marks, etc. in this publication does not imply, even in the absence of a specific statement, that such names are exempt from the relevant protective laws and regulations and therefore free for general use.
The publisher, the authors and the editors are safe to assume that the advice and information in this book are believed to be true and accurate at the date of publication. Neither the publisher nor the authors or the editors give a warranty, expressed or implied, with respect to the material contained herein or for any errors or omissions that may have been made. The publisher remains neutral with regard to jurisdictional claims in published maps and institutional affiliations.

This Springer imprint is published by the registered company Springer Nature Switzerland AG
The registered company address is: Gewerbestrasse 11, 6330 Cham, Switzerland

If disposing of this product, please recycle the paper.

Contents

Part I

Epidemiology and Pathophysiology of Diabetes and Obesity

1

Abby Lennon

Diabetes

Epidemiology

Prevalence

An estimated 529 million people live with all forms of diabetes, according to analysis prepared for the Global Burden of Disease Study 2021. This equates to a global age-adjusted prevalence level of 6.1%. Of the known types of diabetes, type 2 diabetes (T2D) contributes to most cases, with 96% of all cases globally being diagnosed as T2D [6]. The prevalence of diabetes has grown consistently across the globe since the 1990s, and 2050 projections show no meaningful decline in its growth with over 1.3 billion people projected to live with diabetes and global prevalence rate near 10% [1, 6].

In the United States (US), the Centers for Disease Control and Prevention estimates a total of 38.1 million adults diagnosed with diabetes, or 11.3% of the US population, with approximately 8.7

A. Lennon (✉)
Clinical Pharmacy Specialist, Bariatrics, Inova Bariatrics, Fairfax, VA, USA
e-mail: Abby.Lennon@inova.org

© The Author(s), under exclusive license to Springer Nature Switzerland AG 2025

J. Clements (ed.), *The Pharmacist's Pocket Guide for Diabetes and Obesity*, https://doi.org/10.1007/978-3-031-88835-9_1

million of those being undiagnosed [7]. On top of the substantial number of individuals estimated to have diabetes, another 97.6 million adults, or 38% of the US adult population, are estimated to have prediabetes [7]. Prediabetes is a recognizable state that identifies individuals at risk of developing T2D [8].

While T2D is the predominant form of diabetes, pharmacists and providers must be aware of all known forms given the risk of misdiagnosis followed by the potential for inappropriate therapy. Of other known types, the most common are type 1 diabetes (T1D) and gestational diabetes (GD). In the United States an estimated 5.7% of individuals report having T1D, and GD is diagnosed in 8.3% of adult individuals giving birth [5]. Other forms include monogenic diabetes syndromes or maturity-onset diabetes of the young (MODY), with estimates of 1–5% of the total diabetes population; drug-induced diabetes, with variable rates and impact depending on the offending agent; and diseases of the exocrine pancreas (e.g., pancreatitis, cystic fibrosis, neoplasms) [9].

Risk Factors

Type 2 Diabetes

The risk of developing T2D is influenced by factors both intrinsic and extrinsic to a patient. The most common intrinsic factors include age, body mass index (BMI), race/ethnicity, lack of physical activity, and a family history of diabetes in first-degree relatives [8]. It is crucial to note that while race and ethnicity are identified as risk factors, they may be heavily influenced by social determinants of health (SDOH) within an individual country or community. For example, while the American Diabetes Association (ADA) Standards appropriately state that Asian Americans and African Americans are at additional risk, global prevalence rates for diabetes are lowest in Sub-Saharan Africa, East Asia, and the Pacific. Pharmacists and providers should not overgeneralize risk based on characteristics identified within the demographics of an individual's electronic medical chart [1, 8].

Extrinsic factors, most often associated with SDOH, also heavily influence an individual's risk of developing T2D and the outcomes associated with the disease. While there are no strict definitions for SDOH categories or subcategories, categories frequently refer to economic stability, food security, neighborhood and built environment, and health care [10]. Each of these categories has been associated with an increased risk of T2D or an increased risk of associated complications (see Table 1.1). It is important for pharmacists to consider income, housing status and

Table 1.1 Social determinants of health related to diabetes

Economic stability
Income
Prevalence of diabetes increases as income decreases [11, 12]
Adults with an income less than the federal poverty level are at increased risk for diabetes-related mortality [13]
Education
Prevalence of diabetes increases as the highest degree completed decreases, with the greatest prevalence in those with less than a high school education [14]
Adults with less than a high school education have twofold mortality compared to those with a college degree [13]
Occupation
Unemployment associated with higher rates of T2D [15]
Food security
Improved food access has been associated with lower T2D rates [16]
No clear association with food affordability [17]
Neighborhood and built environment
Lack of clarity on the impact of housing instability on diabetes prevalence and outcomes given ties to economic stability [18–21]
Walkability of neighborhood environment is associated with a lower risk of T2D [22]
Environmental exposure to toxins is associated with increased risk of diabetes. Impact on historically marginalized populations is disproportionate [23–25]
Health care
Uninsured adults more likely to have undiagnosed diabetes [26]
Insurance status influences A1C [27]
Cost-related nonadherence is frequently encountered among people with diabetes, particularly those prescribed insulin [28]

Source: Refs. [11–28]

location, occupation, education, access to food and health care as part of their histories when assessing people with diabetes. Research is still developing on measures to counteract the impact of SDOH on patient care, but its impact cannot be overstated.

Type 1 Diabetes

Risk factors associated with the development of T1D include a clear genetic association. Risk factors that are less well understood, but hypothesized, include seasonality, association with viral infections, the intestinal microbiome, vaccinations, dietary factors, numerous vitamins and minerals as well as stress and socioeconomic factors [29]. Given a lower prevalence than T2D and significant differences in their pathophysiology, more research is required to better stratify a person's risk for T1D. Unlike the risk associated with the development of T2D, there is a less clear impact of SDOH factors on developing T1D, but they remain tied to outcomes associated with the condition [30].

Gestational Diabetes

The ADA defines GD as that which is diagnosed in the second or third trimester of pregnancy and was not clearly overt diabetes prior to gestation or other types of diabetes occurring throughout pregnancy [8]. It is important for pharmacists to completely evaluate the risk of people for T2D, T1D, and developing diabetes during the gestational period. Similar to the risk for T2D, age and BMI may influence the risk of developing diabetes during gestation. Additionally, family history of GD, polycystic ovary syndrome (PCOS), diet, and excessive gestational weight gain have been associated with GD risk [31–39].

Type 2 Diabetes

Pathophysiology

The development of T2D is driven by a combination of insulin resistance and a deficit in insulin secretion from pancreatic beta cells. In addition to the pancreas, adipose tissue, brain, liver, kidneys, skeletal muscle, and small intestine play a role in T2D and are colloquially known as the "Ominous Octet" [40]. Given the complexities of diabetes pathophysiology, it is important to have an understanding of how glucose homeostasis is maintained under normal conditions. While glucose at pathophysiologic levels is not harmful, it is an essential element for bodily function, and numerous organs and hormones play a substantial role in maintaining its homeostasis.

Liver

The liver is the primary organ that stores and releases glucose. During times when exogenous glucose is low, the liver breaks down glycogen through glycogenolysis and undergoes gluconeogenesis to maintain glucose homeostasis. When exogenous glucose is high, the liver undergoes glycogen synthesis and lipogenesis with glucose being incorporated into hepatocytes through insulin-independent actions. These pathways of glucose production and storage are primarily regulated by insulin and glucagon secreted by the pancreatic beta and alpha cells, respectively. Second to the pancreatic hormones, catecholamines produced by the adrenal medulla may also stimulate the liver to undergo glycogenolysis and gluconeogenesis [41–43].

Pancreas

Glucagon and insulin signal to the body to produce or store glucose. Insulin is responsible for signaling the liver to decrease glucose production and signals the muscles and adipose tissues to uptake glucose. In addition, insulin suppresses glucagon release in alpha cells and reduces the production of substrates required for gluconeogenesis. Glucagon is the body's natural counter to insulin and is responsible for stimulating the liver to initiate glycogenolysis and gluconeogenesis. Alpha cells produce glucagon in response to reduced glucose levels. In addition to the liver, glucagon is recognized to act in the kidneys. This function of glucagon is less understood, but there are potential impacts on the maintenance of electrolyte balance (e.g., potassium) and gluconeogenesis [44].

Kidneys

The kidneys play an important role in the maintenance of glucose homeostasis. They are responsible for gluconeogenesis, uptake of glucose for energy demands, and the reabsorption of filtered glucose. Similar to hepatic gluconeogenesis, renal gluconeogenesis is suppressed by insulin. During extended fasting states, the kidneys become increasingly responsible for glucose production as glycogen stores in the liver are reduced. The kidney's potential for glucose production is not often discussed, but when liver glucose production is reduced its role may be clinically relevant. What has become increasingly clinically relevant with the approval of sodium glucose cotransporter 2 (SGLT-2) inhibitors is the reabsorption of glucose in the kidneys through the SGLT family. SGLT-2 and SGLT-1 facilitate the reabsorption of glucose in the kidneys, and under normal conditions, all filtered glucose is retained. However, a threshold for reabsorption can be reached due to elevated plasma glucose which will lead to its renal excretion. SGLT-2 is the primary transporter for renal reabsorption, with almost 90% occurring through this protein. SGLT-1 is the next most prevalent transporter in the kidneys but is also found in the intestines and other tissues [45].

Incretins

Incretins are hormones produced within the gut that have a variety of physiologic actions. The two primary incretins are glucagon-like peptide-1 (GLP-1) and glucose-dependent insulinotropic peptide (GIP). Released in response to the ingestion of food, incretins modulate the production of insulin from the pancreas in the fed state. Of the two, the function and impact of GLP-1 on glucose homeostasis is better understood and has resulted in more pharmacotherapeutic options. In addition to increasing insulin release in response to food ingestion, GLP-1 increases pancreatic beta cell proliferation, decreases gastric emptying and GI motility, decreases glucagon secretion, and increases satiety. In contrast, GIP is known to enhance glucagon response in the fed state, facilitate fat deposition in adipose tissue, and promote bone formation. Incretins are readily metabolized by dipeptidyl peptidase 4 (DPP-4) under normal physiologic conditions [46].

Insulin Resistance

One of the two main drivers of T2D is insulin resistance (IR). Those with IR have a reduced ability of muscle and adipose tissue to uptake glucose as well as increased hepatic glucose output due to the inability to respond to insulin. Despite its known role in T2D, reasons for the development of IR within individual people and populations are less well known other than a clear association of obesity with the development of IR. Additionally, IR is present in several clinical conditions including PCOS, metabolic syndrome, nonalcoholic fatty liver disease, cardiovascular disease, and chronic kidney disease [47–49]. The direct measurement of IR is not routinely performed in clinical practice. Instead, glucose tolerance tests (GTT) and insulin sensitivity tests (ITT) are used as markers of IR in an individual patient. While these tests are accessible to most providers, they are not always specific markers of IR given the complex nature of glucose homeostasis within the body.

Reduced Insulin Secretion

People with T2D frequently encounter reductions in beta-cell insulin production. This has been associated with a reduction in the number of beta cells as well as decreased function. A common understanding of this pathway is that as insulin resistance develops, the pancreas and its beta cells will compensate through increased insulin production and beta cell proliferation. However, persistent IR will lead to eventual beta-cell stress, failure, and death. This process shows itself clinically through the initial development of prediabetes followed by a diagnosis of T2D. With the known potential for reduced insulin secretion, markers of insulin production such as the protein c-peptide may provide useful information in the management of people with T2D [43, 50].

This is an ideal time to note how the terminology for diabetes diagnoses has shifted due to improved understanding of the disease process. Historically, T2D has been referred to as "noninsulin-dependent diabetes mellitus" or "adult-onset diabetes" and T1D as "insulin-dependent diabetes mellitus" and "juvenile diabetes." These terms are nonspecific and have led providers and pharmacists to make quick assumptions on the type of diabetes a patient may have. The ADA Standards are increasingly clear that diagnosis should be specific to prevent mistaken diagnoses and to ensure appropriate pharmacotherapy [8].

Type 1 Diabetes

Pathophysiology

T1D is driven by the autoimmune destruction of pancreatic beta cells. It is critical for all providers to understand that the development of T1D is not simply tied to the age of a patient, as it can occur in both children and adults, with adults at high risk of an initial mistaken diagnosis of T2D. However, the primary age of onset of T1D is childhood. It is not well understood if the onset of the autoimmune response is driven by a triggering event or if it is due to random occurrence, and this question is the subject of ongoing research [51–53].

It is typical for people diagnosed with T1D to have expressed antibodies against multiple proteins associated with pancreatic beta cells, including insulin, islet cells, zinc transporter, glutamate decarboxylase, and tetraspanin-7. Typically, a patient will not present with disease-specific symptoms or progress to T1D when antibodies are present against just one protein. However, the risk of a patient developing T1D with two or more autoantibodies present is 84% [54]. The Juvenile Diabetes Foundation, ADA, and the Endocrine Society have proposed stages for people with T1D. The three stages are defined as follows: Stage 1—presence of autoantibodies, normal glycemic levels, and no symptoms; Stage 2—presence of autoantibodies, elevated glycemic levels, and no symptoms; Stage 3—presence of autoantibodies, elevated glycemic levels, and symptoms. While this staging has historically held less clinical relevance, with the advent of treatment options that delay the progression to Stage 3, it is of increasing importance [55].

Gestational Diabetes

Pathophysiology

A diagnosis of GD can be the result of either underlying or undiagnosed IR and beta cell dysfunction that leads to hyperglycemia during pregnancy or the natural physiologic changes that occur during pregnancy and are unable to be compensated for appropriately [8]. During pregnancy there are substantial changes to insulin sensitivity and resistance that occur to support the growth and development of the fetus. Typically, insulin sensitivity increases early in gestation as the body prepares for the future energy demands of the pregnancy. As the pregnancy progresses, insulin resistance increases and therefore, glucose can be readily provided for fetal growth [56–58]. Given the expectation that insulin resistance will occur, there is evidence to support that the body compensates for this through an increase in insulin production. Despite this some people who are pregnant are unable to fully compensate for IR and will develop GD [56]. In these cases, it is likely that GD will resolve after delivery, but people who develop GD are at increased risk of T2D and cardiovascular disease as well as potential negative health consequences for their child [59].

Diabetes Due to Other Causes

Monogenic Diabetes Syndromes

Single gene mutations resulting in beta cell dysfunction are traditionally classified as maturity-onset diabetes of the young (MODY). MODY is a non-autoimmune form of diabetes that may present similarly to T2D. Patients with MODY are typically in their late teens or early 20 s with hyperglycemia. These people may have less weight gain and insulin resistance as well as no autoantibodies. Pharmacists who are evaluating the potential for MODY should consider those presenting with diabetes in their teens or as a young adult who lack positive autoantibodies or those who present with limited obesity and other potential signs of insulin resistance [9].

Diseases of the Exocrine Pancreas

A number of nondiabetes-related conditions can impact the basic functions of the pancreas and result in diabetes of the exocrine pancreas (DEP). Through these people may develop transient or chronic hyperglycemia, resulting in diabetes. Given that most people will present in adulthood, diabetes may first be mistaken as T2D. The most common cause of DEP is pancreatitis, and additional sources include cystic fibrosis, pancreatic ductal adenocarcinoma, obstructions, and pancreatectomies. Distinct to this condition is the potential for a reduction in function of all islet cells, in which people may have both reduced insulin and glucagon secretion [60].

Drug-Induced Diabetes

Numerous medications have been associated with hyperglycemia as a potential side effect and are important for pharmacists to recognize and diminish potential side effects in both people with and without a diagnosis of diabetes. Of these medications, corticosteroids are most frequently associated with hyperglycemia due to their potential to worsen insulin resistance and increase hepatic glucose production. Other common classes of medications that may impact glucose levels included second-generation antipsychotics, protease inhibitors, immunosuppressants for transplant recipients, statins, and beta blockers [61–64]. It is typically expected that drug-induced diabetes may be reversed with the discontinuation of the offending agent, though this may not always be the case. Pharmacists should be readily prepared to evaluate and manage hyperglycemia in people with diabetes who are receiving these medications and consider potential strategies for mitigation when the clinical benefits of the medication outweigh any potential harm of hyperglycemia.

Diabetes-Related Comorbidities

Chronic hyperglycemia is associated with several long-term complications including both macrovascular and microvascular complications.

Macrovascular

Cardiovascular Disease

Diabetes-associated cardiovascular disease (CVD) is a primary cause of death and disability in people with diabetes. Many of the risk factors for the development of T2D are shared as risk factors for the development of CVD, including obesity, dietary choices, and physical inactivity. However, diabetes remains an independent risk factor for the development of CVD including myocardial infarction and stroke. In people with chronic hyperglycemia, there is a noted ongoing inflammatory state mediated by the release of various cytokines. This inflammatory state is associated with changes to cell-signaling pathways, including platelet activation pathways, and may lead to thrombosis. This inflammation also plays a role in the eventual development of atherosclerosis, which is tied to the presence of ongoing hyperlipidemia. The development of pharmacotherapy for the management of diabetes that both improves hyperglycemia and reduces the risk of CVD has been a crucial recent development in reducing the overall burden of disease [65].

Microvascular

Chronic Kidney Disease and Nephropathy

Diabetes-related nephropathy and the associated chronic kidney disease are leading causes of death for people with diabetes and are among the primary causes of end-stage renal disease (ESRD) globally. Chronic hyperglycemia will result in eventual renal fibrosis due to changes in the hemodynamics of the renal system. In a patient with no intervention, a typical pathway to ESRD starts with renal hypertrophy associated with increases in glomerular size. This may not be noticeable clinically due to limited to no albuminuria. As this process continues, and the glomerular basement membrane continues to thicken, microalbuminuria will begin to be identifiable and progress to eventual macroalbuminuria and significant eGFR decline [66].

Retinopathy

Diabetes retinopathy is a leading cause of blindness worldwide. As with the progression of nephropathy, hyperglycemia leads to changes in retinal hemodynamics. In the early stage, known as non-proliferative diabetic retinopathy, there are noticeable increases in vascular permeability and occlusion of the capillaries, leading to potential microaneurysms and hemorrhages. As retinopathy progresses to proliferative diabetes retinopathy, people will begin to experience significant visual impairments. These impairments are common due to diabetes macular edema, which is associated with thickening of the macula, resulting in changes to vision and eventual blindness [67].

Neuropathy

Of the three primary microvascular complications of diabetes, less is understood of the pathophysiology of diabetic peripheral neuropathy. Similar to retinopathy and nephropathy, there is an expected period of inflammation and oxidative stress due to hyperglycemia. This state results in changes in the thickness of blood vessel membranes and results in peripheral nerve ischemia. People may experience a loss of sensation and pain due to this nerve-related damage, and due to risks associated with infection may lead to eventual amputation [68].

Obesity

Epidemiology

Prevalence

Obesity is a global pandemic that, when combined with all other forms of malnutrition, is the leading cause of poor health. The World Health Organization estimates from 2022, based on the 2019 Global Burden of Disease Study, indicate that 890 million adults across the globe or about 16% of the global population are living with obesity. In addition, 160 million children globally live with obesity. In the United States, the prevalence of obesity has increased dramatically to 42.4% among adults. Rates of obesity are most pronounced among those who identify as non-Hispanic Blacks (49.6%), with rates lowest for non-Hispanic Asians (17.4%) [3–5, 69].

Risk Factors

The risk of developing obesity is tied to a variety of factors, many of which intersect with its pathophysiology and social determinants of health (SDOH). Broadly, the following areas have been implicated in individuals being obese: behavior, social and physical environments, health, biology/genetics, and psychological factors. In the next section on pathophysiology, these factors will be discussed in more detail [70].

Pathophysiology

Behavior

Behaviors are actions that are intrinsically and extrinsically motivated. While conscious thoughts drive some of our behaviors, factors such as the environment, learning history, and others may influence one's behavior without one's conscious awareness. Given this understanding of behavior and that obesity is most regularly associated with surplus energy, pharmacists should recognize that altering a person's behavior may be a complex undertaking [71]. Specific behaviors associated with obesity include, but are not limited to, overeating as a coping mechanism, decreased or reduced quality sleep, shift work (circadian misalignment), and a sedentary lifestyle [72–76].

Additional drivers of a patient's eating behavior can be tied to hormones like ghrelin and leptin. Ghrelin is colloquially known as the "hunger hormone," and while it has other effects on glucose homeostasis, its ability to drive hunger may contribute to behavior changes [77]. Leptin is a hormone that increases satiety. Research has shown that individuals living with obesity tend to be leptin resistant, and administration of exogenous leptin may not provide significant weight loss [78]. Alterations in ghrelin and leptin are seen in obesity. In patients who undergo calorie-restrictive diets, changes in their levels can be seen up to a year later and may be associated with the "yo-yo-effect" many patients experience [79]. Glucagon-like peptide-1(GLP-1) is another appetite-regulating hormone secreted from intestinal L-cells. It has a main action in appetite regulation, which slows gastric emptying, although further research has shown that it may act directly in the central nervous system to modulate appetite control centrally [78]. The therapeutic class of GLP-1 receptor agonists have been shown to be highly efficacious for weight management.

Social and Physical Environments

Within the domains of 'economic stability,' 'food security,' and 'neighborhood and built environment', some of the clearest associations with obesity prevalence are noted at the population health level. Table 1.2 describes the impacts of the SDOH domains on obesity and its prevalence.

Table 1.2 Social determinants of health related to obesity

Economic stability
Income
Increased rates of childhood obesity in the United States among families with lower socioeconomic status [80]
Education
When compared to college graduates, people with a high school education or less have higher rates of obesity [81]
Occupation
Employment discrimination and income loss are influenced by obesity status [82]
Food security
Increased grocery store availability and higher prevalence of fast-food restaurants associated with reduced weight gain [83]
Food insecurity is correlated with increased prevalence of obesity [84–86]
Neighborhood and built environment
Perceived safety within the neighborhood has been shown to correlate with reduced obesity [87]
Health care
Limited data on the relationship between being uninsured and rates of obesity

Source: Refs. [80–87]

Health

Health conditions and medications are known to influence the development and maintenance of obesity. Examples of medical conditions include obstructive sleep apnea (OSA), Cushing's syndrome, hypothyroidism, PCOS, and genetic disorders [88–94]. OSA is uniquely problematic due to its bidirectional relationship with obesity. People living with obesity are more likely to develop OSA, but the changes in sleep patterns in patients with OSA may also have a negative impact on weight [88–90]. Common psychological disorders of depression and anxiety are both associated with a higher prevalence of obesity. In addition to diagnosable disorders, stress and stigma associated with weight have been shown to impact one's weight [95–100].

Pharmacists should be aware of the numerous medications that are associated with additional weight gain. Classes of medications typically associated with weight gain include antidepressants, antipsychotics, antiepileptics, corticosteroids, insulins, and sulfonylureas. For medications used in neuropsychiatric disorders, the likelihood of increased weight gain is often associated with differential impact on serotonin, dopamine, histamine, and muscarinic receptors [101, 102]. While the potential for weight gain will be dependent on the specific agent, current lifestyle factors, and other factors, pharmacists should be prepared to actively assess an individual's risk for additional weight gain due to medication use and implement interventions that are therapeutically warranted [103].

Conclusion

Diabetes and obesity are conditions of worldwide concern. Their management and associated complications can present a significant burden to people and the medical community due to their complexity and cost. Pharmacists are readily positioned to impact people with diabetes and obesity through their knowledge of pharmacotherapy and their position in increasing access to care.

References

1. Ong KL, Stafford LK, McLaughlin SA, Boyko EJ, Vollset SE, Smith AE, et al. Global, regional, and national burden of diabetes from 1990 to 2021, with projections of prevalence to 2050: a systematic analysis for the global burden of disease study 2021. Lancet. 2023;402(10397):203–34.
2. Vos T, Lim SS, Abbafati C, Abbas KM, Abbasi M, Abbasifard M, et al. Global burden of 369 diseases and injuries in 204 countries and territories, 1990–2019: a systematic analysis for the global burden of disease study 2019. Lancet. 2020;396(10258):1204–22.
3. WHO. Obesity and overweight; 2024. Available from: https://www.who.int/news-room/fact-sheets/detail/obesity-and-overweight
4. Swinburn BA, Kraak VI, Allender S, Atkins VJ, Baker PI, Bogard JR, et al. The global syndemic of obesity, undernutrition, and climate

change: the lancet commission report. Lancet. 2019;393(10173):791–846.
5. Ward ZJ, Bleich SN, Cradock AL, Barrett JL, Giles CM, Flax C, et al. Projected U.S. state-level prevalence of adult obesity and severe obesity. N Engl J Med. 2019;381(25):2440–50.
6. Flood D, Seiglie JA, Dunn M, Tschida S, Theilmann M, Marcus ME, et al. The state of diabetes treatment coverage in 55 low-income and middle-income countries: a cross-sectional study of nationally representative, individual-level data in 680 102 adults. Lancet Healthy Longev. 2021;2(6):e340–51.
7. CDC. Diabetes; 2024. National Diabetes Statistics Report. Available from: https://www.cdc.gov/diabetes/php/data-research/index.html
8. American Diabetes Association Professional Practice Committee, ElSayed NA, Aleppo G, Bannuru RR, Bruemmer D, Collins BS, et al. 2. Diagnosis and classification of diabetes: *standards of Care in Diabetes—2024*. Diabetes Care. 2024;47(Supplement_1):S20–42.
9. Nkonge KM, Nkonge DK, Nkonge TN. The epidemiology, molecular pathogenesis, diagnosis, and treatment of maturity-onset diabetes of the young (MODY). Clin Diab Endocrinol. 2020;6(1):20.
10. Hill-Briggs F, Adler NE, Berkowitz SA, Chin MH, Gary-Webb TL, Navas-Acien A, et al. Social determinants of health and diabetes: a scientific review. Diabetes Care. 2021;44(1):258–79.
11. Braveman PA, Cubbin C, Egerter S, Williams DR, Pamuk E. Socioeconomic disparities in health in the United States: what the patterns tell us. Am J Public Health. 2010;100(S1):S186–96.
12. Gaskin DJ, Thorpe RJ, McGinty EE, Bower K, Rohde C, Young JH, et al. Disparities in diabetes: the nexus of race, poverty, and place. Am J Public Health. 2014;104(11):2147–55.
13. Saydah S, Lochner K. Socioeconomic status and risk of diabetes-related mortality in the U.S. Public Health Rep. 2010;125(3):377–88.
14. CDC. Centers for Disease Control and Prevention; 2022. Diabetes Report Card. Available from: https://archive.cdc.gov/diabetes/library/reports/reportcard.html
15. Varanka-Ruuska T, Rautio N, Lehtiniemi H, Miettunen J, Keinänen-Kiukaanniemi S, Sebert S, et al. The association of unemployment with glucose metabolism: a systematic review and meta-analysis. Int J Public Health. 2018;63(4):435–46.
16. Ahern M, Brown C, Dukas S. A National Study of the association between food environments and county-level health outcomes: food environments and county-level health outcomes. J Rural Health. 2011;27(4):367–79.
17. Kern DM, Auchincloss AH, Stehr MF, Diez Roux AV, Moore KA, Kanter GP, et al. Neighborhood price of healthier food relative to unhealthy food and its association with type 2 diabetes and insulin resistance: the multi-ethnic study of atherosclerosis. Prev Med. 2018;106:122–9.

18. Keene DE, Guo M, Murillo S. "That wasn't really a place to worry about diabetes": housing access and diabetes self-management among low-income adults. Soc Sci Med. 2018;197:71–7.
19. Quensell ML, Taira DA, Seto TB, Braun KL, Sentell TL. "I need my own place to get better": patient perspectives on the role of housing in potentially preventable hospitalizations. J Health Care Poor Underserved. 2017;28(2):784–97.
20. Gelberg L, Andersen RM, Leake BD. The behavioral model for vulnerable populations: application to medical care use and outcomes for homeless people. Health Serv Res. 2000;34(6):1273–302.
21. Bernstein RS, Meurer LN, Plumb EJ, Jackson JL. Diabetes and hypertension prevalence in homeless adults in the United States: a systematic review and meta-analysis. Am J Public Health. 2015;105(2):e46–60.
22. Smalls BL, Gregory CM, Zoller JS, Egede LE. Assessing the relationship between neighborhood factors and diabetes related health outcomes and self-care behaviors. BMC Health Serv Res. 2015;15(1):445.
23. Kuo CC, Moon K, Thayer KA, Navas-Acien A. Environmental chemicals and type 2 diabetes: an updated systematic review of the epidemiologic evidence. Curr Diab Rep. 2013;13(6):831–49.
24. Gee GC, Payne-Sturges DC. Environmental health disparities: a framework integrating psychosocial and environmental concepts. Environ Health Perspect. 2004;112(17):1645–53.
25. Krometis LA, Gohlke J, Kolivras K, Satterwhite E, Marmagas SW, Marr LC. Environmental health disparities in the central Appalachian region of the United States. Rev Environ Health. 2017;32(3)
26. Danaei G, Friedman AB, Oza S, Murray CJ, Ezzati M. Diabetes prevalence and diagnosis in US states: analysis of health surveys. Popul Health Metrics. 2009;7(1):16.
27. Ngo-Metzger Q, Sorkin DH, Billimek J, Greenfield S, Kaplan SH. The effects of financial pressures on adherence and glucose control among racial/ethnically diverse patients with diabetes. J Gen Intern Med. 2012;27(4):432–7.
28. Kang H, Lobo JM, Kim S, Sohn MW. Cost-related medication non-adherence among U.S. adults with diabetes. Diabetes Res Clin Pract. 2018;143:24–33.
29. Rewers M, Stene LC, Norris JM. Risk factors for type 1 diabetes. In: Cowie CC, Casagrande SS, Menke A, Cissell MA, Eberhardt MS, Meigs JB, et al., editors. Diabetes in America. 3rd ed. Bethesda: National Institute of Diabetes and Digestive and Kidney Diseases; 2018. Available from: http://www.ncbi.nlm.nih.gov/books/NBK567965/.
30. Morone JF, Teitelman AM, Cronholm PF, Hawkes CP, Lipman TH. Influence of social determinants of health barriers to family management of type 1 diabetes in black single parent families: a mixed methods study. Pediatr Diabetes. 2021;22(8):1150–61.

31. Ben-Haroush A, Yogev Y, Hod M. Epidemiology of gestational diabetes mellitus and its association with type 2 diabetes. Diabet Med. 2004;21(2):103–13.
32. Metzger BE, Buchanan TA, Coustan DR, De Leiva A, Dunger DB, Hadden DR, et al. Summary and recommendations of the fifth international workshop-conference on gestational diabetes mellitus. Diabetes Care. 2007;30(Supplement_2):S251–60.
33. Okosun IS, Chandra KMD, Boev A, Boltri JM, Choi ST, Parish DC, et al. Abdominal adiposity in U.S. adults: prevalence and trends, 1960–2000. Prev Med. 2004;39(1):197–206.
34. Durnwald C. Gestational diabetes: linking epidemiology, excessive gestational weight gain, adverse pregnancy outcomes, and future metabolic syndrome. Semin Perinatol. 2015;39(4):254–8.
35. Zhang C, Tobias DK, Chavarro JE, Bao W, Wang D, Ley SH, et al. Adherence to healthy lifestyle and risk of gestational diabetes mellitus: prospective cohort study. BMJ. 2014;349:g5450.
36. Jenum AK, Mørkrid K, Sletner L, Vange S, Torper JL, Nakstad B, et al. Impact of ethnicity on gestational diabetes identified with the WHO and the modified International Association of Diabetes and Pregnancy Study Groups criteria: a population-based cohort study. Eur J Endocrinol. 2012;166(2):317–24.
37. Anghebem-Oliveira MI, Martins BR, Alberton D, Ramos EADS, Picheth G, Rego FGDM. Type 2 diabetes-associated genetic variants of FTO, LEPR, PPARg, and TCF7L2 in gestational diabetes in a Brazilian population. Arch Endocrinol Metab. 2017;61(3):238–48.
38. Lao TT, Ho LF, Chan BCP, Leung WC. Maternal age and prevalence of gestational diabetes mellitus. Diabetes Care. 2006;29(4):948–9.
39. Pettitt DJ, Jovanovic L. Low birth weight as a risk factor for gestational diabetes, diabetes, and impaired glucose tolerance during pregnancy. Diabetes Care. 2007;30(Supplement_2):S147–9.
40. American Diabetes Association. Diagnosis and classification of diabetes mellitus. Diabetes Care. 2014;37(Supplement_1):S81–90.
41. Titchenell PM, Lazar MA, Birnbaum MJ. Unraveling the regulation of hepatic metabolism by insulin. Trends Endocrinol Metab. 2017;28(7):497–505.
42. Cherrington AD, Moore MC, Sindelar DK, Edgerton DS. Insulin action on the liver *in vivo*. Biochem Soc Trans. 2007;35(5):1171–4.
43. Galicia-Garcia U, Benito-Vicente A, Jebari S, Larrea-Sebal A, Siddiqi H, Uribe KB, et al. Pathophysiology of type 2 diabetes mellitus. Int J Mol Sci. 2020;21(17):6275.
44. Betts JG, Young KA, Wise JA, Johnson E, Poe B, Kruse DH, et al. 17.9 The Endocrine Pancreas – Anatomy and Physiology 2e | OpenStax; 2022. Available from: https://openstax.org/books/anatomy-and-physiology-2e/pages/17-9-the-endocrine-pancreas

45. Gerich JE. Role of the kidney in normal glucose homeostasis and in the hyperglycaemia of diabetes mellitus: therapeutic implications. Diabet Med J Br Diabet Assoc. 2010;27(2):136–42.
46. Kim W, Egan JM. The role of incretins in glucose homeostasis and diabetes treatment. Pharmacol Rev. 2008;60(4):470–512.
47. Sharabi K, Tavares CDJ, Rines AK, Puigserver P. Molecular pathophysiology of hepatic glucose production. Mol Asp Med. 2015;46:21–33.
48. Johnson AMF, Olefsky JM. The origins and drivers of insulin resistance. Cell. 2013;152(4):673–84.
49. Samuel VT, Shulman GI. Mechanisms for insulin resistance: common threads and missing links. Cell. 2012;148(5):852–71.
50. Christensen AA, Gannon M. The Beta cell in type 2 diabetes. Curr Diab Rep. 2019;19(9):81.
51. Atkinson MA, Eisenbarth GS. Type 1 diabetes: new perspectives on disease pathogenesis and treatment. Lancet. 2001;358(9277):221–9.
52. Atkinson MA, Eisenbarth GS, Michels AW. Type 1 diabetes. Lancet. 2014;383(9911):69–82.
53. Flier JS, Underhill LH, Eisenbarth GS. Type I diabetes mellitus. N Engl J Med. 1986;314(21):1360–8.
54. Ziegler AG, Rewers M, Simell O, Simell T, Lempainen J, Steck A, et al. Seroconversion to multiple islet autoantibodies and risk of progression to diabetes in children. JAMA. 2013;309(23):2473.
55. Insel RA, Dunne JL, Atkinson MA, Chiang JL, Dabelea D, Gottlieb PA, et al. Staging presymptomatic type 1 diabetes: a scientific statement of JDRF, the Endocrine Society, and the American Diabetes Association. Diabetes Care. 2015;38(10):1964–74.
56. Di Cianni G, Miccoli R, Volpe L, Lencioni C, Del Prato S. Intermediate metabolism in normal pregnancy and in gestational diabetes. Diabetes Metab Res Rev. 2003;19(4):259–70.
57. Catalano PM, Tyzbir ED, Roman NM, Amini SB, Sims EAH. Longitudinal changes in insulin release and insulin resistance in nonobese pregnant women. Am J Obstet Gynecol. 1991;165(6):1667–72.
58. Parsons JA, Brelje TC, Sorenson RL. Adaptation of islets of Langerhans to pregnancy: increased islet cell proliferation and insulin secretion correlates with the onset of placental lactogen secretion. Endocrinology. 1992;130(3):1459–66.
59. Plows JF, Stanley JL, Baker PN, Reynolds CM, Vickers MH. The pathophysiology of gestational diabetes mellitus. Int J Mol Sci. 2018;19(11):3342.
60. Wynne K, Devereaux B, Dornhorst A. Diabetes of the exocrine pancreas. J Gastroenterol Hepatol. 2019;34(2):346–54.
61. Luna B. Drug-induced hyperglycemia. JAMA. 2001;286(16):1945.
62. Anyanwagu U, Idris I, Donnelly R. Drug-induced diabetes mellitus: evidence for statins and other drugs affecting glucose metabolism. Clin Pharmacol Ther. 2016;99(4):390–400.

63. Chen J, Huang XF, Shao R, Chen C, Deng C. Molecular mechanisms of antipsychotic drug-induced diabetes. Front Neurosci. 2017;21(11):643.
64. Jain V, Patel RK, Kapadia Z, Galiveeti S, Banerji M, Hope L. Drugs and hyperglycemia: a practical guide. Maturitas. 2017;104:80–3.
65. Rodriguez-Araujo G, Nakagami H. Pathophysiology of cardiovascular disease in diabetes mellitus. Cardiovasc Endocrinol Metab. 2018;7(1):4–9.
66. Lin YC, Chang YH, Yang SY, Wu KD, Chu TS. Update of pathophysiology and management of diabetic kidney disease. J Formos Med Assoc. 2018;117(8):662–75.
67. Wang W, Lo ACY. Diabetic retinopathy: pathophysiology and treatments. Int J Mol Sci. 2018;19(6):1816.
68. Schreiber AK, Nones CF, Reis RC, Chichorro JG, Cunha JM. Diabetic neuropathic pain: physiopathology and treatment. World J Diabetes. 2015;6(3):432–44.
69. Okunogbe A, Nugent R, Spencer G, Powis J, Ralston J, Wilding J. Economic impacts of overweight and obesity: current and future estimates for 161 countries. BMJ Glob Health. 2022;7(9):e009773.
70. Safaei M, Sundararajan EA, Driss M, Boulila W, et al. A systematic literature review on obesity: understanding the causes & consequences of obesity and reviewing various machine learning approaches used to predict obesity. Comput Biol Med. 2021;136:104754.
71. Romieu I, Dossus L, Barquera S, Blottière HM, Franks PW, et al. Energy balance and obesity: what are the main drivers? Cancer Causes Control. 2017;28(3):247–58.
72. Macht M. How emotions affect eating: a five-way model. Appetite. 2008;50(1):1–11.
73. Cappuccio FP, Taggart FM, Kandala NB, Currie A, Peile E, Stranges S, et al. Meta-analysis of short sleep duration and obesity in children and adults. Sleep. 2008;31(5):619–26.
74. McHill AW, Wright KP. Role of sleep and circadian disruption on energy expenditure and in metabolic predisposition to human obesity and metabolic disease. Obes Rev. 2017;18(S1):15–24.
75. Broussard JL, Van Cauter E. Disturbances of sleep and circadian rhythms: novel risk factors for obesity. Curr Opin Endocrinol Diabetes Obes. 2016;23(5):353–9.
76. Myers A, Gibbons C, Finlayson G, Blundell J. Associations among sedentary and active behaviours, body fat and appetite dysregulation: investigating the myth of physical inactivity and obesity. Br J Sports Med. 2017;51(21):1540–4.
77. Pradhan G, Samson SL, Sun Y. Ghrelin: much more than a hunger hormone. Curr Opin Clin Nutr Metab Care. 2013;16(6):619–24.
78. Schneeberger M, Gomis R, Claret M. Hypothalamic and brainstem neuronal circuits controlling homeostatic energy balance. J Endocrinol. 2014;220(2):T25–46. https://doi.org/10.1530/JOE-13-0398.

79. Heymsfield SB, Harp JB, Reitman ML, Beetsch JW, Schoeller DA, Erondu N, et al. Why do obese patients not lose more weight when treated with low-calorie diets? A mechanistic perspective. Am J Clin Nutr. 2007;85(2):346–54.
80. Singh GK, Kogan MD, Van Dyck PC, Siahpush M. Racial/ethnic, socioeconomic, and behavioral determinants of childhood and adolescent obesity in the United States: analyzing independent and joint associations. Ann Epidemiol. 2008;18(9):682–95.
81. Ogden CL, Fakhouri TH, Carroll MD, Hales CM, Fryar CD, Li X, et al. Prevalence of obesity among adults, by household income and education – United States, 2011–2014. MMWR Morb Mortal Wkly Rep. 2017;66(50):1369–73.
82. Forse RA, Betancourt-Garcia MM, Kissee MC. Epidemiology and discrimination in obesity. In: Nguyen NT, Brethauer SA, Morton JM, Ponce J, Rosenthal RJ, editors. The ASMBS textbook of bariatric surgery. Cham: Springer International Publishing; 2020. p. 3–14. https://doi.org/10.1007/978-3-030-27021-6_1.
83. Buszkiewicz JH, Bobb JF, Kapos F, Hurvitz PM, Arterburn D, Moudon AV, et al. Differential associations of the built environment on weight gain by sex and race/ethnicity but not age. Int J Obes. 2021;45(12):2648–56.
84. Kowaleski-Jones L, Wen M, Fan JX. Unpacking the paradox: testing for mechanisms in the food insecurity and BMI association. J Hunger Environ Nutr. 2019;14(5):683–97.
85. Farrell P, Thow AM, Abimbola S, Faruqui N, Negin J. How food insecurity could lead to obesity in LMICs. Health Promot Int. 2018;33(5):812–26.
86. Moradi S, Mirzababaei A, Dadfarma A, Rezaei S, Mohammadi H, Jannat B, et al. Food insecurity and adult weight abnormality risk: a systematic review and meta-analysis. Eur J Nutr. 2019;58(1):45–61.
87. Powell-Wiley TM, Moore K, Allen N, Block R, Evenson KR, Mujahid M, et al. Associations of neighborhood crime and safety and with changes in body mass index and waist circumference. Am J Epidemiol. 2017;186(3):280–8.
88. Shechter A. Effects of continuous positive airway pressure on energy balance regulation: a systematic review. Eur Respir J. 2016;48(6):1640–57.
89. Shechter A. Obstructive sleep apnea and energy balance regulation: a systematic review. Sleep Med Rev. 2017;34:59–69.
90. Drager LF, Brunoni AR, Jenner R, Lorenzi-Filho G, Bensenor IM, Lotufo PA. Effects of CPAP on body weight in patients with obstructive sleep apnoea: a meta-analysis of randomised trials. Thorax. 2015;70(3):258–64.
91. Laurberg P, Knudsen N, Andersen S, Carlé A, Pedersen IB, Karmisholt J. Thyroid function and obesity. Eur Thyroid J. 2012;1(3):159–67.

92. Nieman LK, Biller BMK, Findling JW, Newell-Price J, Savage MO, Stewart PM, et al. The diagnosis of Cushing's syndrome: an Endocrine Society clinical practice guideline. J Clin Endocrinol Metab. 2008;93(5):1526–40.
93. Bays H, Scinta W. Adiposopathy and epigenetics: an introduction to obesity as a transgenerational disease. Curr Med Res Opin. 2015;31(11):2059–69.
94. Yildiz BO, Bozdag G, Yapici Z, Esinler I, Yarali H. Prevalence, phenotype and cardiometabolic risk of polycystic ovary syndrome under different diagnostic criteria. Hum Reprod. 2012;27(10):3067–73.
95. Van Der Valk ES, Savas M, Van Rossum EFC. Stress and obesity: are there more susceptible individuals? Curr Obes Rep. 2018;7(2):193–203.
96. Tomiyama AJ. Weight stigma is stressful. a review of evidence for the cyclic obesity/weight-based stigma model. Appetite. 2014;82:8–15.
97. Faith MS, Butryn M, Wadden TA, Fabricatore A, Nguyen AM, Heymsfield SB. Evidence for prospective associations among depression and obesity in population-based studies. Obes Rev. 2011;12(5):e438. https://doi.org/10.1111/j.1467-789X.2010.00843.x.
98. De Wit L, Luppino F, Van Straten A, Penninx B, Zitman F, Cuijpers P. Depression and obesity: a meta-analysis of community-based studies. Psychiatry Res. 2010;178(2):230–5.
99. Milaneschi Y, Simmons WK, Van Rossum EFC, Penninx BW. Depression and obesity: evidence of shared biological mechanisms. Mol Psychiatry. 2019;24(1):18–33.
100. Rajan T, Menon V. Psychiatric disorders and obesity: a review of association studies. J Postgrad Med. 2017;63(3):182–90.
101. Fleischhacker WW, Heikkinen ME, Olié JP, Landsberg W, Dewaele P, McQuade RD, et al. Effects of adjunctive treatment with aripiprazole on body weight and clinical efficacy in schizophrenia patients treated with clozapine: a randomized, double-blind, placebo-controlled trial. Int J Neuropsychopharmacol. 2010;13(08):1115–25.
102. Henderson DC, Vincenzi B, Andrea NV, Ulloa M, Copeland PM. Pathophysiological mechanisms of increased cardiometabolic risk in people with schizophrenia and other severe mental illnesses. Lancet Psychiatry. 2015;2(5):452–64.
103. Medici V, McClave SA, Miller KR. Common medications which lead to unintended alterations in weight gain or organ lipotoxicity. Curr Gastroenterol Rep. 2016;18(1):2.

Part II

Clinical Assessment 2

Lourdes Cross

Clinical Presentation of Diabetes

Type 1 Diabetes

Type 1 diabetes (T1D) accounts for 5–10% of adult diabetes cases [1]. Onset peaks during childhood and adolescence but can occur at any age. At diagnosis, individuals with T1D usually have lower body mass index (BMI) measurements, usually <25 kg/m^2, and present as lean or thin [2]. The hallmark symptoms leading up to diagnosis result from insulin deficiency and hyperglycemia. These include:

- Frequent urination (polyuria)
- Excessive thirst (polydipsia)
- Increased appetite (polyphagia)
- Unexpected weight loss
- Fatigue/lethargy
- Blurred vision

L. Cross (✉)
Department of Pharmacy Practice, Sullivan University College of Pharmacy and Health Sciences, Louisville, KY, USA
e-mail: LVCross@sullivan.edu

© The Author(s), under exclusive license to Springer Nature Switzerland AG 2025

J. Clements (ed.), *The Pharmacist's Pocket Guide for Diabetes and Obesity*, https://doi.org/10.1007/978-3-031-88835-9_2

Onset of symptoms ranges from weeks to months. As blood glucose exceeds renal thresholds (~180 mg/dL), glucosuria promotes osmotic diuresis and hypovolemia, causing polyuria and polydipsia [3]. Individuals may also present acutely with diabetic ketoacidosis (DKA) as the initial manifestation. This acute complication reflects deficient insulin combined with increases in counterregulatory hormones (e.g., glucagon, cortisol, catecholamines) and leads to hyperglycemia, ketosis, and metabolic acidosis [4].

Latent autoimmune diabetes in adults (LADA) represents a subtype of T1D with distinct clinical features that appear gradually, typically occurring after age 35. Current estimates suggest LADA may account for up to 10% of adults originally misdiagnosed with type 2 diabetes (T2D) [5]. Individuals with LADA exhibit a lower prevalence of metabolic syndrome compared to those with T2D [6]. The distinguishing characteristic of LADA is the gradual destruction of pancreatic beta cells by autoimmune processes, similar to T1D. This leads to gradual development of insulin deficiency over months to years. Most individuals require insulin therapy as endogenous insulin production declines.

Type 2 Diabetes

T2D accounts for most diabetes cases in adults. It is a complex metabolic disorder characterized by chronic hyperglycemia that commonly occurs in the setting of overweight or obesity. Many individuals with T2D meet the diagnostic criteria for metabolic syndrome and have a family history, highlighting the role of genetic risk. Newly diagnosed individuals may exhibit hyperglycemia-related symptoms, such as polyuria, polydipsia, polyphagia, blurred vision, slow wound healing, recurrent infections, and lack of energy. However, T2D can also develop gradually without clearly identifiable symptoms. Thus, periodic blood glucose screening is vital even in asymptomatic adults. In rare cases, severely uncontrolled hyperglycemia can progress to a hyperosmolar hyperglycemic state—marked by extreme hyperglycemia, dehydration, and neurological changes—in the absence of ketoacidosis. While DKA is atypical for the initial presentation of T2D, acute illnesses or infections can sometimes trigger this emergency complication.

Ketosis-prone diabetes represents an intermediary form of diabetes with features of both T1D and T2D [1]. It is characterized by ketoacidosis occurring in individuals who do not fit the typical clinical presentation of autoimmune T1D. Ketosis-prone diabetes usually affects those of non-Caucasian ethnicity and exhibits intermittent insulin deficiency between ketoacidosis episodes [7]. The presence of autoantibodies and beta cell dysfunction helps distinguish subtypes that may require lifelong insulin therapy from those that can transition to oral agents [8]. The exact mechanisms causing beta cell dysfunction in ketosis-prone diabetes remain unclear.

Diagnostic Criteria

Accurate, timely diagnosis of diabetes relies on established diagnostic criteria that health-care professionals can utilize to guide individuals with prediabetes and diabetes. The primary screening modalities include fasting plasma glucose (FPG), 2-hour oral glucose tolerance test (OGTT), and glycosylated hemoglobin (A1C) [1]. These tests are equally suitable for diagnostic screening (Table 2.1). While OGTT is not often favored due to its inconvenience, it remains a preferred option to diagnose gestational diabetes mellitus (GDM).

In symptomatic individuals, a random blood glucose ≥200 mg/dL can confirm a diagnosis of diabetes [1]. For asymptomatic cases, current criteria are: FPG ≥126 mg/dL, 2-hour glucose during 75-g OGTT ≥200 mg/dL, or A1C ≥6.5% [1]. Repeat testing showing two abnormal results from the same or separate samples is recommended when symptoms are absent. Discordant results should prompt evaluation for interfering conditions such as inadequate fasting, recent illness, or sample mishandling. Specific high-risk groups may also experience A1C variability independent of glycemic status. This includes those with hemoglobinopathies, pregnancy, advanced kidney disease, human

Table 2.1 Diagnostic criteria for prediabetes and diabetes

	Normal/ Euglycemia	Prediabetes	Diabetes
A1C (%)[a]	<5.7	5.7–6.4	≥6.5
Fasting plasma glucose (mg/dL)[a,b]	<100	100–125	≥126
2-h plasma glucose (mg/dL)[a,c]	<140	140–199	≥200
Random plasma glucose (mg/dL)	–	–	≥200 + symptoms[d]

Source: Ref. [1]

[a]Repeat testing showing two abnormal results from the same or separate samples is recommended when symptoms are absent

[b]Fasting defined as no caloric intake for at least 8 h

[c]75-g oral glucose tolerance test

[d]Polyuria, polydipsia, polyphagia, blurred vision, weakness, unexplained weight loss

immunodeficiency virus, and recent blood transfusions. In these cases, only plasma glucose criteria should be used to confirm diagnoses [1].

Screening for Diabetes

Screening for diabetes is critical for early detection and intervention to mitigate long-term complications. Initial risk stratification helps identify individuals needing diagnostic testing, primarily A1C, FPG, or OGTT.

Type 1 Diabetes

At the time of diagnosis, individuals with T1D typically present with acute symptoms, dangerously elevated blood glucose levels, and a significant risk of life-threatening DKA. A family history of autoimmune diabetes, coupled with either a personal background or familial instances of allergic diseases or other autoimmune conditions, elevates the risk of developing T1D compared to that of the general population [1]. Because T1D develops from autoimmune destruction of insulin-producing beta cells, screening involves detecting autoantibodies predictive of future clinical disease. Testing for islet cell autoantibodies (ICA) and autoantibodies to insulin, glutamic acid decarboxylase (GAD), islet tyrosine phosphatases islet antigen 2 (IA-2) and IA-2β, and zinc transporter 8 (ZnT8) can identify those at high risk of developing symptomatic hyperglycemia warranting close monitoring [1]. According to the American Diabetes Association (ADA) Standards, the test for GAD antibodies should be conducted first when screening for antibodies related to diabetes. If negative, it should be followed up by testing for IA-2 or ZnT8 antibodies. In antibody-positive individuals, assessing glycemic indices further stratifies near-term diabetes risk. When multiple autoantibodies are detected, it is advisable to consider additional testing as applicable to determine if the individual meets criteria for therapy that may potentially delay development of clinical diabetes.

Type 2 Diabetes

The ADA Standards recommend screening adults with overweight or obesity (BMI ≥25 kg/m^2 or ≥ 23 kg/m^2 for Asian Americans) if they have additional risk factors such as family history, high-risk ethnicity, hypertension, or history of gestational diabetes (Table 2.2) [1]. Considering that the risk of T2D increases with age, guidelines also advise screening all adults ≥35 years every 3 years. Those with multiple risk markers may benefit from annual screening. Preferred diagnostic tests are A1C, FPG, or 2-hour OGTT. For screening through OGTT, it is essential to ensure adequate carbohydrate intake (≥150 g/day) for 3 days before the test [1].

Due to growing pediatric obesity, screening children and adolescents with overweight (BMI ≥85th percentile) or obesity (BMI ≥95th percentile) plus other risk factors for diabetes is also recommended after the onset of puberty or by age 10 years [1]. Early identification promotes timely lifestyle and pharmaceutical interventions to preserve long-term health in younger, high-risk groups.

Table 2.2 Screening recommendations

Prediabetes or diabetes in adults
1. Consider in adults with BMI ≥25 kg/m^2 (or ≥ 23 kg/m^2 in Asian Americans) with one of the following risk factors: First-degree relative with diabetes High-risk race/ethnicity (e.g., African American, Latino, native American, Asian American, Pacific islander) History of cardiovascular disease Hypertension (≥130/80 mmHg or taking medications for hypertension) HDL cholesterol level <35 mg/dL and/or a triglyceride level >250 mg/dL Polycystic ovary syndrome Physical inactivity Other conditions association with insulin resistance (e.g., acanthosis nigricans)
2. Individuals with prediabetes should be tested annually
3. Individuals who were diagnosed with gestational diabetes should be tested at least every 3 years and should have lifelong testing
4. In the absence of the above criteria, testing should begin at age 35 years
5. Conduct repeat testing at least once every 3 years in individuals with normal blood glucose levels, adjusting the frequency based on blood glucose values and individual risk factors
6. Individuals with HIV: Screen with a fasting glucose test prior to starting ART, at the time of switching ART, and 3–6 months after starting or switching ART If results are normal, fasting glucose should be monitored annually
7. Individuals taking high-risk medications: For individuals prescribed second-generation antipsychotic medications, initially screen for prediabetes and diabetes, then retest 12–16 weeks after starting the medication, or sooner if clinically warranted, followed by annual screenings thereafter Consider screening individuals taking other medications associated with an increased risk of these conditions (e.g., glucocorticoids, statins, thiazide diuretics)
Postpancreatitis diabetes mellitus
1. Screen for diabetes within 3–6 months after an episode of acute pancreatitis, then annually thereafter
2. Individuals with chronic pancreatitis should be screened for diabetes annually

(continued)

Table 2.2 (continued)

Cystic fibrosis-related diabetes
1. Individuals with cystic fibrosis who have not been previously diagnosed with cystic fibrosis-related diabetes should be screened annually, starting at age 10
Posttransplantation diabetes mellitus
1. Individuals should be screened for hyperglycemia after an organ transplant
2. A diagnosis of posttransplantation diabetes mellitus should be confirmed when an individual is stable on an immunosuppressive regimen and does not have an acute infection

Source: Ref. [1]

ART antiretroviral therapy, *BMI* body mass index, *HDL* high-density lipoprotein, *HIV* human immunodeficiency virus

Other Diabetes Classifications

Screening for less common forms of diabetes should be considered in clinical practice (Table 2.2). Specifically, screening for postpancreatitis diabetes mellitus is warranted in those with a history of pancreatic complications. For individuals with cystic fibrosis, where cystic fibrosis-related diabetes stands as a prevalent comorbidity, annual screening starting at age 10 is recommended [1]. While hyperglycemia frequently manifests in the early posttransplant phase, a conclusive diagnosis of posttransplantation diabetes mellitus should be established once the individual is stable on maintenance immunosuppression and is without acute infection. Subsequent screening intervals should be tailored to each individual.

Gestational Diabetes

Screening for gestational diabetes mellitus (GDM) should begin at the initial prenatal visit with glucose assessment in women with preexisting risk factors for T2D. However, all pregnant women

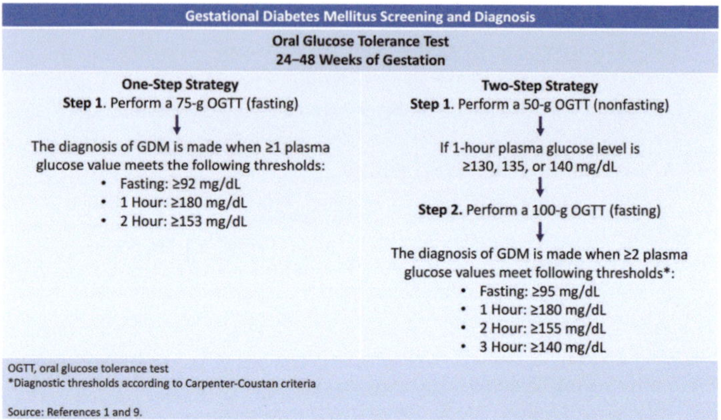

Fig. 2.1 Gestational diabetes mellitus screening and diagnosis

should undergo GDM testing at 24–28 weeks of gestation, even if earlier screening is negative. Preferred diagnostic tests include a one-step 75-g fasting OGTT or a two-step approach with a 50-g nonfasting glucose load test followed by a fasting 100-g OGTT for those exceeding threshold values [1, 9]. Established GDM diagnostic cut points exist for the one-step and two-step methods based on elevated fasting, 1, 2, and 3-h plasma glucose levels during OGTT (Fig. 2.1). Identifying and promptly treating GDM decreases maternal and fetal morbidity including preeclampsia, fetal overgrowth, shoulder dystocia, neonatal hypoglycemia, and perinatal mortality [10]. Furthermore, women with histories of GDM have nearly sevenfold lifetime risks of developing T2D and thus require ongoing monitoring after delivery [11].

Differential Diagnosis

Type 1 Versus Type 2 Diabetes

Distinguishing type 1 versus T2D has implications for treatment plans and diabetes education. Factors favoring T1D include lean body habitus without metabolic syndrome features, acute symptomatic onset, unexplained weight loss, personal/family history of autoimmunity, and presence of DKA. In contrast, factors favoring T2D diagnosis include overweight/obesity, metabolic syndrome comorbidities (e.g., hypertension, dyslipidemia), lack of autoimmunity, gradual symptomatic onset, and the absence of DKA at presentation (Table 2.3) [1]. Testing for autoantibodies (e.g., ICA, GAD-65, IA-2, ZnT8) can confirm an autoimmune pathophysiology indicative of T1D or LADA [1]. Additionally, simultaneous measurement of C-peptide and glucose levels gauges endogenous insulin reserves and helps categorize degrees of insulin deficiency [1]. Low C-peptide predicts insulin requirement and can prompt initiation of replacement therapy. Pursuing diagnostic clarity through autoantibody profiling and C-peptide measurement ensures accurate classification of diabetes subtypes, allowing for individualization of treatment regimens to the underlying pathophysiology.

Table 2.3 Differences in features between T1D and T2D

	T1D	T2D
Age at diagnosis	Usually childhood/ adolescence	Adulthood
Body mass index	Normal (or underweight)	Overweight or obese
Family history of diabetes	Negative or positive	Frequently positive
Onset of symptoms	Weeks to months	Months to years
Acute complications at diagnosis	Increased	Mildly increased
Long-term complications at diagnosis	Low	High
Autoimmunity	Increased	Absent
C-peptide levels at diagnosis	Often nondetectable	Normal to increased
Insulin resistance	Usually absent	Increased
Insulin requirement	At diagnosis	Absent or years after diagnosis

Source: Ref. [1]
T1D type 1 diabetes, *T2D* type 2 diabetes

Drug-Induced Hyperglycemia

Distinguishing drug-induced hyperglycemia from uncontrolled diabetes is vital to prevent improper initiation or intensification of hypoglycemic therapy. Common medications can alter glycemic control through effects on insulin sensitivity, insulin production and secretion, and glucose utilization (Table 2.4). Examples of

Table 2.4 Medications associated with increased blood glucose levels

Medication/drug class[a]	Proposed mechanism	Comment
Atypical antipsychotics[b]	Increase insulin resistance, decrease insulin secretion, weight gain	The greatest risk is associated with olanzapine and clozapine, while aripiprazole and ziprasidone pose a lower risk
Beta blockers	Increase insulin resistance, decrease insulin secretion	Non-vasodilating beta blockers such as atenolol, metoprolol, and propranolol pose the greatest risk, whereas vasodilating beta blockers like carvedilol, labetalol, and nebivolol are not associated with hyperglycemia
Glucocorticoids[b]	Increase insulin resistance, decrease insulin secretion	The greatest risk is associated with parenteral and oral formulations, but topical formulations can occasionally pose a risk as well
HMG-CoA reductase inhibitors (statins)	Increase insulin resistance, decrease insulin secretion	The American Diabetes Association recommends statin therapy for most people with diabetes who have existing cardiovascular disease or cardiovascular risk factors, as the benefits outweigh the risks
Protease inhibitors[b]	Increase insulin resistance, decrease insulin secretion, promote lipodystrophy	The risk does not vary significantly among the different protease inhibitors

(continued)

Table 2.4 (continued)

Medication/drug class[a]	Proposed mechanism	Comment
Thiazide and thiazide-like diuretics	Increase insulin resistance, decrease insulin secretion, secondary to hypokalemia	Hyperglycemia may be dose-related and prevented through management of hypokalemia, although mixed evidence has been reported. A potassium level below 4.0 mmol/L may potentially increase the risk of drug-induced diabetes

Source: Refs. [12–16]

[a]The list includes only ones commonly encountered in primary care settings

[b]In this table, atypical antipsychotics, glucocorticoids, and protease inhibitors have the most significant risk of causing drug-induced hyperglycemia

high-risk drug classes include atypical antipsychotics, glucocorticoids, and protease inhibitors [12–16]. These medications carry risks of triggering hyperglycemic crises ranging from severe sustained hyperglycemia to DKA or hyperosmolar hyperglycemic states, particularly in older individuals with comorbidities. Health-care professionals can educate individuals about the risk of drug-induced hyperglycemia, emphasizing the need for appropriate glucose monitoring and offering therapeutic recommendations to mitigate potential risks associated with medications.

Summary The clinical presentation of diabetes is highly heterogeneous given the diversity of risk factors and underlying pathophysiologic processes involved across type 1, type 2, and other specific subtypes. Key distinguishing features in the symptoms, diagnostic and screening approaches, and risk factor profiles can help guide accurate categorization of diabetes subtypes. Utilizing established criteria and testing methodologies facilitates timely, evidence-based diagnoses. Health-care professionals play critical roles in assessing diabetes risk, interpreting optimal screening modalities, and initiating collaborative treatment plans tailored to individuals with diabetes.

References

1. American Diabetes Association Professional Practice Committee. 2. Diagnosis and classification of diabetes: standards of care in diabetes−2024. Diabetes Care. 2024;47(Suppl 1):S20–42.
2. Holt RIG, DeVries JH, Hess-Fischl A, Hirsch IB, Kirkman MS, Klupa T, et al. The management of type 1 diabetes in adults. A consensus report by the American Diabetes Association (ADA) and the European Association for the Study of diabetes (EASD). Diabetes Care. 2021;44(11):2589–625.
3. Vallon V, Komers R. Pathophysiology of the diabetic kidney. Compr Physiol. 2011;1(3):1175–232.
4. Chiasson J-L, Aris-Jilwan N, Bélanger R, Bertrand S, Beauregard H, Ekoé J-M, et al. Diagnosis and treatment of diabetic ketoacidosis and the hyperglycemic hyperosmolar state. CMAJ. 2003;168(7):859–66.
5. Naik RG, Brooks-Worrell BM, Palmer JP. Latent autoimmune diabetes in adults. J Clin Endocrinol Metab. 2009;94(12):4635–44.
6. Pozzilli P, Pieralice S. Latent autoimmune diabetes in adults: current status and new horizons. Endocrinol Metab (Seoul, Korea). 2018;33(2):147–59.
7. Umpierrez GE, Smiley D, Kitabchi AE. Narrative review: ketosis-prone type 2 diabetes mellitus. Ann Intern Med. 2006;144(5):350–7.
8. Balasubramanyam A, Nalini R, Hampe CS, Maldonado M. Syndromes of ketosis-prone diabetes mellitus. Endocr Rev. 2008;29(3):292–302.
9. Mellitus GD. ACOG practice bulletin no. 190: gestational diabetes mellitus. Obstet Gynecol. 2018;131(2):e49–64.
10. Ornoy A, Becker M, Weinstein-Fudim L, Ergaz Z. Diabetes during pregnancy: a maternal disease complicating the course of pregnancy with long-term deleterious effects on the offspring. A clinical review. Int J Mol Sci. 2021;22(6)
11. Bellamy L, Casas J-P, Hingorani AD, Williams D. Type 2 diabetes mellitus after gestational diabetes: a systematic review and meta-analysis. Lancet (London, England). 2009;373(9677):1773–9.
12. Fathallah N, Slim R, Larif S, Hmouda H, Ben SC. Drug-induced hyperglycaemia and diabetes. Drug Saf. 2015;38(12):1153–68.
13. Zillich AJ, Garg J, Basu S, Bakris GL, Carter BL. Thiazide diuretics, potassium, and the development of diabetes: a quantitative review. Hypertension. 2006;48(2):219–24.
14. De Hert M, Detraux J, van Winkel R, Yu W, Correll CU. Metabolic and cardiovascular adverse effects associated with antipsychotic drugs. Nat Rev Endocrinol. 2011;8(2):114–26.
15. Tsiodras S, Mantzoros C, Hammer S, Samore M. Effects of protease inhibitors on hyperglycemia, hyperlipidemia, and lipodystrophy: a 5-year cohort study. Arch Intern Med. 2000;160(13):2050–6.
16. Lansang MC, Hustak LK. Glucocorticoid-induced diabetes and adrenal suppression: how to detect and manage them. Cleve Clin J Med. 2011;78:748–56.

Non-pharmacologic Interventions for Type 2 Diabetes

3

Alaina Van Dyke and Carly Lacey

Introduction

Importance of Non-pharmacologic Interventions

In the United States, most diagnosed cases of diabetes are classified as type 2 diabetes (T2D) (90–95% of cases) while type 1 diabetes (T1D) is much less common (5–10% of cases) [1]. While T1D is caused by an autoimmune reaction where the body attacks and destroys the cells of the pancreas that produce insulin, T2D is largely a lifestyle-related chronic condition that manifests as insulin resistance, though genetics may play a role as well. Several large, randomized controlled trials (RCTs) have proven that lifestyle and behavioral interventions are particularly effective in preventing and delaying the onset of T2D, as well as improving other cardiometabolic markers (e.g., blood pressure, cholesterol, and inflammation) [2–5]. Evidence also exists suggesting that certain

A. Van Dyke (✉) · C. Lacey
Department of Pharmacy Practice, Jerry H. Hodge School of Pharmacy, Texas Tech University Health Sciences Center, Dallas, TX, USA
e-mail: Alaina.VanDyke@ttuhsc.edu; Carly.Lacey@ttuhsc.edu

© The Author(s), under exclusive license to Springer Nature Switzerland AG 2025

J. Clements (ed.), *The Pharmacist's Pocket Guide for Diabetes and Obesity*, https://doi.org/10.1007/978-3-031-88835-9_3

lifestyle and behavioral interventions have the ability to treat, and in some cases reverse, T2D [6]. Most clinical practice guidelines for diabetes recommend lifestyle interventions as first-line in the prevention and treatment of T2D and should include, at a minimum, personalized prescriptions for a healthy meal plan, regular physical activity and exercise, and healthful behavior practices [7–9]. While engaging in a healthy lifestyle is also important for people living with T1D, focus on non-pharmacologic interventions can prevent and treat T2D in adults.

The Pharmacist's Role in Non-pharmacologic Interventions

Evidence supports the efficacy and cost-effectiveness of lifestyle behavior modification programs for the prevention and treatment of T2D [7, 10]. Therefore, it is important that all members of the health-care team become well versed in providing lifestyle education and counseling to people with T2D and those at high risk. The pharmacist can play a key role in lifestyle-related education and counseling, motivational interviewing to promote behavioral change, and deprescribing pharmacologic therapy as necessary in people who are engaged in intensive lifestyle change.

Lifestyle Modifications as a Cornerstone of Treatment

In June 2020, the American College of Lifestyle Medicine published a position statement that reads: "sufficiently intensive lifestyle intervention (intensive therapeutic lifestyle change), particularly adopting a predominantly whole food, plant-based dietary pattern, exercise, and sleep, may be comparable to bariatric surgery, a commonly recognized means of effectively achieving T2D remission, but without the potential for side effects" [6]. This position statement is the result of an extensive literature review and summarizes the evidence supporting key lifestyle interventions for T2D remission. In this paper, remission is defined as "achieving glycemia below the diabetic range in the absence of active pharmacologic or surgical therapy of at least 1 year's duration." The position statement also serves as a call to action to begin adopting remission as the clinical treatment goal for people with T2D. However, even when remission is not the goal or is unable to be achieved with adequate, intensive lifestyle intervention, evidence strongly supports the use of lifestyle and behavior modifications for the prevention and treatment of T2D [6].

Lifestyle medicine as treatment and prevention for T2D is not a novel concept; rather, it is already embedded within American Diabetes Association (ADA) and American Association of Clinical Endocrinology (AACE) guidelines. The AACE 2023 T2D management algorithm notes that "lifestyle modification underlies all therapy" as step 1 in the treatment algorithm and "includes exercise, healthy dietary changes, smoking cessation, and reduced alcohol intake" [9]. The ADA 2024 Standards of Care in Diabetes not only discusses lifestyle change in the context of management of diabetes, but also in the setting of prevention in people with prediabetes or obesity [7]. Specifically, for people with overweight or obesity, the ADA recommends "an intensive lifestyle behavior change program to achieve and maintain a weight reduction of at least 7% of initial body weight" via healthy eating and physical activity [7]. Evidence for this recommendation derives from the assessment of several major RCTs: the Diabetes Prevention Program (DPP), the Finnish Diabetes Prevention Study (DPS), and the Da Qing Diabetes Prevention Study (Da Qing study) [2–4].

In the DPP, adults at high risk of developing T2D were divided into three groups: standard lifestyle plus metformin, standard lifestyle plus placebo, or intensive lifestyle modification alone [2]. For standard lifestyle participants, change information covering food intake, importance of weight loss, and instructions to increase physical activity was provided in written format as well as in one annual in-person session. In contrast, the intensive lifestyle intervention group participated in 16 lessons in a one-on-one session discussing individualized habits for food intake, exercise, and behavior change. Compared with the standard lifestyle plus placebo group, the lifestyle plus metformin group's incidence of

T2D was 31% lower and the intensive lifestyle group's incidence of T2D was 58% lower after an average follow-up period of 2.8 years. Since the education of pharmacists focuses on pharmacotherapy, additional focus on aspects of lifestyle modification is beneficial for making guideline-directed recommendations for people with diabetes and those at risk for developing diabetes.

Dietary Interventions

As previously mentioned, T2D is considered a lifestyle-related chronic disease in that many lifestyle choices may influence the development and progression of the condition. Nutrition, or dietary pattern, is one such lifestyle factor that has been shown to have a large impact on diabetes. In fact, in adult people with T2D, medical nutrition therapy (MNT) has demonstrated reductions in hemoglobin A1C (A1C) similar to what is seen with pharmacologic treatment options available for T2D, with decreases in A1C up to 2.0% at 3–6 months [11]. In other studies, specific dietary patterns, such as a whole-food, plant-based eating pattern and the Mediterranean diet, have been shown to improve glycemic control, promote weight loss, and improve cardiovascular disease (CVD) risk factors [12, 13]. While there is no consensus on one particular eating pattern for the prevention and treatment of T2D, most guidelines recognize dietary interventions as a vital component of diabetes management [8, 9, 13, 14].

Table 3.1 summarizes several popular dietary patterns that have been investigated for the management of T2D. While all eating patterns described can be used safely in the short term (1–2 years), it is wise to consider long-term maintenance of a Mediterranean-style pattern as this is the only dietary intervention shown to have long-term safety data for protection against CVD morbidity and mortality as well as all-cause mortality [17, 18]. Regardless of the dietary pattern that is followed, there are a few overarching themes that should be applied to all eating patterns for people with T2D to optimize health outcomes, including:

Table 3.1 Summary of dietary patterns for people with diabetes

Dietary pattern	Characteristics	Outcomes in diabetes	Additional comments
Mediterranean	↑ Vegetables, nuts, fruits, beans, and whole grains; uses olive oil as the principal source of dietary fat; moderate consumption of fish, other seafood, dairy products, and wine; ↓ red and processed meat; ↓ sugar	↓ Risk of DM ↓ A1C, BP, and triglycerides ↑ Weight loss and healthy weight maintenance Primary and secondary prevention of major CVD events and mortality	Only meal pattern with RCTs showing long-term benefits regarding CVD events and mortality

(continued)

Table 3.1 (continued)

Dietary pattern	Characteristics	Outcomes in diabetes	Additional comments
Vegan	↑ Plant-based foods × all animal-derived products (dairy, eggs, meat, fish)	↓ Risk of DM ↓ A1C ↑ Weight loss ↓ LDL and non-HDL cholesterol	No long-term safety data; requires supplementation of certain vitamins and minerals Lower risk of T2D than any ovo-vegetarians
Lacto-ovo vegetarian	Plant-based pattern free of all flesh foods but including egg (ovo) and dairy (lactose) products × red meat	↓ Risk of DM ↓ A1C ↑ Weight loss ↓ LDL and non-HDL cholesterol	No long-term safety data
Low fat	↑ Vegetables, fruits, starches (e.g., breads, pasta, whole grains, starchy vegetables), lean protein, and low-fat dairy products (defined as total fat intake ≤30% of total calories and saturated fat intake ≤10%)	↓ Risk of DM ↓ A1C, BP, and triglycerides	No long-term safety data

Very low fat	Typically consists of the following the breakdown of macronutrients: 70–77% carbohydrate, 13–20% protein, and 10% fat	↓ BP ↑ Weight loss	No long-term safety data
Low carbohydrate	Often defined as limiting carbohydrate to 26–45% of total calories ↑ Vegetables low in carbohydrate content, meat, poultry, fish, shellfish, eggs, cheese, nuts, oils, butter, and avocado × foods high in starch and sugar such as pasta, rice, potatoes, bread, and some fruits	↓ A1C, BP, and triglycerides ↑ Weight loss ↑ HDL cholesterol	No long-term safety data. When compared with a low-fat pattern, there are greater benefits early (3–6 months) followed by equilibration at 1–2 years Contraindicated in T1D, simultaneous use of SGLT-2i, pregnancy, breastfeeding, cardiac arrythmias [15]
Paleo	↑ Lean meat, shellfish, vegetables, eggs, nuts, berries × grains, dairy, salt, refined fats, sugar	Mixed results	Inconclusive evidence
Very low carbohydrate (VLC)	Defined as limiting non-fiber carbohydrate to 20–50 g/day (<26% of total calories) to induce ketosis, resulting in >50% of calories from fat	↓ A1C, BP, and triglycerides ↑ Weight loss ↑ HDL cholesterol	No long-term safety data

(continued)

Table 3.1 (continued)

Dietary pattern	Characteristics	Outcomes in diabetes	Additional comments
Dietary approaches to stop hypertension (DASH)	↑ Whole grains, vegetables, fruits, low-fat dairy products, poultry, and fish ↓ Saturated fat, red meat, sweets, and sugar-containing beverages ↓ Sodium intake	↓ Risk of DM ↓ Blood glucose, BP, and lipids in DM	No long-term safety data
Intermittent fasting	Ranges from restricting food for 18–20 h per day to alternating fasting and eating days to longer periods	↓ Weight, BP ± A1C results vary from no change to reduction ↑ Insulin sensitivity	Includes fasting for religious purposes No safety data in pregnancy or people with disordered eating

Adapted from sources: Refs. [8, 10, 12, 16]

A1C hemoglobin A1C, *BP* blood pressure, *CVD* cardiovascular disease, *DM* diabetes mellitus, *HDL* high-density lipoprotein, *LDL* low-density lipoprotein, *RCT* randomized controlled trials, *SGLT-2i*, sodium-glucose transport protein 2 inhibitors

1. Increase intake of whole foods and limit highly processed foods.
2. Emphasize non-starchy vegetables and fruits.
3. Minimize added sugar and refined grains.

Exercise and Physical Activity

Exercise and Physical Activity in Type 2 Diabetes

Although commonly used interchangeably, physical activity and exercise are distinct terms. Physical activity is a broad, all-encompassing phrase referring to increased energy use above the body's baseline through any movement that involves skeletal muscle contraction [19]. More specifically, exercise refers to physical activity intended to improve a person's health or physical fitness that is "planned, structured, [and] repetitive" [19]. Including both physical activity and exercise in discussions with people with T2D is important, as increases in both forms of movement lead to beneficial health implications (see Table 3.2). On the other hand, people should be educated and encouraged to reduce periods of uninterrupted sedentary activity due to increased risk of worsened glycemic control associated with prolonged inactivity over 30 min [14].

Guideline Recommendations

Current T2D guidelines highlight the importance of physical activity and exercise and provide specific recommendations regarding weekly duration goals and type of activities (refer to Table 3.3). Themes from both guidelines (ADA and AACE) include a combination of aerobic and anaerobic activity as well as decreasing sedentary time. Common to both guidelines, breaking up activity throughout the week should be encouraged rather than aggregating all activity into 1 or 2 days. For people with underlying heart, lung, or kidney conditions, consult their respective specialists or an exercise specialist prior to the initiation of exercise.

Table 3.2 Types of physical activity and exercise with selected benefits in people with T2D

Type	Examples	Selected benefits
Aerobic exercise	Walking Cycling Jogging Swimming	↑ Insulin sensitivity ↓ A1C ↓ Triglycerides ↓ BP ↓ Insulin resistance
Resistance exercise	Free weights Weight machines Body weight exercises Elastic resistance band exercises	↑ Glycemic control ↓ Insulin resistance ↓ BP ↓ Fat mass ↑ Lean body mass ↑ Strength
Physical activity	Balance training Stretching Tai chi (flexibility, balance, and resistance) Yoga (flexibility, balance, and resistance)	↑ Balance ↑ Range of motion ↓ Falls ↑ Glycemic control (except stretching →no impact)

Source: Ref. [20]
A1C hemoglobin A1C, *BP* blood pressure

Types and Intensity of Exercise and Person-Specific Considerations

One straightforward way to discuss exercise intensity in a person-friendly manner is to utilize the talk test [19]. During easy activities, a person can sing whereas during vigorous activity, a person may need to catch their breath after only several words. During moderate activities, a person can talk but not sing. By incorporating the talk test into the ADA or AACE guidelines for intensity of activity, people can begin to gauge their own activity level more accurately and potentially document their progress as their physical fitness improves.

Besides the talk test, there are two other common methods for measuring physical activity intensity. The first is via monitoring the heart rate. If a person's maximal (max) heart rate is estimated, it can be utilized to define a relative exercise intensity. To estimate max heart rate, subtract a person's age from 220. Utilizing max

Table 3.3 Selected physical activity and exercise recommendations from ADA and AACE guidelines

Guideline	ADA 2024	AACE 2022
Highly recommended	None	Create individualized prescription for physical activity involving aerobic and resistance exercise and reduction in sedentary behavior Initial prescription for aerobic physical activity may require a progressive increase in the volume and intensity of exercise Goal is 150 min/week of moderate exercise during 3–5 sessions per week with moderate intensity = activity that achieves a heart rate 50–60% higher than one's basal heart rate Include resistance exercises that use the major muscle groups 2–3 times/week Individuals should also incorporate flexibility and range-of-motion training Reduce sedentary behavior by encouraging increase in non-exercise and/or active leisure activity

(continued)

Table 3.3 (continued)

Guideline	ADA 2024	AACE 2022
Moderately recommended	For adults with T2D, recommendations include ≥150 min per week of moderate-to vigorous-intensity aerobic activity spread over at least 3 days/week with ≤2 consecutive days of inactivity Younger or more physically fit individuals could complete shorter durations (≥75 min/week) of vigorous-intensity or interval training Resistance exercise includes 2–3 sessions/week on nonconsecutive days For all people with diabetes, evaluate baseline physical activity and sedentary time (i.e., quiet sitting, lying, and leaning) If not meeting activity guidelines, encourage an increase in physical activities (e.g., walking, yoga, housework, gardening, swimming, and dancing)	None
Conditionally recommended	Older adults with diabetes can be encouraged to complete flexibility and balance training 2–3 times/week. Yoga and tai chi may be included based on individual preferences to increase flexibility, muscular strength, and balance Prolonged sitting should be interrupted every 30 min for blood glucose benefits	None

Selected details	Adults with T2D can be encouraged to complete aerobic activity bouts ≥10 min, with the goal of ≥30 min/day most days of the week Resistance exercises include weights, weight machines, elastic bands, or body weight. Each session should include ≥1 one set of ≥5 different resistance exercises involving the large muscle groups Daily exercise (or ≤ 2 days between sessions) is recommended to decrease insulin resistance in all type of diabetes	Avoid breaks >2–3 days between exercise sessions to retain insulin sensitivity Resistance training session includes single-set repetitions targeting major muscle groups. Recommendation includes either (1) 150 min weekly based on 30 min of moderate intensity exercise for 5 days or (2) 20–25 min of moderate intensity exercise 3 days/week for total of 60–75 min weekly plus resistance training including each major muscle group 2–3 days/week

Adapted from source: Refs. [12, 14]
ADA American diabetes association, *AACE* American association of clinical endocrinology, *min* minutes

heart rate, moderate intensity exercise would be classified as 64–76% of max heart rate and vigorous activity is 77–93% [21]. For example, for a 40-year-old person, max heart rate would be estimated at 180 beats per minute (bpm). After multiplying max heart rate by the specified ranges for moderate and vigorous activity above, the following target heart ranges would result:

- Moderate activity: 115–137 bpm.
- Vigorous activity: 138–167 bpm.

Checking pulse in the neck, wrist, or chest is a free method to monitor exercise intensity, if one is reminded to utilize their index and middle fingers rather than the thumb since the thumb has a pulse. For the technologically savvy person, many wearable heart rate monitors or smartwatches are available to track heart rate, and these can connect to smartphone applications as a method to determine relative exercise intensity. Another method for measuring intensity is via metabolic equivalent of task (MET)-minutes [19]. A MET is a single unit ratio that quantifies an activity's energy expenditure compared to energy expenditure at rest. Thus, when a body is at rest, the energy expended equals 1 MET. On the other hand, running a 10-min mile is equal to 10 METs. By multiplying the METs of an activity by the time the activity is completed over, MET-minutes can be calculated. For example, running 10-min miles (10 METs) for 60 min would equal 600 MET-min (or 10 MET-hours). Exercise intensity is classified as follows: low intensity is less than 3.0 METs, moderate-intensity is 3.0–5.9 METs, and vigorous-intensity activity is 6.0 or more METs. Since the T2D guidelines recommend 75 min of vigorous activity or 150 min of moderate-intensity activity weekly, this is equivalent to 500–1000 MET-min weekly. See Table 3.4 for examples of various exercise intensities.

When discussing recommendations for increased physical activity, consider the FITT (frequency, intensity, time, and type) principle to help people set goals and work toward guideline recommendations for exercise [22]. An example FITT recommendation for a person with diabetes who currently walks their dog once a week for 30 min includes "walk 3 times weekly while able to

Table 3.4 Example activities for each intensity level

Low (Less than 3.0 METs)	Moderate (3.0–5.9 METs)	High (6.0 or more METs)
Walking less than 2.5 mph	Walking 2.5 mph Bicycling less than 10 mph Dancing Yardwork Doubles tennis Yoga	Jogging/running Bicycling over 10 mph Singles tennis HIIT

Source: Ref. [19]
HIIT high intensity interval training, *METs* metabolic equivalent of tasks, *mph* miles per hour

talk to their dog (moderate intensity) for 30 min." By including all four facets of FITT, people with diabetes can leave their medical appointments with structured recommendations rather than vague encouragement to simply increase exercise.

Practical Tips for Incorporating Physical Activity into Daily Life and Overcoming Barriers

When discussing physical activity with people, encourage them to share their personal barriers to allow for individualized goal setting. If a person reports that they only exercise when their significant other can join them, remind them of their own autonomy and explore styles of activity where they can listen to music or a podcast rather than waiting for their significant other. Additionally, you may recommend that this person try group exercise classes if having company or camaraderie during exercise is important to them.

For people with limited time due to family or work obligations, remind them that the diabetes guidelines specifically state that even 10 min of activity at a time will count toward their exercise goal for the day. Encourage people to walk during their lunch breaks, park in the farthest parking spots from the entrance at their destinations, and take the stairs rather than elevators, when possible. For people who are technology savvy, encourage the use of smartphones or watches to track daily step counts. Remind people that the 2024 ADA guidelines cite a 2–9% decrease in cardiovascular morbidity and all-cause mortality with a daily increase of 500 steps [14].

When discussing physical activity, as with all other lifestyle interventions, it is important to set SMART goals for the person, that is, those that are specific, measurable, attainable, relevant, and time bound [23]. In lifestyle medicine, the concept of SMART-EST goals adds to the familiar concept with advice that goals should also be evidence-based, strategic, and tailored. Table 3.5 provides descriptions of each facet of SMART-EST goal setting.

By setting goals using the SMART-EST method, people can start at any level and work toward attaining the guideline-recommended levels of activity [24]. This same strategy can be applied throughout the other non-pharmacologic areas discussed in this chapter.

Table 3.5 SMART-EST goals defined with practical examples

Factor	Description	Example	Avoid
Specific	Include details on type and amount of exercise	Walk 30 min 5 times per week	Vague instructions to "increase activity".
Measurable	Quantify time, amount, or percentage of the activity	Eat entirely plant-based meals for 1 out of 3 meals daily	General instructions to "increase plant-based meals"
Attainable	Set a practical goal based on the person's current status	Begin walking 5 min daily for person who is currently sedentary	Starting with goal of "exercise 150 min per week" in a person who is currently sedentary

(continued)

Table 3.5 (continued)

Factor	Description	Example	Avoid
Relevant	Focus on a behavior the person views as valuable and desires to achieve	If a person smokes and drinks sodas daily but is only interested in focusing on diabetes management today, focus on decreasing sodas	Person who ambulates using a walker due to severe osteoarthritis of the hips is unlikely to run 5 km
Time-bound	Set a determined timeframe for completion of the goal	Expected follow-up in 1 month	Setting a goal without an end date or a check-in date
Evidence based	Select interventions that are beneficial and supported by guidelines and research	Based on ADA recommendations, goal of at least 5% weight loss for people with T2D and obesity	Setting goals based on celebrities or unverified social media personalities online
Strategic	Utilize motivational interviewing to help set goals based on a person's readiness to change	Person reports 0 out of 10 motivation to quit drinking eight sodas daily. Start with a focus on documenting daily added sugar intake to increase awareness	Person reports 2 out of 10 motivation to quit smoking, avoid forcing selection of a quit date
Tailored	Ensure the goals are appropriate for a given person	If a person reports eating fast-food hamburgers 7 times weekly, consider increasing by one home-cooked meal each week rather than starting with a ban on fast food	If a person does not currently drink alcohol, avoid reiterating a goal of drinking less than 2 drinks daily is unnecessary

Source: Ref. [23]
ADA American Diabetes Association

Weight Management

Weight loss has many benefits in T2D management including improvement in insulin resistance, reduction in insulin doses, and reduction in non-insulin therapies [24]. Due to recent approvals in weight loss medications, weight loss goals are now targeted up to 15% of body weight, with sustained weight losses over 10% associated with possible remission in T2D and benefits for cardiovascular outcomes and mortality [24]. Refer to the obesity section and related chapters for more details on weight management strategies.

Sleep Health and Diabetes Control

Understanding the Connection Between Sleep and Diabetes

The impact of sleep disturbances on diabetes is complex, but it is known that sleep disorders are a risk factor for developing T2D. Sleep disturbances, which include insufficient or excess sleep duration, poor quality of sleep, a diagnosed sleep disorder (such as obstructive sleep apnea [OSA] or insomnia), and circadian misalignment, have been linked to insulin resistance, glucose intolerance, increased risk of obesity, diabetes, and poor glycemic control in people with T2D [25–27]. Several proposed mechanisms for these findings include decreased glucose utilization by the brain during waking hours, increased sympathetic nervous system activity (which reduces insulin secretion and promotes insulin resistance), increased systemic inflammatory response, and changes in appetite-regulating hormones [27].

Sleep assessments should be conducted for all people suspected of having sleep disturbances, especially those with T2D or those at high risk, and referrals to sleep medicine specialists and behavioral health professionals should be made as indicated. Below are some common sleep assessments and tools to help identify sleep-related problems.

- Sleep diary: captures typical daily sleep patterns over at least a 1-week period; ideally, it should include data on time in bed, bedtime, wake time, time awake during sleep period, and time out of bed.
- Retrospective mini-sleep assessment: captures average sleep patterns, such as bedtime, waketime, and sleep duration, on weekdays and weekends.
- STOP-BANG (Snoring history, tired during the day, observed stop breathing while sleep, high blood pressure, body mass index more than 35 kg/m^2, age more than 50 years, neck circumference more than 40 cm, and male gender): screens for OSA in people with multiple risk factors.
- Epworth Sleepiness Scale: helps providers recognize daytime sleepiness.
- ASHA (Adolescent Sleep Hygiene Survey): helps providers identify negative beliefs about sleep and behaviors leading to poor sleep quality and quantity in adults and adolescents.

Strategies for Improving Sleep

Despite there being a strong link between sleep disturbance and T2D, there is limited published evidence exploring whether optimizing sleep quality and duration will reduce the risk of diabetes or improve glycemic control in those with established diabetes. Nonetheless, it is important to emphasize healthy sleep behaviors to promote optimal physiological functioning, which can reduce the risk of certain diabetes complications such as CVD and may aid in improved glycemic control. When considering lifestyle-based strategies to implement for improving sleep, several areas should be addressed, including sleep patterns, sleep environments, and daytime and pre-bedtime behaviors [28–30].

Sleep patterns consist of one's typical duration, timing, and quality of sleep. The National Sleep Foundation recommends all adults should get 7–9 h of sleep each night. If an assessment of sleep patterns reveals excessive sleep or time in bed, then limiting time in bed is recommended. If the issue is insufficient sleep duration, then extending the sleep period is recommended. Either way, the most effective strategy for adjusting sleep duration is to do so slowly, increasing or decreasing time in bed by 15–30 min per week. It is also advisable to keep sleep duration consistent on all days of the week, ensuring less than a 1-h difference between weekdays and weekends [28–30].

The optimal sleep environment has been compared to that of a cave—dark, cool, and quiet. Light is a well-known disruptor of sleep, and therefore, it is important to minimize all sources of light, even intermittent sources (e.g., lights from a car passing by the window or flipping on the light to go to the bathroom at night). Black out curtains or an eye mask can aid in reducing light exposure during the night, if necessary. Since light, or lack of light, is an important regulator of the body's circadian rhythm, it is also recommended to reduce late afternoon/early evening light exposure by using dim lights (table lamps versus overhead lights), closing windows and blinds in the late afternoon, and wearing blue-light blocking glasses in the evenings, if needed. Likewise, it is important to introduce bright light upon waking first thing in the morning. Another common sleep disruptor is external noise, which should also be minimized to the extent possible. This can be done with the use of white noise (a consistent, non-variable noise) or a free-standing fan set to medium or high. Avoid sleeping with any noises that are variable in nature, including noise from a television, radio, or other sound machines and devices. Lastly, keeping the environment cool, but not cold, is important as our body cannot regulate temperature during sleep the same way it does during wake periods. The ideal temperature for sleep for most people is between 60 and 67 °F [28–30].

Daytime and pre-bedtime behaviors are often overlooked despite being an important component of sleep health. Light exposure was addressed above with the sleep environment. Some additional daytime behaviors and activities to consider are as follows: limit daytime caffeinated beverages, especially in the late afternoon, and eliminate nighttime caffeinated beverages; avoid alcohol within 3 h of bedtime; eliminate post-dinner snacking and avoid high-sodium foods, especially with dinner; ensure sufficient fluid intake throughout the day; increase daytime physical activity; and discontinue all stimulating activities 60–90 min prior to bedtime. A pre-bedtime routine that promotes sleep should also be established and implemented approximately 15–20 min before bed each night. This may include 3–5 non-stimulating activities that are done outside or in bed, but preferably outside of the bedroom. An example pre-bedtime routine may consist of gentle stretching (5 min), brushing teeth and skin care (5 min), reading a book, journaling, or meditation (10 min). These activities will need to be individualized and may change slightly over time.

Stress Management and Mental Health

As a chronic illness, T2D leads to many stressors including financial, emotional, and social [14]. In fact, the ADA Standards recommend psychosocial screening for anxiety, depression, and disordered eating in all people with T2D and additional focused screening in older adults for cognitive impairment and depression [14]. In people on insulin therapies or sulfonylureas, additional care should be taken to address fear of hypoglycemia as well as a focus on prevention. Diabetes distress, the term given to the unique emotional and negative psychological impact of a chronic illness, can impact not only people with diabetes, but also their family and caregivers. When mental health concerns are identified via screening, referral to a mental health provider is vital to help address concerns and assist people with cognitive behavioral therapy, mindfulness, and potential pharmacotherapy. If a person is deemed to have life-threatening or suicidal thoughts, emergent mental health assistance should be offered. Offer people the suicide help line (#988) as a phone number for mental health emergencies. As a pharmacist, one way to decrease distress for people with diabetes in the clinic or ambulatory setting is to educate them and their caregivers about their disease state and medications to help reduce anxiety due to uncertainty.

Mindfulness is a helpful tool that can be utilized for overall stress reduction in both people with diabetes and their pharmacists. The practice of mindfulness is based on foundational knowledge about stress, which can be divided into positive stress and negative stress [31]. Positive stress helps with motivation and is associated with productivity, such as thought of reaching goals and healthy challenges. Negative stress, otherwise called distress, crosses into unproductive territory, and is associated with common disease states (i.e., obesity, diabetes, and cardiovascular disease). Implementation of mindfulness techniques has been shown to improve mood and coping skills while decreasing distress. Use caution in suggesting mindfulness or meditation practices in people with a past medical history of psychosis, seizures, post-traumatic stress, or severe depression due to risk of triggering episodes of these conditions. Mind and body practices including meditation, yoga, and art and music therapy are emerging areas of evidence. In fact, the American Heart Association has released a statement supporting adjunctive use of meditation to reduce cardiovascular risk given the modality's low cost, low risk, and possible benefit, pending further research [32].

As a pharmacist, mindfulness can be incorporated in appointments to help decrease diabetes distress. The Centers for Disease Control and Prevention (CDC) offers a 15-min scenario to offer to people with diabetes in a group or individual setting (see https://www.cdc.gov/diabetes/professional-info/toolkits/new-beginnings/mindfulness.html) [33]. Meditation topics from the CDC to quickly incorporate into appointments and offer to people with diabetes to utilize in their lives outside the clinic include:

- Create a list of people, pets, events, and things to be thankful for, spending time to dwell on positive thoughts for each item on the list.
- Create a personal mantra and repeat internally or aloud.
- Set aside 10 min to solely focus on breathing; and/or.
- Practice mindfulness prior to and directly following a meal to gain awareness for emotional eating or overeating.

Smoking Cessation

Benefits of smoking cessation are well-characterized throughout the medical literature. In the 2020, US Surgeon General's report on smoking cessation, health benefits of smoking cessation include reduction in cancer (including lung, laryngeal, oral cavity, pharynx, esophagus, pancreas, bladder, colorectal, liver, and kidney) and CVD (reduction of inflammation, improvement in HDL levels, reduction in stroke and cardiovascular morbidity and mortality) [34]. Per the Surgeon General's report, quitting smoking is beneficial no matter a person's age and improves quality of life. The ADA recommends counseling all people who smoke to avoid use of all tobacco products including e-cigarettes and utilize a combination of counseling and pharmacological therapy to assist with quit attempts [14].

Pharmacological therapy includes bupropion, varenicline, and nicotine replacement therapy, each optimized based on availability, pricing, and a person's comorbidities. While advertised as less harmful than combustible cigarettes, e-cigarettes and vapes are associated with lung injury and are not without risk [35]. People with diabetes have elevated risk of macrovascular conditions when compared to healthy people, and smoking serves to amplify this risk and impact morbidity and mortality. Thus, individuals should be advised to quit at every encounter with a health-care professional.

Smoking Cessation Resources

Many resources exist to help people who desire to quit smoking or are considering quitting. The national smoking cessation quit line (1–800-QUIT-NOW) provides counseling and referral to state-specific programs to assist with smoking cessation, no matter where a person is located in the United States. For Spanish-speaking people, 1–855-DÉJELO-YA is available for support in a quit attempt. For people who speak Chinese, Vietnamese, or Korean, the Asian Smokers' Quitline was established to support coaching in these native languages [36]. As part of a CDC campaign to assist with quitting, *Tips from Former Smokers*® draws upon social media, infographics, and videos to provide support for people interested in quitting and aims to provide relatable content by using individuals, who have experienced the quitting process firsthand.

For the veteran population, the US Department of Veterans Affairs has several resources available. A specific quit line is available to the veteran population (1–855-QUIT-VET) as well as a text messaging program (English: text VET to 47848 or sign up at smokefree.gov/VET, or for Spanish text VETesp to 47848 or https://veterans.smokefree.gov/tools-tips-vet/smokefreevetesp). For veterans with smartphones, the Stay Quit Coach 2.0 phone application offers multiple resources for smoking cessation including goal setting, progress tracking, and strategies for coping with stress and nicotine cravings.

Alcohol Consumption

According to the Dietary Guidelines for Americans 2020–2025, there are no additional restrictions for alcohol consumption recommended for people with diabetes; therefore, people with T2D can follow the same recommendations as those without diabetes [14, 37]. There is no evidence demonstrating long-term negative impacts on glycemic management with moderate alcohol consumption. However, acute risks associated with drinking alcohol are hypoglycemia and delayed hypoglycemia. People with diabetes, especially those taking insulin or insulin secretagogue therapy, should be educated on these risks and instructed to monitor blood glucose more frequently during and after alcohol use.

It is also important to be mindful of what is considered "moderate" alcohol use, currently defined as no more than 1 drink a day for women and no more than 2 drinks a day for men. In the United States, a standard drink is equal to any drink containing 14 g of pure ethanol. This equals a 12-ounce beer that is 5% alcohol by volume (ABV), a 5-ounce glass of wine that is 12% ABV, or 1.5 ounces of 80-proof spirits with 40% ABV (a "shot"). People should be educated on the size of a standard drink, as many tend to underestimate their alcohol consumption. Many free smartphone applications exist to help people quantify and track the amount of alcohol they consume, though none are specifically endorsed by prominent health organizations.

Summary and Key Takeaways

Increased counseling on the impact of dietary patterns, increased physical activity, sleep, weight loss, smoking cessation, and stress management on T2D can give people confidence, hope, and feelings of autonomy when living with diabetes. It is often said that pharmacists are one of the most accessible health-care providers; therefore, pharmacists' knowledge on lifestyle interventions can serve as a powerful tool for management, treatment, and possibly even remission of T2D.

References

1. CDC. Centers for Disease Control and Prevention: Diabetes fast facts. https://www.cdc.gov/diabetes/basics/quick-facts.html#:~:text=Type%202%20diabetes%20accounts%20for,become%20more%20overweight%20or%20obese; 2023. Accessed 19 Feb 2024
2. Knowler WC, Barrett-Connor E, Fowler SE, Hamman RF, Lachin JM, Walker EA, Nathan DM. Reduction in the incidence of type 2 diabetes with lifestyle intervention or metformin. N Engl J Med. 2002;346(6):393–403. https://doi.org/10.1056/NEJMoa012512.
3. Lindström J, Ilanne-Parikka P, Peltonen M, Aunola S, Eriksson JG, Hemiö K, et al. Sustained reduction in the incidence of type 2 diabetes by lifestyle intervention: follow-up of the Finnish diabetes prevention study. Lancet. 2006;368(9548):1673–9. https://doi.org/10.1016/s0140-6736(06)69701-8.
4. Li G, Zhang P, Wang J, An Y, Gong Q, Gregg EW, et al. Cardiovascular mortality, all-cause mortality, and diabetes incidence after lifestyle intervention for people with impaired glucose tolerance in the Da Qing diabetes prevention study: a 23-year follow-up study. Lancet Diabetes Endocrinol. 2014;2(6):474–80. https://doi.org/10.1016/s2213-8587(14)70057-9.

5. Nathan DM, Bennett PH, Crandall JP, Edelstein SL, Goldberg RB, Kahn SE, et al. Does diabetes prevention translate into reduced long-term vascular complications of diabetes? Diabetologia. 2019;62(8):1319–28. https://doi.org/10.1007/s00125-019-4928-8.
6. Kelly J, Karlsen M, Steinke G. Type 2 diabetes remission and lifestyle medicine: a position statement from the American College of Lifestyle Medicine. Am J Lifestyle Med. 2020;14(4):406–19. https://doi.org/10.1177/1559827620930962.
7. American Diabetes Association Professional Practice Committee. 3. Prevention or delay of diabetes and associated comorbidities: standards of Care in Diabetes–2024. Diabetes Care. 2023;47(Supplement_1):S43–51. https://doi.org/10.2337/dc24-S003.
8. Diabetes and Nutrition Study Group. Evidence-based European recommendations for the dietary management of diabetes. Diabetologia. 2023;66(6):965–85. https://doi.org/10.1007/s00125-023-05894-8.
9. Samson SL, Vellanki P, Blonde L, Christofides EA, Galindo RJ, Hirsch IB, et al. American association of clinical endocrinology consensus statement: comprehensive type 2 diabetes management algorithm – 2023 update. Endocr Pract. 2023;29(5):305–40. https://doi.org/10.1016/j.eprac.2023.02.001.
10. Evert AB, Dennison M, Gardner CD, Garvey WT, Lau KHK, MacLeod J, et al. Nutrition therapy for adults with diabetes or prediabetes: a consensus report. Diabetes Care. 2019;42(5):731–54. https://doi.org/10.2337/dci19-0014.
11. Franz MJ, MacLeod J, Evert A, Brown C, Gradwell E, Handu D, et al. Academy of nutrition and dietetics nutrition practice guideline for type 1 and type 2 diabetes in adults: systematic review of evidence for medical nutrition therapy effectiveness and recommendations for integration into the nutrition care process. J Acad Nutr Diet. 2017;117(10):1659–79. https://doi.org/10.1016/j.jand.2017.03.022.
12. Blonde L, Umpierrez GE, Reddy SS, McGill JB, Berga SL, Bush M, et al. American association of clinical endocrinology clinical practice guideline: developing a diabetes mellitus comprehensive care Plan-2022 update. Endocr Pract. 2022;28(10):923–1049. https://doi.org/10.1016/j.eprac.2022.08.002.
13. Rosenfeld RM, Kelly JH, Agarwal M, Aspry K, Barnett T, Davis BC, et al. Dietary interventions to treat type 2 diabetes in adults with a goal of remission: An expert consensus statement from the American College of Lifestyle Medicine. Am J Lifestyle Med. 2022;16(3):342–62. https://doi.org/10.1177/15598276221087624.
14. American Diabetes Association Professional Practice Committee. 5. Facilitating positive health behaviors and Well-being to improve health outcomes: standards of care in diabetes – 2024. Diabetes Care. 2023;47(Supplement_1):S77–S110. https://doi.org/10.2337/dc24-S005.

15. Watanabe M, Tuccinardi D, Ernesti I, Basciani S, Mariani S, Genco A, et al. Scientific evidence underlying contraindications to the ketogenic diet: an update. Obes Rev. 2020;21(10):e13053. https://doi.org/10.1111/obr.13053.
16. Pawlak R. Vegetarian diets in the prevention and management of diabetes and its complications. Diabetes Spectr. 2017;30(2):82–8. https://doi.org/10.2337/ds16-0057.
17. Estruch R, Ros E, Salas-Salvadó J, Covas MI, Corella D, Arós F, et al. Primary prevention of cardiovascular disease with a mediterranean diet supplemented with extra-virgin olive oil or nuts. N Engl J Med. 2018;378(25):e34. https://doi.org/10.1056/NEJMoa1800389.
18. de Lorgeril M, Salen P, Martin JL, Monjaud I, Delaye J, Mamelle N. Mediterranean diet, traditional risk factors, and the rate of cardiovascular complications after myocardial infarction: final report of the Lyon diet heart study. Circulation. 1999;99(6):779–85. https://doi.org/10.1161/01.cir.99.6.779.
19. Olson, R. D. (2023) Physical Activity Guidelines for Americans, 2nd edition. Washington, DC2018.
20. Colberg SR, Sigal RJ, Yardley JE, Riddell MC, Dunstan DW, Dempsey PC, et al. Physical activity/exercise and diabetes: a position statement of the American Diabetes Association. Diabetes Care. 2016;39(11):2065–79. https://doi.org/10.2337/dc16-1728.
21. CDC. Centers for Disease Control and Prevention: Target heart rate and estimated maximum heart rate. https://www.cdc.gov/physicalactivity/basics/measuring/heartrate.htm; 2022. Accessed 19 Feb 2024
22. Professional.Heart. Pescatello LS: prescribing exercise prescriptions that FITT for adults with elevated blood pressure and cholesterol in the middle of the cardiovascular disease risk spectrum. https://professional.heart.org/en/science-news/physical-activity-as-a-critical-component-of-first-line-treatment-for-elevated-bp-or-cholesterol/commentary; 2021. Accessed 19 Feb 2024
23. White ND, Bautista V, Lenz T, Cosimano A. Using the SMART-EST goals in lifestyle medicine prescription. Am J Lifestyle Med. 2020;14(3):271–3. https://doi.org/10.1177/1559827620905775.
24. American Diabetes Association Professional Practice Committee. 8. Obesity and weight management for the prevention and treatment of type 2 diabetes: standards of care in diabetes–2024. Diabetes Care. 2023;47(Supplement_1):S145–S57. https://doi.org/10.2337/dc24-S008.
25. Anothaisintawee T, Reutrakul S, Van Cauter E, Thakkinstian A. Sleep disturbances compared to traditional risk factors for diabetes development: systematic review and meta-analysis. Sleep Med Rev. 2016;30:11–24. https://doi.org/10.1016/j.smrv.2015.10.002.
26. Cappuccio FP, D'Elia L, Strazzullo P, Miller MA. Quantity and quality of sleep and incidence of type 2 diabetes: a systematic review and meta-analysis. Diabetes Care. 2010;33(2):414–20. https://doi.org/10.2337/dc09-1124.

27. Reutrakul S, Punjabi NM, Van Cauter E. Impact of sleep and circadian disturbances on glucose metabolism and type 2 diabetes. In: Cowie CC, Casagrande SS, Menke A, Cissell MA, Eberhardt MS, Meigs JB, et al., editors. Diabetes in America. Bethesda: National Institute of Diabetes and Digestive and Kidney Diseases; 2018.
28. Clayton JS, Bonnet J. Foundations of lifestyle medicine board review manual. 4th ed. Chesterfield, MO: American College of Lifestyle Medicine; 2023.
29. Kryger M, Roth T, Dement W. Principles and practice of sleep medicine. 6th ed. Elsevier; 2016.
30. Hirshkowitz M, Whiton K, Albert SM, Alessi C, Bruni O, DonCarlos L, et al. National sleep foundation's updated sleep duration recommendations: final report. Sleep Health. 2015;1(4):233–43. https://doi.org/10.1016/j.sleh.2015.10.004.
31. Priya G, Kalra S. Mind-body interactions and mindfulness meditation in diabetes. Eur Endocrinol. 2018;14(1):35–41. https://doi.org/10.17925/ee.2018.14.1.35.
32. Levine GN, Lange RA, Bairey-Merz CN, Davidson RJ, Jamerson K, Mehta PK, et al. Meditation and cardiovascular risk reduction: a scientific statement from the American Heart Association. J Am Heart Assoc. 2017;6(10) https://doi.org/10.1161/jaha.117.002218.
33. CDC. Centers for Disease Control and Prevention: Mini-lesson: mindfulness strategies for managing diabetes distress. https://www.cdc.gov/diabetes/professional-info/toolkits/new-beginnings/mindfulness.htm; 2022. Accessed 19 Jan 2024
34. U.S. Department of Health and Human Services. Smoking cessation: a report of the Surgeon General; 2020.
35. Kiernan E, Click ES, Melstrom P, Evans ME, Layer MR, Weissman DN, et al. A brief overview of the national outbreak of e-cigarette, or vaping, product use-associated lung injury and the primary causes. Chest. 2021;159(1):426–31. https://doi.org/10.1016/j.chest.2020.07.068.
36. Quitline AS: Asian Smokers' Quitline. https://www.asiansmokersquitline.org/about-asq; 2022. Accessed 19 Feb 2024
37. U.S. Department of Health and Human Services. Dietary Guidelines for Americans, 2020–2025. 9th ed; 2020.

Pharmacological Interventions for Diabetes Management

4

Elizabeth J. Hay-Bradford

The Triumvirate, Ominous Octet, and Beyond

As the pathophysiology for diabetes mellitus continues to evolve, the arsenal of pharmacologic interventions available for the management of this complex disease state continues to expand. Starting with the Triumvirate in 1987, this theory identified pancreatic beta-cell failure and insulin resistance in the muscle and liver as the primary mechanisms of hyperglycemia [1]. The pathogenesis of diabetes has now expanded to include more pathways, leading to the creation of the Ominous Octet, followed by the egregious eleven (Fig. 4.1). Although the final common denominator is beta-cell dysfunction, many pharmacological interventions available have been created to target at least one or more of these proposed 11 mechanisms.

E. J. Hay-Bradford (✉)
Clinical Pharmacy Specialist – Ambulatory Care, Prisma Health Upstate – Ambulatory Care Pharmacy Clinics, Greenville, SC, USA
e-mail: elizabeth.haybradford@prismahealth.org

© The Author(s), under exclusive license to Springer Nature Switzerland AG 2025

J. Clements (ed.), *The Pharmacist's Pocket Guide for Diabetes and Obesity*, https://doi.org/10.1007/978-3-031-88835-9_4

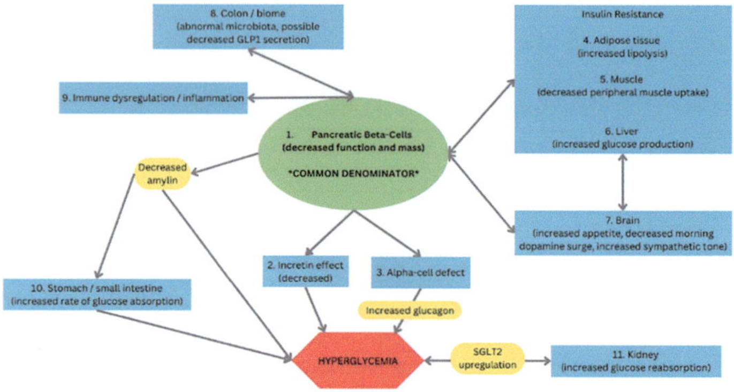

Fig. 4.1 The Egregious Eleven. The egregious eleven contains 11 pathways of hyperglycemia, with a final common denominator of beta-cell dysfunction. These pathways are various targets for pharmacologic interventions approved for management of diabetes and may have effects in the gastrointestinal system, adipose tissue, brain, kidney, liver, muscle, and pancreas. (Adapted from source: Ref. [1])

Management of Diabetes Mellitus

It is recommended that most individuals with type 1 diabetes (T1D) be treated with insulin therapy using multiple daily injections or continuous infusion, ideally mimicking the body's physiological basal and prandial insulin needs [2]. Pramlintide is also approved for use in adults with T1D and will be discussed later in this chapter. Many other glucose-lowering medications discussed in this chapter are currently approved only for type 2 diabetes (T2D).

Although not recognized as a specific type of diabetes by the American Diabetes Association (ADA), awareness of latent autoimmune diabetes in adults (LADA) has increased, and the term is accepted in clinical practice [3]. Although LADA shares features of both T1D and T2D, patients are often managed as if they have T1D; however, due to the condition's slow progressive nature, insulin therapy may not always be necessary upon diagnosis. Some experts recommend the use of an individual's c-peptide level to decide how to best approach LADA therapy, with lower c-peptide levels indicating more beta-cell deterioration and an increased need for insulin therapy [4].

Starting with metformin as a common first-line therapy, moving to alternative oral agents, and then followed by injectable therapies, this chapter will review the mechanism of action, side effects, contraindications, and important clinical considerations of each class of glucose-lowering medication available.

Biguanide (Metformin)

Mechanism of Action

Metformin decreases intestinal glucose absorption and hepatic glucose production while also increasing peripheral glucose uptake and utilization [5]. With its multifold mechanism, metformin enhances insulin sensitivity and lowers both basal and postprandial glucose levels.

Contraindications and Potential Side Effects

Metformin is contraindicated and should be avoided in severe renal impairment [estimated glomerular filtration rate (eGFR) <30 mL/min/1.73 m^2] and acute or chronic metabolic acidosis, including diabetic ketoacidosis (DKA). Metformin also carries a black box warning for lactic acidosis. This condition is rare, but risk tends to be increased in patients with renal impairment, excessive alcohol intake, hepatic impairment, and hypoxic states, such as acute congestive heart failure [5].

The most common side effects are gastrointestinal (GI) related, with the highest incidence of diarrhea and nausea/vomiting at 53.2% and 25.5%, respectively [5]. Some of these side effects can be mitigated by titrating the dose slowly or taking the medication with food. The extended-release (ER) formulation is associated with a lower incidence of diarrhea and nausea/vomiting at 9.6%

and 6.5%, respectively [6]. Other side effects may include abdominal cramping, flatulence, heartburn, and fatigue.

Clinical Considerations

- Metformin is often considered first-line due to its established history for the management of T2D. It is cost-effective, widely available, and may also be considered in prediabetes, antipsychotic-induced weight gain, and polycystic ovarian syndrome (PCOS).
- Renal failure is a common risk factor for metformin-related adverse events and renal function should be assessed prior to metformin initiation and reassessed often while on metformin therapy [5]. Dose and monitoring frequency should be adjusted accordingly, as shown in the chart below.

Metformin renal dosing and monitoring		
eGFR [mL/min/1.73 m^2]	Daily dose (max)	Monitoring frequency (min)
eGFR >60	2000 mg	6 months–1 year
eGFR 45–60	2000 mg	3–6 months
eGFR 30–45	1000 mg[a]	
eGFR <30	Use is contraindicated	

[a]Initiation not recommended eGFR <45 mL/min/1.73 m^2

- Long-term metformin use has been associated with vitamin B12 deficiency, with an average of 6%–30% of individuals having vitamin B12 deficiency due to metformin, and there is an increased risk with doses greater than or equal to 1500 mg/day [7]. Vitamin B12 concentrations should be assessed every 1–2 years while on metformin therapy, especially in people with anemia, peripheral neuropathy, or malabsorption syndromes, and health-care providers should consider screening for vitamin B12 deficiency prior to metformin initiation [8].

– The use of intravenous contrast dye can increase the risk of acute renal failure and metformin therapy is typically held starting the day of a procedure and up to 2–3 days later, or once normal renal function is verified. As a precaution, metformin is often held for patients admitted to the hospital for surgery or acute conditions.

Dosing and Advantages/Disadvantages

Metformin should be titrated slowly and taken with a meal to reduce the risk of GI side effects.

Medication	Starting dose	Usual maintenance dose	Max daily dose
Metformin (IR)	500 mg once daily or twice daily or 850 mg once daily	1000–2000 mg daily	2550 mg
Metformin ER	500–1000 mg once daily		

ER extended release, *IR* immediate release

Advantages	Disadvantages
Cost-effective Weight loss or neutral Low hypoglycemia risk Available "off-label" for other conditions	GI side effects Caution in impaired renal function Risk of B12 deficiency long term

Insulin Secretagogues

Sulfonylureas and Meglitinides

There are two classes of insulin secretagogues, sulfonylureas and meglitinides. These classes are structurally different and act on different beta-cell receptors while having a similar mechanism of action.

Mechanism of Action

Insulin secretagogues inhibit adenosine triphosphate (ATP)-sensitive potassium channels (K-ATP channels) in pancreatic beta cells, causing an influx of calcium, which stimulates insulin release. Sulfonylureas also reduce glucose output from the liver and increase insulin sensitivity [9].

Insulin Secretagogues: Sulfonylureas

Initially divided into first-generation and second-generation agents, second-generation agents have replaced first-generation due to increased potency and less side effects [9].

Contraindications and Potential Side Effects

Sulfonylureas are contraindicated in DKA and are not a viable choice for individuals with T1D due to the need for functioning beta cells [10].

Select sulfonylureas carry precautions and warnings for individuals with sulfonamide allergies and potentially increased cardiovascular (CV) risk. Despite these initial concerns, sulfonylureas have been commonly used in this population without issue, and the warning is no longer listed as a contraindication for immediate-release glipizide. As for potential CV risk, the Food and Drug Administration (FDA) added a warning of increased risk of CV mortality, up to 2.5× higher, based on a study conducted by the University Group Diabetes Program [11]. Interpretation of the results has been controversial and the increase in mortality was not significant. In other trials, second-generation sulfonylureas have not been associated with increased CV risk, but the warning remains on all labels.

Stimulation of the beta cells from sulfonylurea therapy is independent of blood glucose levels, increasing the risk of hypoglycemia. Although incidence of severe hypoglycemia is low, incidence is often higher with sulfonylurea add-on therapy compared to add-on therapy of liraglutide, glargine, or sitagliptin [12]. Hypoglycemia that did not require the aid of others and defined as 56 mg/dL occurred in 10.1% of individuals on sulfonylurea therapy. Overall, the risk of hypoglycemia is greater with sulfonylureas than metformin [12].

Sulfonylurea-associated weight gain can vary among individuals. The incidence of a gain of 10% or more was higher with sulfonylurea or insulin add-on therapy compared to sitagliptin or liraglutide therapy [12]. If the weight gain does not stabilize or causes worsening glucose management, discontinuation of the sulfonylurea is recommended.

Clinical Considerations

- Individuals may experience "primary failure," defined as less than 10% reduction in fasting blood glucose after at least four weeks of therapy. As beta cells become fatigued due to continued stimulation, "secondary failure" can also occur within a few years of initiating therapy, often leading to decreased glucose control and the need for additional therapy. Approximately 53% of individuals on sulfonylurea therapy alone required additional insulin therapy after 6 years [13].
- In individuals with decreased kidney function and chronic kidney disease (CKD), conservative initial and maintenance dosing is recommended to avoid hypoglycemia. In this patient population, glipizide is the preferred sulfonylurea due to its shorter half-life and inactive metabolites, lowering the risk of hypoglycemia. In contrast, glyburide should be avoided in individuals with eGFR <60 mL/min/1.73 m^2.
- In individuals with increased CV risk, a medication from another therapeutic class would be preferred. If no other medications are available, glimepiride is recommended due to evidence showing no difference in CV outcomes compared to linagliptin, a DPP4-inhibitor [14].

– While individuals with LADA may benefit from medications indicated for T2D, experts suggest avoiding use of sulfonylureas due to the potential for further deterioration of beta-cell function [4].

Dosing and Advantages/Disadvantages

Sulfonylureas should be titrated to glycemic effect, taken with or before the first main meal of the day, and could be divided into two doses for improved control. Hypoglycemia risk increases when added to other glucose-lowering medications.

Medication	Starting dose	Usual maintenance dose (mg/day)	Max dose (mg/day)
Glipizide (IR)	2.5–5 mg once daily	2.5–10	20
Glipizide ER	2.5–5 mg once daily	5–10	20
Glyburide	0.75–3 mg once daily	0.75–6	12
Glimepiride	1–2 mg once daily	2–4	8

ER extended release, *IR* immediate release

Advantages	Disadvantages
Inexpensive Well tolerated	Hypoglycemia Weight gain

Insulin Secretagogues: Meglitinides

Contraindications and Potential Side Effects

Meglitinides are associated with similar weight gain and potentially less hypoglycemia compared to sulfonylureas. Less hypoglycemia may be due to stimulation of the beta cells being dependent on the presence of glucose.

There is no concern with utilizing meglitinides if there is a known or documented sulfonamide allergy. While there are no long-term trials assessing CV outcomes with meglitinide therapy, there are some concerns due to their similar mechanism of action as sulfonylureas.

Clinical Considerations

- Compared to sulfonylureas, meglitinides are associated with similar efficacy and may be considered as an alternative therapy for individuals unable to use metformin or sulfonylureas [15]. Use is typically limited by their frequent dosing with meals and short duration of action, but this can be a benefit for people with inconsistent meal timing or schedules.
- In individuals with renal dysfunction, repaglinide is preferred due to primarily hepatic metabolism; however, there is an increased risk for drug interactions associated with various hepatic enzymes, such as CYP2C8 and CYP3A4 [16].

Dosing and Advantages/Disadvantages

Due to their rapid onset and short duration of action, meglitinides are typically dosed multiple times a day prior to each meal. These medications should be started on a low dose and increased to achieve glycemic goals with appropriate monitoring of prandial blood sugars.

Medication	Starting dose	Usual maintenance dose	Max dose (mg/day)
Repaglinide	A1C <8%: 0.5 mg before each meal A1C >8%: 1–2 mg before each meal	0.5–1 mg before each meal	4
Nateglinide	60–120 mg before each meal	60–120 mg before each meal	360

Advantages	Disadvantages
Reduction of postprandial levels Well tolerated	Frequent dosing Hypoglycemia (less than sulfonylureas) Weight gain Generics available, but more costly compared to sulfonylureas and metformin

Thiazolidinediones

Thiazolidinediones, such as pioglitazone, are insulin sensitizers and rely on the presence of insulin for its primary mechanism, but it is not an insulin secretagogue. These medications are not utilized as initial therapy, and use is often limited due to potential side effects and contraindications.

Mechanism of Action

Thiazolidinediones act on the peroxisome proliferator-activated receptor γ (PPARγ) receptors found in adipose tissue, skeletal muscle, and the liver, leading to decreased insulin resistance in the periphery and liver, increased glucose disposal, and decreased hepatic glucose output [9].

Contraindications and Potential Side Effects

Thiazolidinediones have several contraindications and should not be used in individuals with heart failure, history or elevated risk of fractures, active liver disease, active or history of bladder cancer, pregnancy, or T1D [17].

Potential side effects associated with thiazolidinediones may include weight gain, edema and heart failure, skeletal fractures, and a small risk of bladder cancer (pioglitazone). Although the risks of fractures and bladder cancer appear to be low with conflicting results, these concerns should be discussed prior to starting therapy [9].

Clinical Considerations

- In the 2023 ADA Standards of Care, pioglitazone received more attention than in previous years, earning consideration to lower the risk of stroke or myocardial infarction in individuals with a history of stroke and evidence of insulin resistance. This recommendation was based on evidence resulting in a lower risk of stroke, myocardial infarction, and diabetes in the pioglitazone group 4.8 years after a recent stroke, compared to placebo [2].
- Without an FDA-approved treatment available for nonalcoholic steatohepatitis (NASH) – now known as metabolic dysfunction-associated steatohepatitis (MASH), pioglitazone has also gained attention for its ability to improve glucose and lipid metabolism and improve fibrosis and steatosis. In a meta-analysis, pioglitazone was associated with resolution of NASH and may improve or halt progression of fibrosis [2].
- These newer benefits, lower risk of stroke and improvement in liver fibrosis, still need to be weighed against the risks of weight gain, fracture, and edema associated with this medication class.

Dosing and Advantages/Disadvantages

The only thiazolidinedione currently available in the United States is pioglitazone. Pioglitazone is often dosed once daily and the dose may be increased to achieve glycemic goals, but side effects may affect tolerability of higher doses.

Medication	Starting dose	Usual maintenance dose	Max dose (mg/day)
Pioglitazone	15–30 mg once daily	15–30 mg once daily	45

Advantages	Disadvantages
Once daily dosing Potential benefits in NASH Potential benefits poststroke	Contraindicated in heart failure Weight gain and edema Fracture risk

Alpha-Glucosidase Inhibitors

Mechanism of Action

The α-glucosidase inhibitors target specific enzymes called α-glucosidases in the brush border of the small intestine. These enzymes are critical for the release of glucose from complex carbohydrates, and inhibition prevents postprandial glucose peaks [18].

Contraindications and Potential Side Effects

Alpha-glucosidase inhibitors have many contraindications, such as DKA, cirrhosis, inflammatory bowel disease (IBD), colonic ulceration, partial intestinal obstruction, and chronic intestinal diseases. Use is not recommended in individuals with hepatic impairment, renal impairment, or stress-related states, such as fever, trauma, or infection [19].

Significant GI side effects and abdominal discomfort can affect up to 50% of individuals on this class of medications, often limiting their use in practice. These effects can include bloating, flatulence, cramping, and diarrhea, so this medication is not an ideal choice for individuals with acute or chronic GI conditions [20].

Clinical Considerations

- Hypoglycemia with this class of medications must be treated with simple carbohydrates only, such as those in fruit juices, milk, or glucose tablets. This is due to the absorption of disaccharides and polysaccharides, found in table sugar, candy, and soft drinks, being delayed [20].

Dosing and Advantages/Disadvantages

Alpha-glucoside inhibitors should be taken with the first bite of each main meal.

Medication	Starting dose	Usual maintenance dose	Max dose (mg/day)
Acarbose	25 mg three times a day	50–100 mg three times a day	150–300
Miglitol	25 mg three times a day	50 mg three times a day	300

Advantages	Disadvantages
Drug is not absorbed	Frequent dosing GI side effects Minimal efficacy

Sodium-Glucose Cotransporter 2 Inhibitors (SGLT-2i)

Mechanism of Action

The SGLT-2i block SGLT-2 receptors in the proximal tubule, lowering the renal threshold for glucose reabsorption and preventing the kidneys from reabsorbing glucose into the bloodstream [9]. This class can lower both fasting and prandial blood glucose levels.

Contraindications and Potential Side Effects

This specific class is contraindicated in individuals on dialysis; however, there are multiple risk factors and considerations to discuss when initiating therapy. Patient education is critical for mitigation of side effects.

While this class of medications has renal and CV benefits in addition to blood glucose management, this class also comes with unique risks, such as genital infections, urinary tract infections (UTIs), lower limb amputations (LLAs), bone fractures, and euglycemic diabetes-related ketoacidosis (euDKA).

Genital infections and UTIs are side effects that typically appear early in treatment and are often self-limiting or manageable with antibiotic or antifungal treatment [21]. While manageable, recurrent infections may be bothersome and lead to discontinuation of therapy. Patients should be educated on practical hygiene to lessen infection risk. Fournier's gangrene, a rare urological emergency, has also been associated with this class and patients should be advised to report any pain in the external genitalia, perineum, and perianal region [9].

While a class effect of LLAs and bone fracture risk cannot be ruled out by available data, these concerns primarily came from evidence with canagliflozin, which included a high-risk population. Regarding LLAs, other SGLT-2i have had similar incidence in other trials but were often not significant compared to placebo [21]. Individuals with previous amputation or active foot ulcer are at an increased risk and should be educated on monitoring and advice for preventative footcare. Bone fracture risk is inconsistent among trials and were not demonstrated with empagliflozin and dapagliflozin. This side effect was also not replicated in the kidney outcome trial with canagliflozin [21]. While patients should be monitored for this risk, it is not often seen as a reason to avoid, hold, or discontinue therapy.

Due to the risk of euDKA with SGLT-2i therapy, a warning was added to all labels within this drug class. Unlike most DKA cases, the DKA associated with this class often occurs with euglycemic glucose levels (blood glucose <250 mg/dL) in the presence of severe anion gap metabolic acidosis (pH <7.3) and ketonemia or ketonuria (elevated ketones in blood or urine). Although rare, there are certain risk factors associated with euDKA, such as insulin deficiency, commonly associated with a low c-peptide or LADA diagnosis, sudden reductions in insulin doses, increased requirements for insulin due to illness or surgery, carbohydrate and food restriction, severe dehydration, and heavy alcohol consumption [21].

SGLT-2i have an insulin-independent mechanism, causing a lower risk of hypoglycemia compared to other glucose-lowering medications. Due to their "diuretic-like effect," SGLT-2i can also cause polyuria, dehydration, dizziness, or hypotension. Patients should be monitored and educated on adequate hydration and this class should only be started in a euglycemic, euvolemic state. If SGLT-2i and diuretics are taken concomitantly, then kidney function should be closely monitored, and doses may be adjusted based on monitoring and blood pressure measurements. Older patients are at significantly greater risk for dehydration [21].

Clinical Considerations

- As eGFR declines, the amount of glucose reaching the proximal tubule also decreases, leading to lower glucose-lowering efficacy of this class of medications. Due to this, it is not recommended to start or continue SGLT-2i therapy at eGFR <45 mL/min/1.73 m^2 for glycemic benefit; however, they can be added or continued for cardiorenal benefits as low as eGFR of 20–25 mL/min/1.73 m^2, depending on the agent utilized [9].
- SGLT-2i therapy is strongly encouraged for individuals with indicators of elevated risk for established atherosclerotic cardiovascular disease (ASCVD), heart failure (HF), or CKD [9]. Success of CV in individuals with T2D led to more trials in renal disease and CV disease (CVD), including HF, regardless of diabetes status. Empagliflozin has been shown to reduce the risk of cardiovascular events, as well as HF hospitalizations and all-cause mortality [22]. Dapagliflozin showed positive results among people with T2D and at high risk of CV events by reducing the risk of CV death and HF hospitalizations [22]. SGLT-2i therapy, specifically canagliflozin, dapagliflozin, and empagliflozin, is preferred for people with T2D and renal disease due to its positive results, such as reduction in end-stage renal disease, renal death, and CV death [22]. In addition, dapagliflozin and empagliflozin can be recommended among individuals with renal disease without diabetes.
- Prior to initiation, any hypovolemia should be corrected. If eGFR dips after initiation of therapy, often within the first month, eGFR is expected to stabilize over time. It is recommended to check eGFR within 4 weeks of starting therapy, and if there is a 30% increase in serum creatinine, maintain therapy and address other non-related factors to continue SGLT2i therapy [23].

- Due to additional warnings for euDKA in the perioperative period, it is recommended to hold SGLT-2i therapy for 3 days (canagliflozin, dapagliflozin, empagliflozin) or 4 days (ertugliflozin) prior to surgery. If euDKA is diagnosed, SGLT-2-i therapy should be discontinued [24].
- As of 2023, sotagliflozin was approved by the FDA for CV risk reduction and HF. Sotagliflozin is unique due to its dual inhibition of both SGLT-1 and SGLT-2. Although improvements in body weight and A1C have been shown in various analyses, it is important to note that this medication does not yet have an indication for diabetes management alone. It is also associated with an eightfold increase in DKA compared with placebo [2].

Dosing and Advantages/Disadvantages

Due to their diuretic-like effect, it is typically recommended that SGLT-2i be taken in the morning.

Medication	Starting dose (mg)	Usual maintenance dose	Maximum daily dose (mg/day)	eGFR limit (mL/min/1.73 m²)
Empagliflozin (Jardiance®)	10	10–25 once daily	25	<20
Dapagliflozin (Farxiga®)	5	5–10 mg once daily	10	<25
Canagliflozin (Invokana®)	100	100–300 mg once daily	300	<30
Ertugliflozin (Steglatro®)	5	5–15 mg once daily	15	<45
Bexagliflozin (Brenzavvy®)	20	20 mg once daily	20	<30
Sotagliflozin[a] (Inpefa®)	200	200–400 mg once daily, no more than 1 h prior to first meal of the day	400	<25

[a]Indicated for cardiovascular risk reduction and heart failure only

Advantages	Disadvantages
HF, CKD, and CV benefits (select medications only) Once daily dosing Potential weight loss Low risk of hypoglycemia	Brand name only (expensive) Less effective at lower eGFR (for glycemic benefit) Risk of dehydration Risk of UTI/yeast infections Risk of DKA

Glucagon-Like Peptide-1 (GLP-1)-Based Therapies

Role of GLP-1

In healthy individuals, the ingestion of food leads to the release of incretin hormones from the intestine, called GLP-1 and glucose-dependent insulinotropic polypeptide (GIP). These hormones are released in addition to pancreatic beta-cell hormones, insulin, and amylin. These hormones and peptides have effects on gastric emptying, glucagon release, and appetite. After food absorption, GLP-1 and GIP promote insulin secretion, also called the "incretin effect," but in individuals with diabetes these steps can be disrupted.

Dipeptidyl Peptidase 4 Inhibitors (DPP-4i)

Mechanism of Action

The class of DPP-4i is a GLP-1-based therapy, often used as an add-on therapy for people needing additional glucose lowering for postprandial excursions. Unlike other glucose-lowering therapies, they do not have additional CV or kidney benefits. Medications in this class work by inhibiting the DPP-4 enzyme, which is expressed on the surface of many cell types that deactivate bioactive peptides. By inhibiting this enzyme, these peptides will not be deactivated.

Contraindications and Potential Side Effects

Compared to other medications, DPP-4i have a low risk of hypoglycemia and appear to have an overall neutral effect on body weight.

Although data is insufficient to determine a causal relationship, DPP-4i are not recommended in individuals with a history of pancreatitis. If an individual complains of persistent, severe abdominal pain, pancreatitis should be considered and any DPP-4i should be discontinued.

Clinical Considerations

- Due to similar mechanisms, use of DPP-4i with other GLP-1 type therapies should be avoided. When prandial insulin is initiated, the use of DPP-4i should be limited or discontinued, as these medications do not have additional benefits on outcomes and may increase medication burden.
- In individuals with kidney dysfunction, linagliptin is recommended due to primary elimination in the enterohepatic system and it does not require dose adjustment. In addition, use of DPP-4i is limited due to lack of benefits for individuals with CVD, renal disease, obesity, or liver disease.

Dosing and Advantages/Disadvantages

Medication	Starting dose (mg)	Usual maintenance dose	Max daily dose (mg/day)
Sitagliptin (Januvia®, Zituvio®)	100	100 mg once daily	100
Linagliptin (Tradjenta®)	5	5 mg once daily	5
Saxagliptin (Onglyza®)	2.5–5	2.5–5 mg once daily	5
Alogliptin	25	25 mg once daily	25

Advantages	Disadvantages
Once daily dosing Low risk of hypoglycemia Less expensive GLP1-based therapy	Risk of pancreatitis Weight neutral Limited to postprandial excursions

Monoincretin (GLP-1) and Dual-Incretin (GLP-1/GIP) Therapy

Mechanism of Action

These classes mimic the action of one or both endogenous GLP-1 and GIP hormones by stimulating insulin secretion from pancreatic beta cells, reducing elevated levels of glucagon, and slowing gastric emptying [9]. GLP-1 and GLP-1/GIP receptor agonists are resistant to the rapid degradation of the DPP-4 enzyme. These therapies can impact glycemic control through multiple mechanisms, as shown in Table 4.1 at the end of this chapter.

Contraindications and Potential Side Effects

GLP-1 therapies are contraindicated in individuals with a personal or family history of medullary thyroid carcinoma (MTC) or with multiple endocrine neoplasia syndrome type 2 [25]. Typical warnings include pancreatitis, diabetic retinopathy complications, hypoglycemia (if used with insulin secretagogue or insulin), acute kidney injury.

Gastrointestinal side effects are most common, affecting 10 to 50% of individuals [9]. GI side effects typically improve as the medication is continued, but side effects may worsen due to poor dietary patterns, skipping titrations, or when increasing doses. Education should be provided on the risk of GI side effects and ways to mitigate them, which include:

- Nausea/vomiting: Have clear and cold liquids, avoid overeating, slow eating pattern.
- Diarrhea: Avoid fried, greasy, and fatty food.
- Constipation: Increase fiber intake with dietary intake or fiber supplement, water intake, exercise.

Table 4.1 Properties and consideration of glucose-lowering therapies is meant to be a summary chart at the end of the chapter as a quick reference. monoincretin and dual incretin therapy

Medication class	Mechanism / Effects (Egregious Eleven)	Efficacy	Average change in A1C	Hypoglycemia	Weight	Average change in	Oral / Injectable	Typical dosing	Cost	CV Effects (Key trials)		Renal effects (Key trials)	
										MACE	HF	Progression of CKD	Dosing considerations
Metformin	4, 5, 6, 8	High	(-) 1.5-2%	No	Neutral/loss	(-) 2 - 3kg	Oral	QD - BID	Low	Potential benefit (DDPOS)	Neutral	Neutral	Contradindicated at eGFR <30 ml/min
SGLT2 inhibitors	11	Intermediate - High	(-) 0.5 - 1%	No	Loss (intermediate)	(-) 1 - 5kg	Oral	QD	High	Benefit: canagliflozin (CANVAS), empagliflozin (EMPA-REG)	Benefit: canagliflozin (CHIEF-HF), dapagliflozin (DAPA-HF), empagliflozin (EMPEROR), ertugliflozin (VERTIS-CV)	Benefit: canagliflozin (CREDENCE), dapagliflozin (DAPA-CKD), empagliflozin (EMPA-KIDNEY)	Glucose-lowering effect is lower at lower eGFR. May have transient lowering after initiation of therapy
GLP-1 RAs	1,2,3, 7, 8, 9, 10	High - Very High	(-) 0.8 - 1.6% (product and dose dependent)	No	Loss (intermediate - very high)	(-) 1 - 10kg	Oral/ Injectable	BID, QD, QW	High	Benefit: dulaglutide (REWIND), liraglutide (LEADER), semaglutide (SELECT)	Neutral	Benefit for renal endpoints in CVOTs (albuminuria outcomes): dulaglutide (AWARD-7), liraglutide (LEADER), semaglutide (FLOW)	No dose adjustment for dulaglutide, liraglutide, semaglutide

GIP / GLP-1 RA	1,2,3, 7, 8, 9, 10	Very High	(-) 1.06 - 1.94% (product and dose dependent)	No	Loss (very high)	(-) 15.7%	Injectable	QW	High	TBD	TBD	TBD	No dose adjustment
DPP-4 inhibitors	1,2,3, 7, 8, 9, 10	Intermediate	(-) 0.5 - 0.9%	No	Neutral/loss	0	Oral	QD	High	Neutral	Neutral, potential risk (saxagliptin)	Neutral	No dose adjustment for linagliptin
Thiazolidin-ediones	4, 5, 6	High	(-) 1 - 1.5%	No	Gain	(+) 4kg	Oral	QD	Low	Potential benefit (stroke): Pioglitazone (IRIS)	Increased risk	Neutral	No dose adjustment, but generally not recommended in renal impairment
Sulfonylureas (2nd gen.)	1	High	(-) 1.5 - 2%	Yes	Gain	(+) 1 - 2kg	Oral	QD	Low	Neutral	Neutral	Neutral	Glipizide and glimepiride may be cautiously considered, but avoid glyburide in CKD
Insulin (human)	management of hyperglycemia with reduced insulin secretion	High to Very High	(-) 1.4% (product and dose dependent)	Yes	Gain	(+) 1.7 - 2.5kg	Injectable	TID, BID, QD	Low	Neutral	Neutral	Neutral	Titrate based on clinical response
Insulin (analog)		High to Very High		Yes	Gain		Injectable		High	Neutral	Neutral	Neutral	

The "Mechanism/Effects" column identifies the numbered mechanisms of the Egregious Eleven from Fig. 4.1
Adapted from source: Refs. [2, 9, 38–41]

Clinical Considerations

- GLP-1 therapies should be stopped on the day of an elective procedure or surgery if dosed once daily. If the prescribed therapy is dosed once weekly, it should be stopped at least a week prior to elective surgeries [26].
- GLP-1 therapies may potentially preserve beta-cell function and protect against apoptosis [9].
- Semaglutide (subcutaneous), dulaglutide, and liraglutide are recommended for those with clinical ASCVD due to positive CV outcome results [9]. Liraglutide can reduce the risk of cardiovascular events and all-cause mortality among people with T2D and at high risk of CV events; semaglutide and dulaglutide have shown reductions in major CV events [27].
- For the treatment of obesity, semaglutide had positive CV results, but the trials did not include individuals with diabetes [27].
- Semaglutide 1 mg, as a once-weekly injection, was studied in people with T2D and CKD; the trial was halted early due to overwhelming efficacy with semaglutide reducing the risk of clinically important kidney outcomes and death from CV causes [28].
- Tirzepatide has anticipated CV trials, as one trial will compare tirzepatide to dulaglutide for the primary outcome of time to first occurrence of any major adverse cardiovascular event (MACE), assessing for both noninferiority and superiority [29]. In addition, other trials are in progress or upcoming for incretin therapies in other disease states (e.g., peripheral arterial disease, obstructive sleep apnea) [26].
- Currently, tirzepatide is the only dual-acting GLP-1/GIP therapy and is associated with the greatest glucose-lowering effect and weight loss compared to other GLP-1 therapies, such as semaglutide [30].

– Tirzepatide may impact oral contraceptives (OCPs), delaying gastric emptying and affecting absorption, potentially leading to decreased efficacy during initiation and titration of tirzepatide. The same results have not been found with other GLP-1 therapies at this time; however, due to a similar mechanism, patient education is critical [31]. Information on this interaction and education on appropriate management should be provided.

Dosing and Advantages/Disadvantages

Medication	Starting dose	Usual maintenance dose	Max dose
Semaglutide (oral) (Rybelsus®)	3 mg	7–14 mg once daily	14 mg/day
Semaglutide* (inj.) (Ozempic®)	0.25 mg	0.5–2 mg once weekly	2 mg/ week
Dulaglutide* (Trulicity®)	0.75 mg	1.5–4.5 mg once weekly	4.5 mg/ week
Exenatide (Byetta®)	5 mcg	5–10 mcg twice daily	20 mcg/ day
Exenatide (ER) (Bydureon BCise®)	2 mg	2 mg once weekly	2 mg/ week
Liraglutide* (Victoza®)	0.6 g	1.2–1.8 mg daily	1.8 mg/ day
Tirzepatide (Mounjaro®)	2.5 mg	5–15 mg once weekly	15 mg/ week

ER extended release

Advantages	Disadvantages
CV benefits for selected GLP-1 agents Weight loss May aid in decreasing insulin needs Once daily or once weekly (except Byetta®)	Brand name only (expensive) GI side effects MTC risk (in animals) Risk of pancreatitis and gallstones Caution in gastroparesis

Interchangeability of Incretin Therapies

Multiple interchanges between incretin therapies are not encouraged in clinical practice, but may be necessary for several reasons such as medication availability, insurance coverage, or treatment goals. There are limited head-to-head trials available and there is limited evidence on equivalent doses; however, clinical experience has allowed us to determine similar comparative doses.

Medication (units) (route/ interval)	Comparative doses									
Exenatide (μg) (SC twice daily)	5	10								
Semaglutide (mg) (PO daily)	3	7	14							
Liraglutide (mg) (SC weekly)	0.6	1.2	1.8							
Dulaglutide (mg) (SC weekly)		0.75	1.5	3						
Semaglutide (mg) (SC weekly)		0.25	0.5		1	2				
Exenatide XR (mg) (SC weekly)			2							
Tirzepatide (mg) (SC weekly)			2.5			5	7.5	10	12.5	15

PO oral(ly), *SC* subcutaneous(ly), *XR* extended release
Adapted from source: Ref. [32]

Insulin

Mechanism of Action

Insulin acts in target tissues (liver, skeletal muscle, and adipose tissue) to regulate metabolism of macronutrients, carbohydrates, proteins, and fats. Insulin is the "key" to allow glucose into cells to provide the necessary energy to function, and exogenous insulin is used to control fasting hyperglycemia by replacing the patient's insulin production.

Contraindications and Potential Side Effects

Insulin is contraindicated during acute episodes of hypoglycemia. All insulin contains a warning for hypoglycemia as a potential side effect, especially in combination with other agents. In addition to shifting glucose, insulin causes potassium to shift into the cell, potentially leading to hypokalemia. With long-term therapy and high doses, insulin may also be associated with weight gain. Individuals with hepatic or renal impairment should be monitored closely due to an increased risk of hypoglycemia.

Clinical Considerations

- Due to its efficacy in reducing blood sugars rapidly, insulin is typically the drug of choice for A1C >10%, blood glucose >300 mg/dL or if signs of catabolism or hyperglycemia are present [2]; however, when available, monoincretin (GLP-1) or dual-incretin therapy (GLP-1/GIP) may be considered for individuals with T2D.
- While not everyone with T2D will require use of insulin, exogenous insulin is necessary for people with T1D due to having little to no endogenous production of insulin. Insulin is also the recommended treatment for diabetes in pregnancy due to its safety, efficacy, and individualized dosing in pregnancy compared to other diabetes agents.
- Insulins are available as "human" or "analog." Human insulin, such as NPH and regular, is derived from recombinant DNA human insulin. Analogs have an amino acid substitution that can change the onset or duration of action. While they are widely used, analog insulins tend to be more expensive [9].
- Education on appropriate injection technique and management of hypoglycemia is critical when initiating insulin therapy; technique should be regularly monitored for safety and

efficacy. Regular dose adjustments to reach glycemic goals are recommended to avoid therapeutic inertia.

– Signs of overbasalization may include basal insulin greater than 0.5 units/kg/day, high differential (>50 mg/dL) in bedtime-to-morning or postprandial-to-preprandial glucose, hypoglycemia, and glycemic high variability [33].

Dosing and Advantages/Disadvantages

Insulin is commonly injected subcutaneously via a syringe, pen, or pump. Common injection sites include the abdomen, thigh, and back of the upper arm. There are many insulin types available, varying in formulations, concentrations, and pharmacokinetics. The cost of insulin products may vary based on insurance coverage and product formulation. A comparison of the products available and recommended dosing and steps to initiating or intensifying injection therapy are shown in Table 4.1 and Fig. 4.2.

Advantages	Disadvantages
Individualized dosing Rapid decrease in A1C/glucose levels	Risk of hypoglycemia and weight gain Cost of certain products Injection burden

Insulin type	Insulin preparation (U-100 unless otherwise noted)	Onset	Peak	Duration
Ultra-rapid acting	Insulin aspart (Fiasp®)	15–20 min	90–120 min	5–7 h
	Insulin lispro (Lyumjev®)	15–17 min	120–174 min	4.6–7.3 h

(continued)

Insulin type	Insulin preparation (U-100 unless otherwise noted)	Onset	Peak	Duration
Rapid-acting	Insulin aspart (Novolog®)	10–20 min	30–90 min	3–5 h
	Insulin lispro U-100, U-200 (Humalog®, Admelog®)			
	Insulin glulisine (Apidra®)			
Short-acting/ intermediate-acting*	Regular (Humulin R®, Novolin R®)	30–60 min	2–4 h	5–8 h
	NPH* (Humulin N, Novolin N)	2–4 h	4–10 h	10–24 h
	Regular* U-500 (Humulin R 500®)	15–30 min	4–8 h	13–24 h
Long-acting	Insulin glargine (Lantus®, Basaglar®, Semglee®, Rezvoglar®)	2–4 h	No peak	20–24 h
	Insulin glargine U-300 (Toujeo)	6 h		36 h
	Insulin degludec U-100, U-200 (Tresiba®)	1 h		42 h

Adapted from source: Ref. [34]

Safe Insulin Use

In addition to patient education on proper administration of insulin and standard management of hypoglycemia, glucagon is recommended for all individuals taking insulin due to risk of hypoglycemia, especially when combined with other therapies for glucose management [2]. Initially, standard treatment of hypoglycemia is recommended, and glucagon products are intended to be used in cases of a hypoglycemic emergency where standard treat-

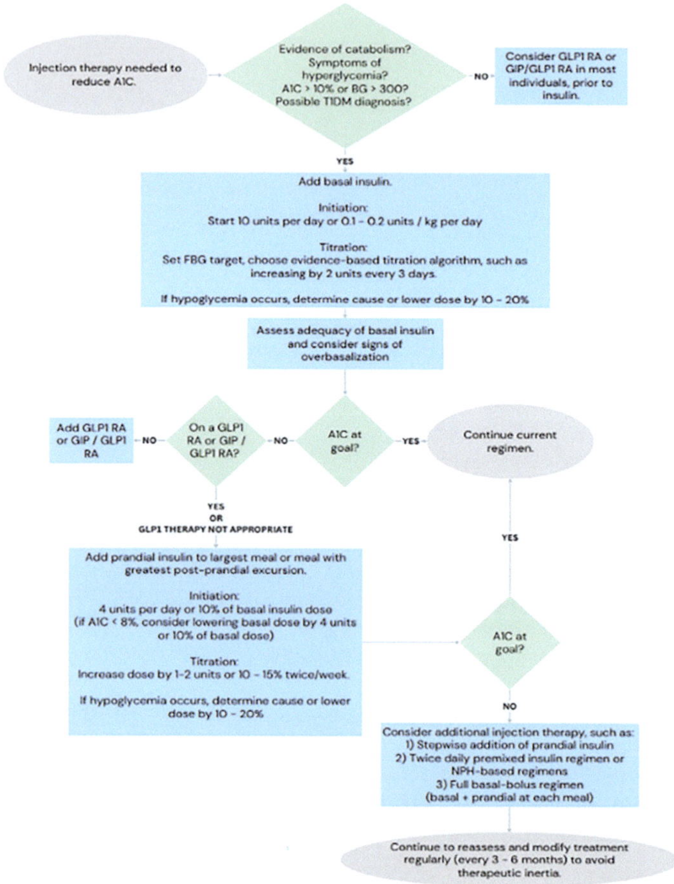

Fig. 4.2 This flowchart shows the recommended procedure for intensifying injectable therapies, considering GLP1-therapy and insulin, in Type 2 Diabetes. Adapted from Elsayed NA et al. [2])

ment is ineffective or not possible (i.e., unresponsive). There are multiple glucagon products available for use, and family, caregivers, or others providing support need to be aware of its location and how to administer it properly in case of emergency.

Medication	Product dosing
Gvoke HypoPen (subcutaneous)	Inject 1 mg as needed. May repeat in 15 min if little to no response
Baqsimi (nasal spray)	Inject 3 mg (one actuation) into a single nostril May repeat in 15 min if little to no response
Zegalogue (dasiglucagon subcutaneous)	Inject 0.6 mg as needed May repeat in 15 min if little to no response

Other Pharmacological Agents

Bromocriptine

A new formulation of the dopamine agonist more commonly used in Parkinson's disease, bromocriptine mesylate, was FDA approved for treatment of T2D. The dopamine agonist is thought to improve hepatic insulin sensitivity and decrease hepatic glucose, but the exact mechanism for glycemic control is unknown and so is its role in treatment [9].

Colesevelam

Colesevelam, a once daily bile acid sequestrant, binds bile acid in the intestinal lumen, decreasing the bile acid pool for reabsorption. This medication is weight neutral and has a small risk for hypoglycemia. It can cause a decrease in LDL-C but also lead to an increase in triglycerides, especially when used in combination with sulfonylureas and insulins. The role of colesevelam is not clear, but it may be beneficial for patients that require A1C and LDL-C reduction as an add-on agent [9]. This medication should be avoided in patients at risk of bowel obstruction and may interfere with absorption of other medications and fat-soluble vitamins. Other medications should be separated by 4 h between administrations [35].

Pramlintide

Co-secreted from pancreatic beta cells, amylin regulates glucose by reducing secretion of glucagon, increasing satiety, and slowing gastric emptying, similar to GLP-1 therapies. Pramlintide was the first non-insulin agent for T1D and is effective at lowering A1C overall and postprandial levels. Pramlintide may be effective as add-on therapy in people with T1D with elevated postprandial blood sugars despite maximum prandial insulin doses. It can be associated with some weight loss and primarily nausea, occurring in 20 to 50% of patients. Dosing is different in people with T1D and T2D; however, this medication has fallen out of favor due to GI side effects, risk of hypoglycemia with insulin, and required frequent dosing and adjustments with meals [9].

Combination Products

Patients with diabetes often take multiple medications for diabetes alone and may have additional medications for comorbid disease states. On average, people with diabetes were found to be taking 4.8 chronic medications a day, with 17% taking seven or more medications per day. Glucose-lowering medications contributed to almost 30% of the average total medication burden [36].

To aid in decreasing medication burden, it can be beneficial to consider combination products available for diabetes management. Combination medications may help increase compliance by lowering the number of physical tablets or injections a patient administers per day or help standardize their dosing regimen. Unfortunately, combination products are fixed dosing that cannot be modified, and some are only available as a brand name product, making them an expensive therapy option. There are many combination products available, with the majority containing two medications.

Oral combination products	
Actoplus Met; Actoplus Met XR	Pioglitazone + Metformin
Avandamet	Rosiglitazone + Metformin
Avandaryl	Rosiglitazone + Glimepiride
Duetact	Pioglitazone + Glimepiride
Glucovance	Glyburide + Metformin
Glyxambi	Empagliflozin + Linagliptin
Invokamet; Invokamet XR	Canagliflozin + Metformin
Janumet; Janumet XR	Sitagliptin + Metformin
Jentadueto; Jentadueto XR	Linagliptin + Metformin
Kazano	Alogliptin + Metformin
Kombiglyze XR	Saxagliptin + Metformin
Metaglip	Glipizide + Metformin
Oseni	Alogliptin + Pioglitazone
PrandiMet	Repaglinide + Metformin
Qtern	Saxagliptin + Dapagliflozin
Segluromet	Ertugliflozin + Metformin
Steglujan	Ertugliflozin + Sitagliptin
Synjardy; Synjardy XR	Empagliflozin + Metformin
Trijardy; Trijardy XR	Empagliflozin + Linagliptin + Metformin
Xigduo	Dapagliflozin + Metformin
Injectable combination products	
Novolog Mix 70/30	Insulin aspart protamine (70%) + insulin aspart (30%)
Humalog Mix 50/50	Insulin lispro protamine (50%) + insulin lispro (50%)
Humalog Mix 75/25	Insulin lispro protamine (75%) + insulin lispro (25%)
Humulin 70/30; Novolin 70/30	Insulin NPH (70%) + insulin regular (30%)
Soliqua	Lixisenatide + insulin glargine
Xultophy	Liraglutide + insulin degludec

Putting it into Practice

The ADA and AACE have provided professional guidance, following evidence-based medicine, and suggested algorithms for diabetes management. Product selection is usually determined considering anticipated A1C effects, side effects, dosage form, cost/coverage, and comorbid disease states. See Figs. 4.3, 4.4 and Table 4.1 for therapeutic recommendations based on comorbid conditions and considerations for glucose-lowering medications.

The ADA Standards of Care 2024 guidelines provide many "A" level recommendations based on clear or supportive evidence from randomized controlled trials that are adequately powered. Other recommendations are indicated as a B through E, based on evidence ranging from well-conducted cohort studies to expert consensus or clinical experience.

Type 1 Diabetes

For individuals with T1D, insulin therapy via continuous infusion or multiple daily doses, such as a basal-bolus regimen, is strongly recommended. The ADA also encourages use of available diabetes technology early in management, such as automated insulin delivery systems and continuous glucose monitoring. Due to the high risk of hypoglycemia with insulin therapy, glucagon products may also be considered, and patients should receive extensive diabetes education, consisting of lifestyle modifications, glycemia targets and management, and sick-day management. The ADA also recommends choosing an insulin plan based on the needs of each individual and in consideration of dosing flexibility, medication costs, and risk of hypoglycemia.

Type 2 Diabetes

Unlike T1D, there are many other pharmacologic options available for people with T2D. In many ADA recommendations, CV

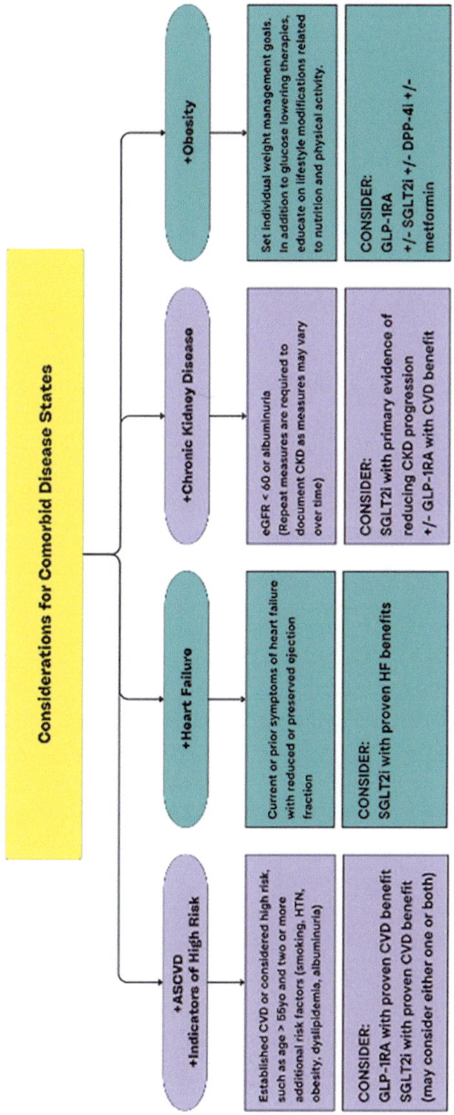

Fig. 4.3 Therapeutic recommendations when considering comorbid disease states in addition to Type 2 diabetes. Adapted from Elsayed NA et al.

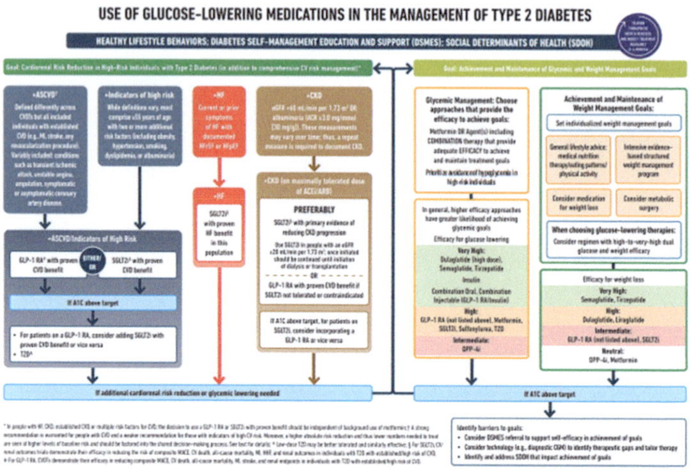

Fig. 4.4 Therapeutic recommendations for Type 2 Diabetes and the use of glucose-lowering agents per the 2024 ADA Standards of Care. Adapted from source: Refs. Elsayed NA et al. and [37]

risk, CKD risk, and weight management are considered along with glycemic management when choosing an appropriate therapy, as the published algorithm for the management of T2D. In addition to pharmacologic therapy, healthy lifestyle behaviors are also strongly recommended. Recommended as an expert consensus, treatment plan and therapies should also be reevaluated at regular intervals and adjusted as necessary to prevent therapeutic inertia.

For individuals with established or high risk of CVD, heart failure, or CKD, an agent that reduces risk for CV and kidney disease is highly recommended, such as an SGLT-2i or GLP-1 RA. These medications are recommended independent of A1C due to their additional benefits. In the 2024 Standards of Care, the ADA reminds health-care providers that if an SGLT-2i is utilized in individuals with an eGFR less than 45 mL/min/1.73 m^2, glycemic benefits will be reduced, and additional agents may be required. When eGFR is less than 30 mL/min/1.73 m^2, a GLP-1 RA is preferred. While insulin can be used for T2D, it is often

Medication Class	Mechanism / Effects (Egregious Eleven)	Efficacy	Average Change in A1C	Hypoglycemia	Weight	Average Change in	Oral / Injectable	Typical Dosing	Cost	CV Effects (Key Trials)		Renal Effects (Key Trials)	
										MACE	HF	Progression of CKD	Dosing Considerations
Metformin	4, 5, 6, 8	High	(-) 1.5-2%	No	Neutral/loss	(-) 2 - 3kg	Oral	QD - BID	Low	Potential benefit (DDPOS)	Neutral	Neutral	Contradindicated at eGFR < 30 ml/min
SGLT2 inhibitors	11	Intermediate - High	(-) 0.5 - 1%	No	Loss (intermediate)	(-) 1 - 5kg	Oral	QD	High	Benefit: canagliflozin (CANVAS), empagliflozin (EMPA-REG)	Benefit: canagliflozin (CHIEF-HF), dapagliflozin (DAPA-HF), empagliflozin (EMPEROR), ertugliflozin (VERTIS-CV)	Benefit: canagliflozin (CREDENCE), dapagliflozin (DAPA-CKD), empagliflozin (EMPA-KIDNEY)	Glucose-lowering effect is lower at lower eGFR. May have transient lowering after initiation of therapy.
GLP-1 RAs	1,2,3, 7, 8, 9, 10	High - Very High	(-) 0.8 - 1.6% (product and dose dependent)	No	Loss (intermediate - very high)	(-) 1 - 10kg	Oral/ Injectable	BID, QD, QW	High	Benefit: dulaglutide (REWIND), liraglutide (LEADER), semaglutide (SELECT)	Neutral	Benefit for renal endpoints in CVOTs (albuminuria outcomes): dulaglutide (AWARD-7), liraglutide (LEADER), semaglutide (FLOW)	No dose adjustment for dulaglutide, liraglutide, semaglutide
GIP / GLP-1 RA	1,2,3, 7, 8, 9, 10	Very High	(-) 1.06 - 1.94% (product and dose dependent)	No	Loss (very high)	(-) 15.7%	Injectable	QW	High	TBD	TBD	TBD	No dose adjustment
DPP-4 inhibitors	1,2,3, 7, 8, 9, 10	Intermediate	(-) 0.5 - 0.9%	No	Neutral/loss	0	Oral	QD	High	Neutral	Neutral, potential risk (saxagliptin)	Neutral	No dose adjustment for linagliptin
Thiazolidinediones	4, 5, 6	High	(-) 1 - 1.5%	No	Gain	(+) 4kg	Oral	QD	Low	Potential benefit (stroke): Pioglitazone (IRIS)	Increased risk	Neutral	No dose adjustment, but generally not recommended in renal impairment
Sulfonylureas (2nd gen.)	1	High	(-) 1.5 - 2%	Yes	Gain	(+) 1 - 2kg	Oral	QD	Low	Neutral	Neutral	Neutral	Glipizide and glimepiride may be cautiously considered, but avoid glyburide in CKD
Insulin (human)	management of hyperglycemia with reduced insulin secretion	High to Very High	(-) 1.4% (product and dose dependent)	Yes	Gain	(+) 1.7 - 2.5kg	Injectable	TID, BID, QD	Low	Neutral	Neutral	Neutral	Titrate based on clinical response.
Insulin (analog)		High to Very High		Yes	Gain		Injectable		High	Neutral	Neutral	Neutral	

Table 4.2 Summary of properties and considerations of diabetes therapies recommended in the 2024 ADA Standards. Adapted from ElSayed NA et al. [2, 9, 37, 38, 39, 40, 41]. The "Mechanism/Effects" column identifies the numbered mechanisms of the Egregious Eleven (referring to Figure 1 at the beginning of this chapter [34].

reserved for individuals with an A1C >10% or blood glucose over 300 mg/dL, signs of catabolism, or symptoms of hyperglycemia. Insulin may also be used as part of initial combination therapy to shorten the time to meeting treatment goals. With the introduction and further development of GLP-1 therapy, GLP-1 and GLP-1/GIP RA have become a strong recommendation over insulin when feasible. GLP-1 RAs are also recommended for individuals who have not yet met their weight goal and desire weight loss.

Based on clinical experience and expert consensus, when lower-cost medications are utilized the ADA cautions health-care providers to select an affordable option while also considering risks associated with each class of therapy, such as hypoglycemia, CV and kidney events, and weight gain.

Conclusion

From the first commercial insulin therapy in 1923 to the most recent approval of tirzepatide in 2022, the last century has been a period of significant growth and evolution for diabetes management. With so many new medications available, health-care providers need to understand the clinical considerations, dosing, and side effects of each medication to tailor a safe and effective plan for each individual with diabetes. In addition to pharmacologic therapy, individuals should also be educated on non-pharmacological and lifestyle modifications to aid in glycemic control.

For people with T1D, insulin is the therapy of choice and multiple daily doses are often required due to the insulin-dependent nature of T1D. The amount of evidence and guidance for the management of LADA is lacking in comparison to T1D and T2D, but similar medications may be utilized. Select medications indicated for T2D may be effective upon diagnosis; however, insulin may eventually become necessary due to progression of beta-cell dysfunction.

Many glucose-lowering medications are indicated for T2D, and management has changed from a predominantly glucose-centric approach to a holistic, person-centered approach, focused on addressing underlying causes of diabetes and preventing diabetes-related complications. Metformin continues to be a first-line recommended therapy for prediabetes and diabetes based on both cost and efficacy. Despite their higher cost, SGLT-2i and GLP-1-based therapies have become key players in diabetes management with evidence of cardiorenal and metabolic benefits. Alternative therapies, such as DPP-4i, sulfonylureas, and pioglitazone, may be utilized for certain individuals but have fallen out of favor due to side effects, lack of efficacy, or potential cardiorenal concerns. Insulin remains a key player in diabetes management when necessary for glycemic control; however, insulin therapy continues to evolve with possible approval of once-weekly insulin in the future. Glucose-lowering medication continues to expand in the number of therapeutic classes and specific products, offering more evidence, guidance, and hope for the future of diabetes management.

References

1. Suits A, Gudoor R, Shubrook J. Achieving remission in the era of clinical inertia: what is preventing us from treating type 2 diabetes? Diabetology. 2023;4(1):93–107. https://doi.org/10.3390/diabetology4010011.
2. El Sayed NA, Aleppo G, Aroda VR, American Diabetes Association, et al. 9. Pharmacologic approaches to glycemic treatment: standards of Care in Diabetes—2024. Diabetes Care. 2024;47(Suppl. 1):S158–78.
3. El Sayed NA, Aleppo G, Aroda VR, American Diabetes Association, et al. 2. Classification and diagnosis of diabetes: standards of Care in Diabetes—2023. Diabetes Care. 2023;46(Suppl. 1):S19–40.
4. Buzzetti R, Tuomi T, Mauricio D, et al. Management of latent autoimmune diabetes in adults: a consensus statement from an International Expert Panel. Diabetes. 2020;69(10):2037–47.
5. Glucophage (metformin) [prescribing information]. Princeton, NJ: Bristol-Myers Squibb; 2018.
6. Glumetza (metformin) [prescribing information]. Bridgewater, NJ: Salix Pharmaceuticals; 2019.
7. Kim J, Ahn CW, Fang S, Lee HS, Park JS. Association between metformin dose and vitamin B12 deficiency in patients with type 2 diabetes. Medicine (Baltimore). 2019;98(46):e17918.
8. El Sayed NA, Aleppo G, Aroda VR, American Diabetes Association, et al. 3. Prevention or delay of type 2 diabetes and associated comorbidities: standards of Care in Diabetes—2023. Diabetes Care. 2023;46(Suppl. 1):S41–8.

9. Trujillo J, Haines S. Diabetes Mellitus. In: JT DP, Yee GC, Posey L, Haines ST, Nolin TD, Ellingrod V, editors. Pharmacotherapy: a pathophysiologic approach. 11th ed. McGraw Hill; 2020. Accessed 27 Nov 2023.
10. Glipizide tablets [prescribing information]. Baudette, MN: ANI Pharmaceuticals Inc; 2022.
11. A study of the effects of hypoglycemia agents on vascular complications in patients with adult-onset diabetes. VI. Supplementary report on nonfatal events in patients treated with tolbutamide. Diabetes. 1976;25(12):1129–53.
12. GRADE Study Research Group, Nathan DM, Lachin JM, Balasubramanyam A, et al. Glycemic reduction in type 2 diabetes—Glycemic outcomes. N Engl J Med. 2022;387(12):1063–74.
13. Wright A, Felix Burden AC, Paisey RB, U.K. Prospective Diabetes Study Group, et al. Sulfonylurea inadequacy: efficacy of addition of insulin over 6 years in patients with type 2 diabetes in the U.K. Prospective Diabetes Study (UKPDS 57). Diabetes Care. 2002;25(2):330–6.
14. Rosenstock J, Kahn SE, Johansen OE, CAROLINA Investigators, et al. Effect of linagliptin vs glimepiride on major adverse cardiovascular outcomes in patients with type 2 diabetes: The CAROLINA randomized clinical trial. JAMA. 2019;322(12):1155–66.
15. Hasslacher C, Multinational Repaglinide Renal Study Group. Safety and efficacy of repaglinide in type 2 diabetic patients with and without impaired renal function. Diabetes Care. 2003;26(3):886–91.
16. Meneilly GS. Effect of repaglinide versus glyburide on postprandial glucose and insulin values in elderly patients with type 2 diabetes. Diabetes Technol Ther. 2011;13(1):63–5.
17. Actos (pioglitazone) [prescribing information]. Lexington, MA: Takeda Pharmaceuticals America, Inc; 2020.
18. Ghosh S, Collier A. Section 3 - Management of diabetes. In: Ghosh S, Collier A, editors. Churchill's Pocketbook of Diabetes. 2nd ed. Churchill Livingstone; 2012. p. 83–125., ISBN 9780443100819. https://doi.org/10.1016/B978-0-443-10081-9.00010-5.
19. Acarbose tablets, USP [prescribing information]. Congers, NY: Chartwell RX, LLC. 2023.
20. Schmeltz L, Metzger B. 6.19 - Diabetes/Syndrome X. In: Taylor JB, Triggle DJ, editors. Comprehensive medicinal chemistry II. Elsevier; 2007. p. 417–58., ISBN 9780080450445. https://doi.org/10.1016/B0-08-045044-X/00179-6.
21. Wilding J, Fernando K, Milne N, et al. SGLT2 inhibitors in type 2 diabetes management: Key evidence and implications for clinical practice. Diabetes Ther. 2018;9(5):1757–73.
22. Chan JCH, Chan MCY. SGLT2 inhibitors: the next blockbuster multifaceted drug? Medicina. 2023;59(2):388.

23. Meraz-Muñoz AY, Weinstein J, Wald R. eGFR decline after SGLT2 inhibitor initiation: the tortoise and the hare reimagined. Kidney360. 2021;2(6):1042–7.
24. Kumar S, Bhavni SP, Goyal P, et al. Preoperative cessation of SGLT2i. Am Coll Cardiol. https://www.acc.org/Latest-in-Cardiology/Articles/2022/10/07/17/21/Preoperative-Cessation-of-SGLT2i
25. Ozempic (semaglutide) [prescribing information]. Plainsboro, NJ: Novo Nordisk Inc; 2022.
26. Ushakumari DS, Sladen RN. ASA Consensus-based guidance on preoperative management of patients (adults and children) on glucagon-like peptide-1 receptor agonists. Anesthesiology. 2024;140(2):346–8.
27. Modarressi T, Pillai P. GLP1RAs in clinical practice: therapeutic advances and safety perspectives. American College of Cardiology; 2024. https://www.acc.org/Latest-in-Cardiology/Articles/2024/04/15/11/19/GLP1RAs-in-Clinical-Practice
28. Perkovic V, Tuttle KR, Rossing P, FLOW Trial Committees and Investigators, et al. Effects of semaglutide on chronic kidney disease in patients with type 2 diabetes. N Engl J Med. 2024;391(2):109–21.
29. Nicholls SJ, Bhatt DL, Buse JB, SURPASS-CVOT investigators, et al. Comparison of tirzepatide and dulaglutide on major adverse cardiovascular events in participants with type 2 diabetes and atherosclerotic cardiovascular disease: SURPASS-CVOT design and baseline characteristics. Am Heart J. 2024;267:1–11.
30. Frías JP, Davies MJ, Rosenstock J, SURPASS-2 Investigators, et al. Tirzepatide versus semaglutide once weekly in patients with type 2 diabetes. N Engl J Med. 2021;385:503–15.
31. Skelley JW, Swearengin K, York AL, Glover LH. The impact of tirzepatide and glucagon-like peptide 1 receptor agonists on oral hormonal contraception. J Am Pharm Assoc. 2003). 2024;64(1):204–211.e4.
32. Whitley HP, Trujillo JM, Neumiller JJ. Special report: potential strategies for addressing GLP-1 and dual GLP-1/GIP receptor agonist shortages. Clin Diabetes. 2023;41(3):467–73.
33. Cowart K, Carris NW. Practicable measurement and identification of overbasalization. Clin Diabetes. 2022;40(1):75–7.
34. Schroeder EB. Management of type 2 diabetes: selecting amongst available pharmacological agents. [Updated 2022 Jul 28]. In: Feingold KR, Anawalt B, Blackman MR, et al., editors. Endotext [Internet]. South Dartmouth (MA): MDText.com, Inc.; 2000. Available from: https://www.ncbi.nlm.nih.gov/books/NBK425702/.
35. Welchol (colesevelam) [prescribing information]. South Plainfield, NJ: Cosette Pharmaceuticals Inc; 2022.
36. Ab Rahman N, Lim MT, Thevendran S, Ahmad Hamdi N, Sivasampu S. Medication regimen complexity and medication burden among patients with type 2 diabetes mellitus: a retrospective analysis. Front Pharmacol. 2022;21(13):808190.

37. American Diabetes Association Professional Practice Committee. 9. Pharmacologic approaches to glycemic treatment: standards of care in diabetes-2024 [published correction appears in Diabetes Care. 2024;47(7):1238. https://doi.org/10.2337/dc24-er07a.]. Diabetes Care. 2024;47(Suppl 1):S158–S178. https://doi.org/10.2337/dc24-S009.
38. Hinnen D. Glucagon-like peptide 1 receptor agonists for type 2 diabetes. Diabetes Spectr. 2017;30(3):202–10.
39. Rizvi AA, Rizzo M. The emerging role of dual GLP-1 and GIP receptor agonists in glycemic management and cardiovascular risk reduction. Diabetes Metab Syndr Obes. 2022;15:1023–30.
40. Dailey G, Admane K, Mercier F, Owens D. Relationship of insulin dose, A1c lowering, and weight in type 2 diabetes: comparing insulin glargine and insulin detemir. Diabetes Technol Ther. 2010;12(12):1019–27.
41. Garvey WT, Frias JP, Jastreboff AM, SURMOUNT-2 Investigators, et al. Tirzepatide once weekly for the treatment of obesity in people with type 2 diabetes (SURMOUNT-2): a double-blind, randomised, multicentre, placebo-controlled, phase 3 trial. Lancet. 2023;402(10402):613–26.

Management of Complications

5

Emily M. Scopelliti and Nicole Cheung

Introduction

One of the main treatment goals of diabetes is preventing chronic complications related to the condition. Landmark trials, including the United Kingdom Prospective Diabetes Study (UKPDS), the Diabetes Control and Complications Trial (DCCT), and the Action to Control Cardiovascular Risk in Diabetes (ACCORD) trial, have demonstrated the association between achieving glycemic goals through lower A1C levels and the prevention of diabetes-related complications [1–3]. The degree of prevention is related to the magnitude of glycemic control, which emphasizes the importance of early and aggressive diabetes management.

E. M. Scopelliti (✉)
Department of Pharmacy Practice, Jefferson College of Pharmacy,
Thomas Jefferson University, Philadelphia, PA, USA
e-mail: emily.scopelliti@jefferson.edu

N. Cheung
Northwell, New Hyde Park, NY, USA

Department of Science Education, Zucker School of Medicine
at Hofstra/Northwell, Hempstead, NY, USA
e-mail: Nicole.c.cheung@hofstra.edu

© The Author(s), under exclusive license to Springer Nature
Switzerland AG 2025

J. Clements (ed.), *The Pharmacist's Pocket Guide for Diabetes and Obesity*, https://doi.org/10.1007/978-3-031-88835-9_5

A comprehensive diabetes management strategy should focus on glycemic control and include early monitoring, identification, and treatment of diabetes complications to improve quality of life and promote overall well-being.

Microvascular Complications

Diabetic Retinopathy

Background

Diabetic retinopathy is the leading cause of blindness in adults. Its prevalence and progression is related to the duration of disease and the extent of glycemic control [4]. Other major risk factors for the development of diabetic retinopathy include hypertension (HTN), dyslipidemia, kidney disease, and pregnancy [5].

Diabetic retinopathy is often asymptomatic and progresses from nonproliferative diabetic retinopathy (NPDR) to proliferative diabetic retinopathy (PDR) (Table 5.1). It can also lead to other ophthalmic complications including diabetic macular edema (DME) and earlier incidence and progression of glaucoma and cataracts [5].

Screening and Monitoring

Screening and monitoring for ocular abnormalities are vital given the typically asymptomatic nature of the disease. People with type 1 diabetes (T1D) often do not present with retinopathy until at least 5 years after disease onset, supporting the recommendation of initiating annual dilated and comprehensive eye examination within 5 years of diagnosis. People with type 2 diabetes (T2D) may have experienced years of undiagnosed hyperglycemia and should therefore undergo an annual dilated and comprehensive eye examination immediately upon diagnosis. People with risk factors including hyperglycemia, the presence of DME or advanced retinopathy at baseline or those with progressive retinopathy will require more frequent monitoring [6].

Table 5.1 Characteristics, monitoring frequency and treatment of diabetic retinopathy

Type	Characteristics	Monitoring	Treatment
Mild NPDR	Microaneurysms Fluid leakage into the retina	Annually	None
Moderate NPDR	Blood vessel abnormalities Retinal changes DME may be present	Every 6–9 months	None
Severe NPDR	Blood vessel blockage Growth factor signaling blood vessel proliferation	Every 3–6 months	Consider early PRP in T2D
PDR	Blood vessel proliferation increasing risk for hemorrhaging Vision loss Retinal detachment risk leading to permanent vision loss	Every 3 months	First line: PRP in high risk Alternative: Anti-VEGF
CIDME	Edema present within the center of the macula caused by fluid leakage from retinal blood vessels	Every 1–4 months	First line: Anti-VEGFadjunctive: Macular photocoagulation Alternative: Intravitreal corticosteroid therapy

Adapted from source: Ref. [5]
CIDME central-involved diabetic macular edema, *DME* diabetic macular edema, *NPDR* nonproliferative diabetic retinopathy, *PDR* proliferative diabetic retinopathy, *PRP* panretinal laser photocoagulation, *T2D* type 2 diabetes

Due to the increased risk for acceleration and progression of the disease during pregnancy, people with diabetes who are of childbearing age and are planning pregnancy or those who become pregnant should be monitored closely. In these cases, screening with a comprehensive eye exam is recommended before pregnancy, during each trimester, and for 1-year postpartum as indicated depending on the severity of retinopathy during pregnancy [6, 7].

Management Strategies

Management of diabetic retinopathy is inclusive of risk factor management to prevent occurrence and progression. Improving glycemia is the principal management strategy for preventing and delaying diabetic retinopathy. Additionally, appropriate management of dyslipidemia and HTN are also important strategies to prevent risk and slow progression [6].

With appropriate screening and risk factor management, people who develop diabetic retinopathy may require pharmacologic intervention. Those with severe NPDR, PDR and central-involved DME should be immediately referred to an ophthalmologist for consideration of intraocular treatments including panretinal laser photocoagulation (PRP) therapy and intravitreal injections of anti-vascular endothelial growth factor (anti-VEGF) agents. The diabetic retinopathy study (DRS) demonstrated that PRP decreased the risk of severe visual loss by more than 50% in people with high-risk PDR, while the Early Treatment Diabetic Retinopathy Study (ETDRS) demonstrated efficacy in high-risk PDR, severe NPDR in select people, and clinically significant macular edema (CSME) [8, 9]. Anti-VEGF agents have been shown to improve visual acuity. These agents are considered alternatives to PRP in high-risk people and first-line treatment options in central-involved DME (Table 5.1). Available anti-VEGF agents include bevacizumab, ranibizumab, aflibercept, brolucizumab, and faricimab [6].

Diabetic Neuropathy

Background

Diabetic neuropathy significantly impacts quality of life for people with diabetes and is associated with various complications including psychosocial and sleep disorders, pain, falls, and fractures [7]. Diabetic neuropathy is considered a diagnosis of exclusion; therefore, other causes of neuropathy should be ruled out and treated prior to diagnosis [10]. Diabetic neuropathy spans a wide range of clinical presentations and anatomical locations. Examples of common neuropathies related to diabetes include diabetic peripheral neuropathy (DPN) and autonomic neuropathies affecting the cardiovascular, gastrointestinal, and genitourinary systems [6].

DPN may present asymptomatically in up to half of the people affected; therefore, early screening, identification, education, and management are important to prevent future complications [6]. Clinical symptoms of DPN are dependent on nerve fiber involvement (Table 5.2). Small nerve fibers responsible for symptoms of neuropathic pain characterized as burning sensations, known as dysesthesias and "shooting pain," are most often affected first. Neuropathic pain may also present with allodynia, hyperalgesia, and paresthesia. Large fibers are responsible for symptoms related to numbness, loss of protective sensation, and tingling [7].

Cardiovascular autonomic neuropathy (CAN) is independently associated with cardiovascular mortality and may present asymptomatically in the preliminary stages of the disease [11]. Clinical presentation of advanced disease includes resting tachycardia and orthostatic hypotension. Autonomic neuropathies affecting the gastrointestinal tract include constipation, diarrhea, and gastroparesis and are characterized by symptoms, such as nausea, early satiety, vomiting, and fullness [10]. Neuropathies affecting the genitourinary system include neurogenic bladder presenting as urinary incontinence, urgency, frequency, hesitancy, and nocturia. Sexual dysfunction is another common genitourinary disturbance presenting as erectile dysfunction and retrograde ejaculation in

Table 5.2 Sensory examination of DPN

	Small nerve fibers	Large nerve fibers
Symptoms	Neuropathic pain	Tingling, numbness
Examination	Pinprick sensation using disposable pin Temperature sensation (hot/cold) using cold tuning fork	Vibration sensation using 128 Hz tuning fork Ankle reflexes 10-g monofilament measuring protective sensation

Adapted from source: Ref. [10]
Examination results that are absent or reduced are considered clinically diagnostic for DPN

men and dyspareunia and decreased libido in women. Lastly, impaired awareness of hypoglycemia is another complication related to autonomic neuropathy [6].

Screening and Monitoring

Initial screening for DPN is recommended within 5 years of T1D diagnosis and immediately after diagnosis of T2D. Subsequent screenings are recommended at least annually. Screening for DPN entails a clinical history that focuses on symptoms and physical examination to determine the presence of DPN and risk of future complications [6]. The various clinical examinations for DPN evaluate both small and large nerve fibers associated with a variety of functions (Table 5.2).

Management Strategies

Intensive glycemic control is the primary management strategy to prevent diabetic neuropathies. Data supporting glycemic control for prevention is strongest for people with T1D, with a more modest effect demonstrated in the (Action to Control Cardiovascular Risk in Diabetes) trial for people with T2D [12]. Management is critically important given its detrimental effects on quality of life. In addition to pharmacologic treatment options, it is recommended to implement non-pharmacologic approaches that focus on psychosocial aspects of the disease, including sleep and mood disorders, given their strong correlation with DPN [13].

There are currently no available treatments that directly reverse underlying nerve damage. After differential diagnoses are excluded, the symptomatic treatment of neuropathic pain may be considered using a variety of drug classes that have been found to be equally effective in reducing pain. It is important to set appropriate person-centered expectations regarding treatment efficacy as they often do not result in complete pain resolution [13]. Gabapentinoids, serotonin-norepinephrine reuptake inhibitors (SNRIs), tricyclic antidepressants (TCAs), sodium channel blockers, and capsaicin are evidence-based treatment options for pain associated with DPN according to the American Academy of Neurology's guideline update on the treatment of painful diabetic polyneuropathy (Table 5.3). Initial therapy choice should be based

Table 5.3 Pharmacologic treatment of DPN

Pharmacologic therapy	Clinical considerations
Gabapentinoids Gabapentin Pregabalin	Lower doses and slower titration may improve tolerability in elderly May contribute to peripheral edema and should be used in caution with existing peripheral edema related to heart failure, liver, and renal disease May be an appropriate choice for coexisting diagnosis of seizure disorders Require renal dose adjustments Use with caution in those with substance use disorders due to abuse potential and dependence Use caution as pregabalin is a controlled substance (C-V)
SNRIs Duloxetine Venlafaxine Desvenlafaxine	Less likely to be tolerated in patients with symptoms of nausea, dizziness, and fatigue due to common adverse effects Lower doses and slower titration may improve duloxetine tolerability in elderly May be an appropriate choice for coexisting diagnosis of depression or anxiety May cause elevations in blood pressure (venlafaxine and desvenlafaxine)
TCAs Amitriptyline Nortriptyline	Limit use in ≥65 years of age due to anticholinergic side effects Less likely to be tolerated in patients with orthostatic hypotension, urinary retention, and constipation. May be an appropriate choice for coexisting diagnosis of depression or anxiety
Sodium channel blockers Lamotrigine Lacosamide Carbamazepine Oxcarbazepine Valproic acid	Less likely to be tolerated in patients with symptoms of nausea, dizziness, and fatigue due to common adverse effects Avoid valproic acid in pregnancy May be an appropriate choice for coexisting diagnosis of seizure disorders
Capsaicin	Available as 8% patch (FDA approved), 0.075% cream (off-label) and in various over-the-counter products Useful for patients preferring topical treatment

Source: Refs [6, 13]

on specific factors including drug-drug interactions, adverse effects, and comorbidities [10]. If symptom improvement is not experienced after 12 weeks of therapy at appropriate doses, switching to an alternative agent or trying a combination of agents is appropriate and often necessary. Opioids are not recommended for the treatment of DPN due to their addictive potential. People should be referred to a specialty pain clinic if symptoms persist or medications are intolerable [10, 13].

Management of autonomic neuropathies is related to symptomatic treatment according to individual presentation. People experiencing orthostatic hypotension related to CAN should be evaluated for medication-induced causes that may be exacerbating the condition. People may benefit from physical activity to prevent deconditioning related to worsening orthostasis. Fluid replacement and salt supplementation may also be helpful to promote volume repletion. Low-dose fludrocortisone is a pharmacological option for the treatment of orthostatic hypotension; however, dosing is limited by supine HTN [10].

Gastroparesis is often difficult to manage. Dietary recommendations including smaller, more frequent meals that are rich in fiber and low in fat are beneficial. Identifying drug-induced causes may be useful to avoid exacerbating the condition. Common drug classes include TCAs, glucagon-like peptide 1 receptor agonists (GLP-1 RA), and opioids [10]. Metoclopramide is a prokinetic agent used to increase intestinal motility in people with gastroparesis; however, the risk-benefit ratio is not favorable due to extrapyramidal adverse effects and should only be considered for no more than 12 weeks in severe cases of gastroparesis that are not relieved by other treatments [6].

Foot Care

Background

DPN, in addition to foot deformities and peripheral arterial disease (PAD), are common risk factors associated with diabetes-related foot ulcers and amputations, the latter of which has significant effects on all aspects of life, including emotional, psychological, and physical well-being. In addition to foot deformities (e.g., Charcot foot, hammertoe, bunions) and PAD, poor glycemic control, corns, calluses, loss of protective sensation (LOPS) related to DPN, prior ulceration, or amputation, smoking, retinopathy, and significant nephropathy are also risk factors associated with foot complications. Early identification of risk factors and treatment of ulcers are important in preventing complications including amputations [6].

Screening and Monitoring

A comprehensive foot exam to evaluate risk is recommended at least annually. Comprehensive foot evaluations are inclusive of neurological exams as described in Table 5.2 to identify DPN and LOPS, inspection of the skin, identification of foot deformities, and vascular assessment including peripheral pulses. In addition to physical examination, a complete history tailored to identify risk factors is important to stratify risk and recommend appropriate foot exam frequency (Table 5.4). Patients play a vital role in monitoring foot complications and should be educated on how to perform daily foot inspections, skin, and nail care. Patients should

Table 5.4 International Working Group on the Diabetic Foot (IWGDF) Risk Stratification System

Category	Ulcer risk	Characteristics	Screening frequency
0	Very low	No LOPS or PAD	Annually
1	Low	LOPS or PAD	Every 6 to 12 months
2	Moderate	LOPS + PAD or either LOPS or PAD with foot deformity	Every 3 to 6 months
3	High	LOPS or PAD with at least one of the following: History of a foot ulcer Amputation of lower extremity ESRD	Every 1 to 3 months

Adapted from source: Ref. [14]

ESKD end-stage kidney disease, *LOPS* loss of protective sensation, *PAD* peripheral arterial disease also be educated to identify abnormalities such as cuts, sores, blisters, corns, calluses, skin changes (e.g., temperature, color), pain, swelling, and signs or symptoms of infection [6].

Management Strategies

Education on appropriate self-care is one of the most important methods to prevent foot complications in people with diabetes. Specific foot care recommendations are dependent on risk stratification (Table 5.4). Education on appropriate self-care is often appropriate for people with no risk or low risk. People determined to be moderate to high-risk, including those with foot deformities, LOPS, and/or PAD, should be referred to foot care specialists for routine management and follow-up [6].

Important self-care recommendations for proper foot care include daily foot inspections; the use of moisturizers and emollients to prevent dry, cracked skin, wearing socks and shoes consistently to protect feet from injury; and proper cutting of toenails (straight across) to avoid complications. People who are stratified as risk category 1 or higher with LOPS should acquire footwear evaluated for appropriate fit and adaptations for foot deformities if applicable [14]. These adaptations can include orthoses that relieve plantar pressures in those presenting with plantar calluses, custom-made insoles, or extra-depth footwear [6, 14].

Diabetic Nephropathy

Background

Diabetes, especially in combination with uncontrolled HTN, is among the leading causes of end-stage kidney disease (ESKD) in the United States [15]. Up to 40% of people with diabetes will develop chronic kidney disease (CKD) [16]. Risk factors for the development of diabetic nephropathy include duration of disease, poor glycemic control, and HTN. The presence of CKD in diabetes is associated with a variety of acute and chronic complications. Acutely, there is a higher risk of diabetic ketoacidosis and hypoglycemia. In the long term, there is an increased risk for cardiovascular complications, as well as neuropathy, retinopathy, and ESKD, resulting in dialysis or transplantation [17]. A comprehensive approach that is person-centered and multidisciplinary is necessary for optimal management of diabetic nephropathy, including regular assessment and management of cardiovascular risk factors, such as HTN, dyslipidemia, smoking, and obesity [18].

Screening and Monitoring

Diabetic nephropathy is defined by reduced estimated glomerular filtration rate (eGFR) and/or the presence of albuminuria without signs and symptoms indicative of other causes of kidney disease [19]. Initial screening of eGFR and urine albumin to creatinine ratio (ACR) is recommended starting 5 years after diagnosis of T1D and immediately after diagnosis of T2D. The diagnosis of CKD is confirmed by persistent eGFR <60 mL/min/1.73 m^2, persistent urine ACR ≥30 mg/g, or other signs of kidney damage [18]. Suggested monitoring frequency is dependent on CKD progression and risk and may vary from annual follow-up to more than 4 times per year (Table 5.5).

Table 5.5 Risk categorization of diabetic nephropathy based on GFR and albuminuria

<table>
<tr><td colspan="3" rowspan="3"></td><td colspan="3">Albuminuria categories</td></tr>
<tr><td>A1</td><td>A2</td><td>A3</td></tr>
<tr><td><30 mg/g</td><td>30–299 mg/g</td><td>≥300 mg/g</td></tr>
<tr><td rowspan="6">GFR categories (mL/min/1.73 m^2)</td><td>G1</td><td>≥90</td><td rowspan="2">Low risk 1</td><td rowspan="2">Moderate risk 1</td><td rowspan="2">High risk 3</td></tr>
<tr><td>G2</td><td>60–89</td></tr>
<tr><td>G3a</td><td>45–59</td><td>Moderate risk 1</td><td>High risk 2</td><td rowspan="2">Very high risk 3</td></tr>
<tr><td>G3b</td><td>30–44</td><td>High risk 2</td><td rowspan="2">Very high risk 3</td></tr>
<tr><td>G4</td><td>15–29</td><td>Very high risk 3</td><td rowspan="2">Very high risk 4+</td></tr>
<tr><td>G5</td><td><15</td><td>Very high risk 4+</td><td>Very high risk 4+</td></tr>
</table>

Adapted from source: Ref. [18]
GFR glomerular filtration rate

Management Strategies

Given the correlation between diabetic nephropathy and cardiovascular risk, a comprehensive management strategy focuses on optimizing glycemic control as well as improving cardiovascular outcomes [17]. All people with diabetes should be educated on appropriate lifestyle modifications targeting nutrition, physical activity, smoking cessation, and weight loss. A variety of pharmacologic agents have been shown to improve outcomes in people with diabetes and CKD. These therapies target multiple pathways that protect the heart and kidneys and decrease risk by optimizing glucose, blood pressure, and lipid control [18].

In terms of glycemic control and at the time of writing this chapter, sodium-glucose cotransporter-2 inhibitors (SGLT-2i) and metformin are considered first line in people with T2D with CKD. An SGLT-2i should be initiated in patients with an eGFR ≥20 mL/min/1.73 m^2 and may be continued until dialysis or transplant, while metformin may be initiated or continued based on eGFR (refer to chapter 4 for more details). A GLP-1 RA with proven cardiovascular benefit is recommended if further glycemic control is needed despite SGLT-2i and/or metformin therapy [17]; however, emerging evidence indicates that GLP-1 RA with proven benefit could be an option as first-line therapy, rather than metformin for those with T2D and CKD.

First-line agents for HTN in people with diabetes and CKD with albuminuria include angiotensin-converting enzyme inhibitors (ACEi) or angiotensin II receptor blockers (ARB) titrated to the highest tolerable approved doses. There is no clear benefit demonstrated with an ACEi or ARB in people without albuminuria; therefore, dihydropyridine calcium channel blockers (CCB) may be considered to treat HTN in this population [17]. A nonsteroidal mineralocorticoid receptor antagonist (ns-MRA) with proven cardiovascular and kidney benefits is specifically recommended in CKD associated with T2D with persistently elevated urine ACR (≥30 mg/g) despite maximally tolerated doses of an ACEi or ARB. Currently, finerenone is the only drug within the class that has demonstrated cardiovascular and kidney benefits. An ns-MRA should only be recommended if potassium levels are within normal limits and eGFR is ≥25 mL/min/1.73 m^2 [18]. A steroidal

MRA such as spironolactone or eplerenone is recommended for people with T1D or T2D with resistant HTN, heart failure (HF), or hyperaldosteronism in the setting of normal potassium levels and an eGFR ≥45 mL/min/1.73 m^2 [17].

Another first-line therapy included in the comprehensive approach for improving outcomes in people with diabetes and CKD is moderate or high-intensity statins. Statins have been shown to decrease cardiovascular risk in CKD stages 1–4 and kidney transplant. However, this benefit does not appear to extend to those on chronic dialysis [17]. Additional lipid lowering agents may be required based on atherosclerotic cardiovascular disease (ASCVD) risk and lipid goals. Antiplatelet agents should also be recommended as indicated for people with clinical ASCVD [18].

Macrovascular Complications

Hypertension

Background

Over 73% of adults with diabetes mellitus have been diagnosed with HTN, which is a disease that impacts over one billion people worldwide [20, 21]. The pathophysiology of HTN in people with diabetes is due to several factors, including: (1) insulin resistance increasing vascular oxidative stress and inflammation; (2) increased intravascular volume due to increased serum osmolality from hyperglycemia; and (3) increased sympathetic activity and activation of the renin-angiotensin-aldosterone system (RAAS) from autonomic nervous system dysregulation from central obesity and insulin resistance [22]. Diabetes, HTN, and hyperlipidemia are cardiovascular risk factors that contribute to metabolic syndrome and result in macrovascular complications, such as cardiovascular, cerebrovascular, and peripheral vascular disease (PVD) [23].

People with HTN usually are asymptomatic and may experience chest pain or shortness of breath in severe cases contributing to organ damage [24]. Diagnosis is based on at least two blood pressure measurements, in which systolic blood pressure (SBP) is ≥130 millimeters of mercury (mm Hg) or diastolic blood pressure (DBP) is ≥80 mm Hg in the medical office on at least two separate occasions [25, 26]. If an individual with cardiovascular disease presents with a blood pressure reading ≥180/110 mm Hg, then HTN can be diagnosed at a single visit [26]. Additional blood pressure measurements outside the office are recommended to confirm the diagnosis and assist with ruling out masked HTN (in-office blood pressure is normal but out-of-office blood pressure is elevated) and white coat HTN (in-office blood pressure is elevated but out-of-office blood pressure is normal) [25]. The classification of HTN in adults can be found in Table 5.6.

Screening

Due to the mostly asymptomatic nature of HTN, it is recommended to measure blood pressure for people with diabetes at every routine visit, and at least annually in adults 40 or older with risk factors for HTN [26, 27]. It is recommended to be mindful of potential inaccuracies in blood pressure measurements by the patient, health-care professional's technique, and equipment [28]. In preparation for a blood pressure reading, patients should avoid caffeine consumption and physical activity within 30 min of measurement, empty their bladder, and remain seated quietly for at least 5 min. Health-care professionals should ensure cuff deflation is at an appropriate rate and patients should be appropriately positioned with their arm at heart level with legs uncrossed. The appropriate blood pressure cuff size should be used and cover about 80% of the upper arm circumference [24].

Table 5.6 Classification of hypertension

Classification	SBP		DBP
Normal blood pressure	<120 mm hg	AND	<80 mm hg
Elevated blood pressure	120–129 mm hg	AND	<80 mm hg
Stage 1 hypertension	130–139 mm hg	OR	80–89 mm hg
Stage 2 hypertension	≥140 mm hg	OR	≥90 mm hg

Adapted from source: Ref. [25]
DBP diastolic blood pressure, *SBP* systolic blood pressure

Management Strategies

Goals

As per the American Diabetes Association (ADA) Guidelines, the recommended blood pressure goal for people with diabetes or CKD is less than 130/80 mm Hg, which coincides with the recommendation by the 2017 American College of Cardiology (ACC) / American Heart Association (AHA) and Seventh Joint National Committee (JNC 7) Guidelines [25, 29]. The Eighth Joint National Committee (JNC 8) Guidelines recommend a less conservative blood pressure target of less than 140/90 mm Hg [30]. A stricter goal of SBP 110–135 mm Hg and DBP 85 mm Hg is recommended in pregnancy to reduce the risk of accelerated HTN [26]. The American Association of Clinical Endocrinology (AACE) recommends a blood pressure goal of less than 130/80 mm Hg for most people with diabetes, with consideration of implementing a higher goal in people experiencing medication adverse effects, autonomic neuropathy, acute coronary syndrome, frailty, or orthostatic hypotension. A goal of less than 120/70 mm Hg may be considered to prevent progression of complications in people with albuminuria, coronary heart disease (CHD), moderate-to-high risk of CHD, PVD, or retinopathy [7].

Non-Pharmacological Management

Lifestyle modifications are recommended for people with elevated blood pressure >120/80 mm Hg. Options include: (1) promoting weight loss, when indicated, (2) encouraging the Dietary Approaches to Stop Hypertension (DASH) diet to increase fruits and vegetable intake (8–10 servings/day), reduce sodium (<2300 mg/day), and increase potassium intake, (3) limiting alcohol intake to no more than 1 serving/day for women and 2 servings/day for men, and (4) increasing physical activity to at least 150 min of moderate-intensity aerobic exercise per week [24].

Pharmacological Management

Pharmacological treatment for HTN should be indicated in people with diabetes with blood pressure that is persistently elevated

≥130/80 mm Hg. If the office-based blood pressure is ≥160/100 mm Hg, then at least two medications are indicated. The blood pressure threshold is 140/90 mm Hg for initiation of pharmacological treatment in pregnancy [26].

Treatment for HTN includes ACEi or ARB as first-line therapy in coronary artery disease (CAD) or albuminuria, defined as urine ACR >30 mg/g, to reduce cardiovascular events. The combination of an ACEi and ARB is not recommended due to the lack of clinical benefit and increased risk of hyperkalemia and renal impairment. Other options include non-dihydropyridine CCB and thiazide-like diuretic where long-acting agents, such as chlorthalidone and indapamide, have been shown to reduce cardiovascular events. Those uncontrolled on maximum doses or maximally tolerated doses of these classes (with at least one being a thiazide-like diuretic) may be initiated on an MRA [26]. To promote medication adherence, consideration of pills with a combination of antihypertensive medications is recommended.

Second-line agents for HTN include beta blockers, loop diuretics, potassium-sparing diuretics, alpha-1 blockers, alpha-2 agonists, and direct arterial vasodilators. Beta blockers are recommended for concomitant ischemic heart disease, HF, atrial fibrillation, and migraines. Only bisoprolol, carvedilol, and metoprolol succinate are recommended for HF with reduced ejection fraction (HFrEF). Beta blockers can be categorized based on the specific mechanism of action: alpha- and beta-receptor antagonism, beta-1 and beta-2 receptor antagonism (non-cardioselective), and beta-1 receptor antagonism (cardioselective). Caution is advised due to its ability to mask symptoms of hypoglycemia from norepinephrine blockage, such as tachycardia and tremors. Loop diuretics such as furosemide are preferred for symptomatic HF management, and higher doses may be needed when eGFR is less than 30 mL/min/1.73 m^2. Caution is advised for adults aged 65 years and older due to the risk of syndrome of inappropriate antidiuretic hormone secretion and hyponatremia. Caution is advised for those with CKD, elevated baseline serum potassium levels greater than 5.5 mEq/L, or concomitant use of potassium supplements due to the risk of hyperkalemia and resulting cardiac arrhythmias. Alpha-1 blockers, such as terazosin, may be used as adjunct therapy for benign prostatic hyperplasia but use in older adults is not recommended due to the considerable risk of orthostatic hypotension. Alpha-2 agonists are associated with central nervous system effects, bradycardia, and orthostatic hypotension, and similar to beta blockers, their use cannot be discontinued abruptly due to the risk of rebound HTN. Direct arterial vasodilators, such as hydralazine, are also not considered first-line therapies due to reflex tachycardia, fluid retention, and unpredictable blood pressure-lowering effects.

Dyslipidemia

Background

Dyslipidemia, or abnormal lipid profile, affects about 70–85% of people with T2D with the most common presentation being high triglycerides (TG) and low high-density lipoprotein (HDL-C) [31, 32]. The pathophysiology of dyslipidemia in people with diabetes is related to insulin resistance that causes compensatory hyperinsulinemia, which increases free fatty acid levels and hepatic secretion of very low-density lipoproteins (VLDL) and TG [32]. Dyslipidemia is usually asymptomatic, and diagnosis depends on the lipid panel (Table 5.7).

Screening and Monitoring

The ADA recommends that people with diabetes who are not taking a statin or lipid-lowering therapy receive a lipid panel at the time of diabetes diagnosis, at initial medical evaluation, then at least annually. If lipid-lowering treatments are initiated, a lipid panel should be obtained approximately 4–12 weeks after therapy initiation of dose adjustments to guide management [33]. Similarly, AACE guidelines recommend a lipid panel for all individuals with prediabetes, T1D aged 40 years and older, and T2D at diagnosis, then annually as indicated to reach lipid goals. Monitoring of statins with a lipid panel is recommended 6–12 weeks after initiation or dose titration [7].

Table 5.7 Classification of LDL, HDL, and TG Levels

LDL level: Optimal: <100 mg/dL Near optimal/above optimal: 100–129 mg/dL Borderline high: 130–159 mg/dL High: 160–189 mg/dL Very high: ≥190 mg/dL
HDL level: Low: <40 mg/dL High: ≥60 mg/dL
Fasting TG level: Normal: <150 mg/dL Borderline high: 150–299 mg/dL High: 200 to 499 mg/dL Very high: ≥500 mg/dL

Source: Ref. [35]
HDL high-density lipoprotein, *LDL* low-density lipoprotein, *TG* triglycerides

Management Strategies

Non-pharmacological Management

Lifestyle modifications to prevent dyslipidemia include Mediterranean and DASH dietary patterns, weight loss, and increased physical activity. Additional dietary recommendations include increasing dietary n-3 fatty acids, viscous fiber, and plant stanols/sterols [33].

Pharmacological Management

Primary Prevention

For primary prevention, adults between 40 and 75 with diabetes are recommended to receive a moderate-intensity statin regardless of estimated 10-year ASCVD risk. If these adults had multiple ASCVD risk factors, it is reasonable to use a high-intensity statin with the goal of reducing the low-density lipoprotein (LDL-C) by at least 50% from baseline to target an LDL of <70 mg/dL. For those with diabetes and a 10-year ASCVD risk that is 20% or higher, it is reasonable to initiate ezetimibe or a PCSK9 inhibitor despite being on a maximally tolerated statin therapy [33, 34]. Table 5.8 includes additional information regarding LDL goals stratified by risk. As per the Adult Treatment Panel III, LDL is the primary target of therapy because LDL-lowering treatments have been associated with reduced risk for CHD and reduced total mortality among people with existing CHD [35]. Moderate-intensity and high-intensity statin therapies can be found in Table 5.9.

Although uncommon, adults 20–39 years of age may require statin therapy depending on their risk, such as: long duration of diabetes mellitus (≥10 years of T2D, or ≥ 20 years for T1D), albuminuria (≥30 mcg of albumin/mg creatinine), eGFR less than 60 mL/min/1.73 m^2, retinopathy, neuropathy, or ankle-brachial-index (ABI <0.9) [34]. For adults 75 years of age and older, clinical decision-making is advised as it is reasonable to continue or

Table 5.8 LDL-C goals based on risk category

Risk category	Risk factors and estimated 10-year ASCVD risk	LDL-C goal (mg/dL)
Extreme risk	Progressive ASCVD after achieving an LDL-C <70 mg/dL Established clinical cardiovascular disease in people with DM, CKD stage 3 or 4, or HeFH History of premature ASCVD (in years: <55 male, <65 female)	<55
Very high risk	Established or recent hospitalization for ACS, coronary, carotid or PVD, 10-year risk >20% DM or CKD stage 3 or 4 with 1 or more risk factor(s) HeFH	<70
High risk	>2 risk factors and 10-year risk 10–20% DM or CKD stage 3 or 4 with no other risk factors	<100
Moderate risk	<2 risk factors and 10-year risk <10%	<100
Low risk	No risk factors	

Adapted from source: Ref. [34]

ACS acute coronary syndrome, *ASCVD* atherosclerotic cardiovascular disease, *CKD* chronic kidney disease, *HeFH* heterozygous familial hypercholesterolemia, *LDL* low-density lipoprotein, *PVD* peripheral vascular disease

Table 5.9 Moderate-intensity and high-intensity statin therapy

Moderate-intensity statin therapy LDL-C lowering: 30–49%	High-intensity statin terapy LDL-C lowering: ≥ 50%
Atorvastatin 10 or 20 mg Rosuvastatin 5 or10 mg Simvastatin 20 or 40 mg Pravastatin 40 or 80 mg Lovastatin 40 mg Fluvastatin XL 80 mg Pitavastatin 1 or 4 mg	Atorvastatin 40–80 mg Rosuvastatin 20–40 mg

Adapted from source: Ref. [34]
LDL low-density lipoprotein, *XL*, extended release

initiate statin therapy [34]. Of note, statin therapy is contraindicated in pregnancy. Therefore, it is recommended that women of childbearing age who are on statin therapy and sexually active should use contraception and be educated to discontinue statin therapy for at least 1– 2 months before pregnancy is attempted [33, 34].

Secondary Prevention

A high-intensity statin should be used to target an LDL reduction of at least 50% from baseline and an LDL goal of <55 mg/dL in all people with diabetes and concurrent ASCVD. Ezetimibe or PCSK9 inhibitors may be initiated if maximally tolerated statin therapy is not enough to reach target goals [33].

Hypertriglyceridemia

In adults 40–75 years of age with severe hypertriglyceridemia (fasting TG ≥500 mg/dL), and an ASCVD risk of 7.5% or higher, it is reasonable to initiate statin therapy. If triglycerides are persistently elevated or increasing despite lifestyle modifications, omega-3 fatty acids and fibrate therapy may be recommended to prevent acute pancreatitis [34].

Heart Failure

Background

Diabetes and HF are frequent comorbid conditions that increase the risk of the other disease state independently. Diabetes is associated with a nearly twofold and fourfold increase in the risk of HF in men and women, respectively. For each 1% increase in A1C, the risk of developing HF increases by 8% to 36% [36]. The pathophysiology of HF in people with diabetes is multifactorial. Hyperglycemia and hyperinsulinemia are associated with vascular smooth muscle inflammation and atherosclerosis. Cardiomyopathy related to diabetes may also present in the absence of typical risk factors such as HTN or CAD [37]. Signs and symptoms of HF may include shortness of breath, nocturnal cough, tachycardia, third heart sound, fatigue, reduced exercise tolerance, peripheral edema, pulmonary congestion, or ascites [38, 39].

Screening and Monitoring

For those with suspected HF, initial assessment includes clinical history, physical examination, laboratory assessments including natriuretic peptide and a 12-lead electrocardiogram. Since natriuretic peptide can be influenced by factors other than HF, consideration must be taken for those with advanced age, renal impairment, cardiac arrhythmia, and obesity. A transthoracic echocardiography (TTE) is recommended to diagnose HF: (1) HFrEF with a left ventricular ejection fraction (LVEF) ≤40%; (2) HF with mildly reduced ejection fraction (HFmrEF) with an LVEF of 41–49%; or (3) HF with preserved ejection fraction (HFpEF) with an LVEF ≥50% [40].

Routine screening for HF is not recommended. However, those at risk of developing HF may be screened for NT-proBNP and BNP lab values along with care by a multidisciplinary health-care team including a cardiovascular specialist for prevention of new-onset HF. Multivariable risk scores may also be used to calculate and estimate the risk for HF [40].

Management Strategies

Pharmacological management of HF depends on American College of Cardiology/American Heart Association (ACC/AHA) staging, left ventricular ejection fraction (LVEF), and many other factors. Given that diabetes is a risk factor for HF, all people with a diagnosis of diabetes are considered stage A (high risk for HF). Risk factor modification is of critical importance, such as improving glycemic control, weight loss and optimizing management of HTN, dyslipidemia, and cardiovascular disease [37].

Management of HFrEF

Many people with diabetes are considered stage B (asymptomatic with structural heart disease, abnormal cardiac function or elevated natriuretic peptide) [37]. Individuals in stage B with HFrEF should receive an ACEi, an ARB if ACEi-intolerant, and an evidence-based beta blocker (bisoprolol, carvedilol, or metoprolol succinate) to prevent symptomatic HF [40].

Guideline-directed medical therapy (GDMT) is recommended for people with HFrEF in stage C with current or previous symptoms of HF. The goal of GDMT is to titrate medications to target doses that have demonstrated mortality benefit, even when symptoms or lab values improve at lower doses. GDMT includes the following: (1) angiotensin receptor/neprilysin inhibitor (ARNI), ACEi, or ARB; (2) evidence-based beta blocker; (3) MRA; and (4) SGLT-2i. A loop diuretic is also indicated when needed for fluid retention [37, 40]. Sacubitril/valsartan (ARNI) is preferred to ACEi and ARB therapy [40].

African American people with class II–IV HFrEF on optimal GDMT are recommended to receive a combination of hydralazine and isosorbide dinitrate to reduce morbidity and mortality. Once GDMT is optimized, additional agents including ivabradine, vericiguat, digoxin, and potassium binders may be recommended depending on New York Heart Association Class, LVEF, symptoms, vital signs, and laboratory values. For those who progress to stage D (refractory HF), it is recommended to consider alternative options, such as durable mechanical circulatory support (MCS) devices, cardiac transplant, and palliative care [40].

Management of HFpEF

The incidence of HFpEF continues to increase and is associated with over 50% of HF cases in hospitalized patients [41]. Emerging evidence has expanded upon the traditional strategy of exclusively focusing on the management of comorbid conditions. In addition to evaluating risk and treating comorbidities (e.g., atrial fibrillation, CAD, CKD, diabetes, HTN, obesity, and obstructive sleep apnea), symptomatic treatment with loop diuretics is recommended to reduce fluid overload as well as GDMT with SGLT-2i, MRA, ARNI, and ARB [42].

SGLT-2i including empagliflozin and dapagliflozin have been shown to decrease hospitalizations in patients with HFpEF and are therefore indicated in all people without contraindications [42–44]. Women with a relatively higher LVEF demonstrated favorable outcomes with spironolactone and sacubitril/valsartan comparatively to men. ARB are reserved for individuals who are not able to take sacubitril/valsartan due to tolerability or cost [42]. ACEi are not considered an acceptable alternative in HFpEF due to the lack of benefit with perindopril in a clinical trial of elderly individuals with a LVEF >40% [45].

Management of Hyperglycemia in People with HF

Treatment choices for diabetes are dependent on patient-specific cardiovascular risk factors, including HF. Drug classes used for the treatment of diabetes have a variety of effects on HF risk; therefore, close consideration of patient-specific factors is warranted. SGLT-2i are recommended for all individuals with current symptomatic HF as well as those at high risk for HF (stage B). GLP-1 RA are well known for their beneficial cardiovascular outcomes and are considered a favorable add-on therapy when needed for additional glycemic control. Metformin may also be considered as an add-on therapy to SGLT-2i and GLP-1 RA in patients with or at risk for HF. Insulin therapy may also be considered if additional glycemic control is needed despite the aforementioned therapies [37].

Sulfonylureas are not a preferred drug class given their propensity to cause fluid retention and weight gain. Similarly, thiazolidinediones (TZD) are associated with similar effects in addition to evidence demonstrating an increased risk of HF and associated morbidity and mortality. Therefore, TZD should be avoided in HF stage B-D. Dipeptidyl peptidase 4 (DPP-4) inhibitors are also not recommended in HF stage B-D given the association with increased HF hospitalizations with saxagliptin and alogliptin use [37].

Peripheral Vascular Disease

Background

PVD is caused by reduced blood circulation to areas outside of the heart and brain. The most common types include PAD, carotid artery disease, and aortic aneurysmatic disease (AAA). PAD is a condition with atherosclerotic narrowing of the arteries, mostly in the lower extremities. In the United States, it affects 6.5 million adults aged 40 and older and is associated with a 2–4 times increased risk of mortality [41, 46]. Risk factors include hyperlipidemia, HTN, smoking, age greater than 60, and diabetes mellitus with a twofold increase in prevalence. Although about 50% of people are asymptomatic, others may experience intermittent claudication, where exercise-induced ischemia and reduced arterial occlusion cause mild-to-severe pain, mostly in the calf [46].

Diagnosis requires an initial history and physical examination to assess for abnormal lower extremity pulse or vascular bruit, ankle brachial index (ABI), duplex ultrasound, and computed tomography and magnetic resonance angiography [46]. The ABI is a ratio between the systolic ankle blood pressure and the systolic brachial blood pressure and can be conducted at rest or upon exertion. For resting ABI, abnormal is ABI less than or equal to 0.90; borderline is ABI between 0.91 and 0.99, normal is ABI between 1 and 1.40, and noncompressible is ABI >1.40. When the resting ABI is noncompressible, a toe-brachial index should be conducted to further assess the suspected PAD, whereas those with normal or borderline ABI and exertional symptoms should conduct exercise treadmill ABI. Other imaging tools would be recommended to further assess the location and severity of stenosis in symptomatic PAD when revascularization is considered [47].

Screening and Monitoring

People with diabetes age 50 and older are recommended to be screened for PAD using the ABI. Screening may also be recommended in people with diabetes <50 years old in the presence of significant risk factors such as diabetes with a duration of more than 10 years, smoking, HTN, and dyslipidemia [47].

Management Strategies

The goals of therapy are to improve functioning and quality of life due to significant physical activity limitations that may cause functional and mobility loss [48]. People with PAD and claudication should be referred to exercise programs such as supervised treadmill exercise therapy and other modalities to improve walking performance [48]. The program can be at the hospital or in the outpatient setting, with a minimum of 30–45-min sessions at least 3 times a week for a minimum of 12 weeks [47]. People with diabetes and PAD should also be counseled on proper foot care as described previously.

For people with symptomatic PAD, it is recommended to initiate single antiplatelet therapy (SAPT) with either aspirin 75–325 mg once daily or clopidogrel 75 mg once daily to reduce the risk of atherosclerotic events such as myocardial infarction (MI) and cerebrovascular accident (CVA). The efficacy of dual antiplatelet therapy in symptomatic PAD is not well established, and anticoagulation is not recommended to reduce risk of cardiovascular ischemic events. For asymptomatic PAD, SAPT may be reasonable, and for asymptomatic borderline PAD, there is limited evidence to support the use of SAPT [47].

Statins should be started in all people with PAD, and antihypertensive treatment should be optimized in those with concomitant HTN. Cilostazol is recommended to improve symptoms of claudication and increase walking distance. For those with peripheral extremity pain at rest, this may be an indicator of critical limb ischemia where revascularization should be completed to minimize tissue loss [47].

Conclusion

The management of diabetes-related complications is an essential component of comprehensive diabetes care. The significant health consequences related to microvascular and macrovascular complications highlight the complexities of diabetes management beyond A1C lowering. Preventative measures related to glycemic control and risk factor mitigation are important in preventing and delaying the progression of complications that significantly affect the quality of life and overall health of people with diabetes. Effective management requires a collaborative care plan implemented by a multidisciplinary team while engaging patients in self-management strategies and behaviors to attain positive health outcomes.

References

1. UK Prospective Diabetes Study (UKPDS) Group. Intensive blood-glucose control with sulphonylureas or insulin compared with conventional treatment and risk of complications in patients with type 2 diabetes (UKPDS 33). Lancet. 1998;352:837–53.
2. Diabetes Control and Complications Trial Research Group, Nathan DM, Genuth S, Lachin J, et al. The effect of intensive treatment of diabetes on the development and progression of long term complications in insulin-dependent diabetes mellitus. N Engl J Med. 1993;329:977–86.
3. The Action to Control Cardiovascular Risk in Diabetes Study Group. Effects of intensive glucose lowering in type 2 diabetes. N Engl J Med. 2008;358:2545–59.
4. Stratton IM, Kohner EM, Aldington SJ, et al. UKPDS 50: risk factors for incidence and progression of retinopathy in type II diabetes over 6 years from diagnosis. Diabetologia. 2001;44:156–63.

5. Solomon SD, Chew E, Duh EJ, et al. Diabetic retinopathy: a position statement by the American Diabetes Association. Diabetes Care. 2017;40:412–8.
6. American Diabetes Association Professional Practice Committee. 12. Retinopathy, neuropathy, and foot care: standards of Care in Diabetes-2024. Diabetes Care. 2024;47(Suppl 1):S231–43.
7. Blonde L, Umpierrez GE, Reddy SS, et al. American Association of Clinical Endocrinology clinical practice guideline: developing a diabetes mellitus comprehensive care plan-2022 update. Endocr Pract. 2022;28(10):923–1049.
8. The Diabetic Retinopathy Study Research Group. Preliminary report on effects of photocoagulation therapy. Am J Ophthalmol. 1976;81:383–96.
9. Early Treatment Diabetic Retinopathy Study research group. Photocoagulation for diabetic macular edema. Early treatment diabetic retinopathy study report number 1. Arch Ophthalmol. 1985;103:1796–806.
10. Pop-Busui R, Boulton AJ, Feldman EL, et al. Diabetic neuropathy: a position statement by the American Diabetes Association. Diabetes Care. 2017;40(1):136–54.
11. Pop-Busui R, Evans GW, Gerstein HC, et al. Effects of cardiac autonomic dysfunction on mortality risk in the action to control cardiovascular risk in diabetes (ACCORD) trial. Diabetes Care. 2010;33:1578–84.
12. Ismail-Beigi F, Craven T, Banerji MA, et al. Effect of intensive treatment of hyperglycaemia on microvascular outcomes in type 2 diabetes: an analysis of the ACCORD randomised trial. Lancet. 2010;376:419–30.
13. Price R, Smith D, Franklin G, et al. Oral and topical treatment of painful diabetic polyneuropathy: practice guideline update summary: report of the AAN guideline subcommittee. Neurology. 2022;98(1):31–43.
14. Schaper NC, van Netten JJ, Apelqvist J, et al. Practical guidelines on the prevention and management of diabetes-related foot disease (IWGDF 2023 update). Diabetes Metab Res Rev. 2023;40:e3657. https://doi.org/10.1002/dmrr.3657.
15. Johansen KL, Chertow GM, Gilbertson DT, et al. US renal data system 2022 annual data report: epidemiology of kidney disease in the United States. Am J Kidney Dis. 2023;81(3 Suppl1):A8–A11.
16. Alicic RZ, Rooney MT, Tuttle KR. Diabetic kidney disease: challenges, progress, and possibilities. Clin J Am Soc Nephrol. 2017;12(12):2032–45.
17. Kidney Disease: Improving Global Outcomes (KDIGO) Diabetes Work Group. KDIGO 2022 clinical practice guideline for diabetes management in chronic kidney disease. Kidney Int. 2022;102(5S):S1–S127.
18. de Boer IH, Khunti K, Sadusky T, et al. Diabetes management in chronic kidney disease: a consensus report by the American Diabetes Association (ADA) and kidney disease: improving global outcomes (KDIGO). Diabetes Care. 2022;45:3075–90.
19. American Diabetes Association Professional Practice Committee. 11. Chronic kidney disease and risk management: standards of Care in Diabetes-2024. Diabetes Care. 2024;47(Suppl 1):S219–30.

20. Centers for Disease Control and Prevention (2023). National diabetes statistics report. https://www.cdc.gov/diabetes/data/statistics-report/index.html. Accessed 13 Nov 2023.
21. NCD Risk Factor Collaboration (NCD-RisC). Worldwide trends in blood pressure from 1975 to 2015: a pooled analysis of 1479 population-based measurement studies with 19.1 million participants. Lancet. 2017;389(10064):37–55.
22. Liamis G, Liberopoulos E, Barkas F, Elisaf M. Diabetes mellitus and electrolyte disorders. World J Clin Cases. 2014;2(10):488–96.
23. Oparil S, Zaman MA, Calhoun DA. Pathogenesis of hypertension. Ann Intern Med. 2003;139(9):761–76.
24. Iqbal AM, Jamal SF. Essential Hypertension. In: StatPearls, Treasure Island; 2023. https://www.ncbi.nlm.nih.gov/books/NBK539859. Accessed 13 Nov 2023.
25. Whelton PK, Carey RM, Aronow WS, et al. 2017 ACC/AHA/AAPA/ABC/ACPM/AGS/APhA/ASH/ASPC/NMA/PCNA guideline for the prevention, detection, evaluation, and management of high blood pressure in adults: executive summary: a report of the American College of Cardiology/American Heart Association task force on clinical practice guidelines. Hypertension. 2018;71(6):1269–324.
26. ElSayed NA, Aleppo G, Aroda VR, et al. American Diabetes Association 2. Classification and diagnosis of diabetes: standards of care in diabetes. Diabetes Care. 2023;46(Suppl 1):S19–40.
27. U.S. Preventative Services Task Force (USPSTF). Hypertension in adults: screening. 2021. https://uspreventiveservicestaskforce.org/uspstf/recommendation/hypertension-in-adults-screening. Accessed 13 Nov 2023.
28. Berg, S. Four big ways BP measurement goes wrong, and how to tackle them. 2023. https://www.ama-assn.org/delivering-care/hypertension/4-big-ways-bp-measurement-goes-wrong-and-how-tackle-them. Accessed 13 Nov 2023.
29. Chobanian AV, Bakris GL, Black HR, et al. The seventh report of the joint National Committee on prevention, detection, evaluation, and treatment of high blood pressure: the JNC 7 report. JAMA. 2003;289(19):2560–71.
30. James PA, Oparil S, Carter BL, et al. 2014 evidence-based guideline for the management of high blood pressure in adults: report from the panel members appointed to the eighth joint National Committee (JNC 8). JAMA. 2014;311(5):507–20.
31. Verges B. Pathophysiology of diabetic dyslipidaemia: where are we? Diabetologia. 2015;58(5):886–99.
32. Hirano T. Pathophysiology of diabetic dyslipidemia. J Atheroscler Thromb. 2018;25(9):771–82.
33. American Diabetes Association Professional Practice Committee. 10. Cardiovascular disease and risk management: standards of Care in Diabetes-2024. Diabetes Care. 2024;47(Suppl 1):S179–218.

34. Grundy SM, Stone NJ, Bailey AL, et al. 2018 AHA/ACC/AACVPR/AAPA/ABC/ACPM/ADA/AGS/APhA/ASPC/NLA/PCNA guideline on the management of blood cholesterol: executive summary: a report of the American College of Cardiology/American Heart Association task force on clinical practice guidelines. J Am Coll Cardiol. 2019;73(24):3168–209.
35. Expert Panel on Detection, Evaluation, and Treatment of High Blood Cholesterol in Adults. Executive summary of the third report of the National Cholesterol Education Program (NCEP) expert panel on detection, evaluation, and treatment of high blood cholesterol in adults (adult treatment panel III). JAMA. 2001;285(19):2486–97.
36. Dunlay SM, Givertz MM, Aguilar D, et al. Type 2 diabetes mellitus and heart failure: a scientific statement from the American Heart Association and the Heart Failure Society of America: this statement does not represent an update of the 2017 ACC/AHA/HFSA heart failure guideline update. Circulation. 2019;140(7):e294–324.
37. Pop-Busui R, Januzzi JL, Bruemmer D, et al. Heart failure: an underappreciated complication of diabetes. A consensus report of the American Diabetes Association. Diabetes Care. 2022;45(7):1670–90.
38. King M, Kingery J, Casey B. Diagnosis and evaluation of heart failure. Am Fam Physician. 2012;85(12):1161–8.
39. Watson RD, Gibbs CR, Lip GY. ABC of heart failure. Clinical Features Complications BMJ. 2000;320(7229):236–9.
40. Heidenreich PA, Bozkurt B, Aguilar D, et al. 2022 AHA/ACC/HFSA guideline for the Management of Heart Failure: a report of the American College of Cardiology/American Heart Association joint committee on clinical practice guidelines. Circulation. 2022;145(18):e895–e1032.
41. Virani SS, Alonso A, Aparicio HJ, et al. Heart disease and stroke statistics-2020 update: a report from the American Heart Association. Circulation. 2021;143(8):e254–743.
42. Kittleson MM, Panjrath GS, Amancherla K, et al. 2023 ACC expert consensus decision pathway on management of heart failure with preserved ejection fraction: a report of the American College of Cardiology Solution set Oversight Committee. J Am Coll Cardiol 9. 2023;81(18):1835–78.
43. Solomon SD, McMurray JJV, Claggett B, et al. Dapagliflozin in heart failure with mildly reduced or preserved ejection fraction. N Engl J Med. 2022;387:1089–98.
44. Anker SD, Butler J, Filippatos G, et al. Empagliflozin in heart failure with a preserved ejection fraction. N Engl J Med. 2021;385:1451–61.
45. Cleland JG, Tendera M, Adamus J, et al. The perindopril in elderly people with chronic heart failure (PEP-CHF) study. Eur Heart J. 2006;27:2338–45.
46. Soyoye DO, Abiodun OO, Ikem RT, Kolawole BA, Akintomide AO. Diabetes and peripheral artery disease: a review. World J Diabetes. 2021;12(6):827–38.

47. Gerhard-Herman MD, Gornik HL, Barrett C, et al. 2016 AHA/ACC guideline on the management of patients with lower extremity peripheral artery disease: executive summary: a report of the American College of Cardiology/American Heart Association task force on clinical practice guidelines. Circulation. 2017;135:e686–725.
48. Treat-Jacobson D, McDermott MM, Bronas UG, et al. Optimal exercise programs for patients with peripheral artery disease: a scientific statement from the American Heart Association. Circulation. 2019;139(4):e10–33.

Diabetes Technology

6

Katelyn O'Brien and Diana Isaacs

Introduction

Diabetes technology is the term used to describe the hardware, devices, and software that people with diabetes use to assist with self-management, ranging from lifestyle modifications to glucose monitoring and therapy adjustments. This technology includes insulin pumps, also called continuous subcutaneous insulin infusion (CSII), blood glucose monitors (BGM), continuous glucose monitors (CGM), connected insulin pens (CIP), automated insulin delivery (AID) systems, and mobile applications (apps) that assist with diabetes self-management support [1].

Pharmacists have a role in assisting with the selection of the technology that best suits the individual person, educating people with diabetes on use of technology, and interpreting data from devices. The Identify, Configure, Collaborate (ICC) Framework is an approach that supports technology-enabled decision-making to

K. O'Brien (✉)
Department of Pharmacy, Boston Medical Center, Boston, MA, USA
e-mail: katelyn.o'brien@bmc.org

D. Isaacs
Endocrinology and Metabolism Institute, Cleveland Clinic, Cleveland, OH, USA

© The Author(s), under exclusive license to Springer Nature Switzerland AG 2025

J. Clements (ed.), *The Pharmacist's Pocket Guide for Diabetes and Obesity*, https://doi.org/10.1007/978-3-031-88835-9_6

improve outcomes and decrease therapeutic inertia [2, 3]. The hope is that this standardized framework will also enable healthcare professionals to avoid bias in the provision of technology to people with diabetes. In general, no device used in diabetes management works optimally without education, training, and follow-up. Multiple resources are available for online tutorials and training videos, as well as written material on the use of devices. People with diabetes vary in terms of their comfort level with technology, and some prefer in-person training and support. People with more education regarding device use have better outcomes; therefore, the need for additional education should be periodically assessed, particularly if outcomes are not being met.

Continuous Glucose Monitors

CGM measures glucose levels in the interstitial fluid and displays numeric and graphic data regarding current glucose status, together with current and projected trends in the glucose. The directional arrows allow users to proactively respond to glucose data. Depending on the CGM, users may get glucose values every 1–5 min. CGM is different from BGM which requires the person with diabetes to perform a finger stick and gives only one glucose value as measured in the blood. The interstitial glucose and blood glucose values may vary depending on recent food ingestion, medication administration, or physical activity. BGM is still common in people living with diabetes, particularly those on non-insulin regimens. BGM supplies should be prescribed as monitoring should still be encouraged in those using CGM, for calibrations, when sensor glucose does not correlate with symptoms or for when sensors fail or fall off. Currently, there are four different manufacturers of personal CGM on the market in the United States: Dexcom, Abbott, Medtronic, and Ascensia. Abbott and Dexcom also offer professional CGM.

A professional CGM (Table 6.1) is owned by the clinic, and the sensor is placed in the office by staff and can be blinded or unblinded. A blinded CGM collects glucose data without the patient seeing the information in real time; the data are thus less likely to influence patient behaviors and are commonly used in

Table 6.1 Comparison of professional continuous glucose monitors

Features	Abbott Libre Pro	Dexcom G6 Pro
Blinded or unblinded	Blinded	Blinded and unblinded
Maximum wear time	14 days	10 days
Calibrations	None required	None required
Components	Combined disposable sensor/transmitter Touchscreen reader device, owned by clinic	Disposable sensor and separate disposable transmitter Touchscreen reader device, owned by clinic
Care between use	None, disposable	None, disposable
Insertion	Single-step process with auto-inserter	Two-step process: Inserting sensor and attaching transmitter
Body site with FDA approval	Upper arm	Abdomen
System for downloading data and reports	LibreView	CLARITY
Interfering substances	Vitamin C, salicylic acid	Hydroxyurea

Adapted from source: Ref. [4]

research studies. An unblinded CGM allows the user to see the data and has optional alarms in real time. Professional CGM devices are worn for up to 10–14 days depending on the device, although a minimum of 3 days is required for billing. For evaluation and interpretation of glucose data, the patient usually returns to the clinic for sensor download and review of any nutrition and activity logs as well as medication administration history. In general, professional CGM are often used when a patient's insurance does not cover a personal CGM, when a patient wants to evaluate wearing the technology before committing to a personal device, or when glucose data do not correlate with A1C.

Personal CGM are prescribed to the patient and obtained either at a pharmacy or a durable medical equipment (DME) supplier and owned by the user. There are two types of personal CGM: intermittently scanned (isCGM) or real time (rtCGM). An isCGM is a type of personal CGM that requires the patient to scan the sensor using a reader or smart device to obtain a glucose level, whereas an rtCGM monitors glucose levels continuously without the need for scanning. The isCGM products must be scanned at least every 8 h to capture all the data. Ascencia's Eversense CGM is the only implantable CGM on the market. The Eversense E3 CGM received FDA approval for a 6-month wear and can only be inserted by a trained health-care professional at an office visit. A 365-day version was also FDA approved and will be available in the near future. Table 6.2 compares personal CGM devices. The FDA has approved all these personal CGM devices for the capability to make treatment decisions based on the glucose readings. For any cases in which the patient's symptoms do not match the glucose reading, a confirmatory finger stick is recommended with any device. Mean absolute relative difference (MARD) is a marker of accuracy, with a lower MARD value indicating greater accuracy; however, the research approach to how each device is studied varies, so direct comparisons should not be made unless the devices are studied in the same clinical trial. A MARD value less than 10% is sufficiently accurate to make dosing decisions. There is a distinction of integrative CGM (iCGM) which allows the device to integrate with compatible insulin pumps for automated insulin delivery. The iCGM must meet higher accuracy standards. The Libre 2+, Libre 3+, Dexcom G6, Dexcom G7, and Eversense are all considered iCGM. They can all share data in real time with others remotely using shared mobile apps.

There are now 2 over-the-counter CGM options as well designed for people not taking insulin that may not have coverage for personal CGM. This includes the Dexcom Stelo and the Abbott Linto.

	Dexcom Stelo	Abbott Lingo
Wear time	15.5 days	14 days
Ability to share data	Yes, Dexcom clarity	No
Glucose range	70–250 mg/dL	55–200 mg/dL
Real-time alerts	Yes, spike detection only	No
Frequency of glucose readings	15 min	1 min
Education within app	Yes	Yes
Patient age	≥18 yr	≥18 yr

Table 6.2 Comparison of personal CGMs

Features	Freestyle Libre 2	Freestyle Libre 3	G6	G7	Guardian 4	Eversense
CGM type	isCGM	rtCGM	rtCGM	rtCGM	rtCGM	rtCGM
Calibrations	None	None	None, optional	None, optional	None, optional	Twice daily for 3 week, then once daily
Maximum sensor wear	14 days. Libre 2+: 15 days	14 days, libre 3 +: 15 days	10 days	10.5 days	7 days	180 days
iCGM	Yes	Yes	Yes	Yes	No	Yes
Warm up	60 min	60 min	120 min	30 min	Up to 2 hr	Up to 24 h
Body sites with FDA approval	Upper arm	Upper arm	Abdomen, butt*ocks (pediatrics)	Upper arm, buttocks (pediatrics)	Abdomen or arm	Implanted in upper arm
Available applications (apps)	Libre 2, LibreLink up	Libre 3, LibreLink up	Dexcom G6, Dexcom CLARITY, Dexcom follow	Dexcom G7, Dexcom CLARITY, Dexcom follow	Guardian connect, MiniMed Mobile, CareLink	Eversense app, Eversense NOW
Compatible software	LibreView	LibreView	Dexcom CLARITY	Dexcom CLARITY	CareLink	Eversense data management system

(continued)

Table 6.2 (continued)

Features	Freestyle Libre 2	Freestyle Libre 3	G6	G7	Guardian 4	Eversense
Compatible display device	Reader, smart phone	Reader, smart phone	Receiver, smart phone	Receiver, smartphone	Smartphone	Smartphone
Drug interactions	Vitamin C (>500 mg) Libre 2+ (>1000 mg)	Vitamin C (>500 mg) Libre 3+ (>1000 mg)	Hydroxy-urea	Hydroxyurea	Acetaminophen, hydroxyurea	Tetracycline, mannitol
Patient age	≥4 yr Libre 2+ ≥ 2 yr	≥4 yr Libre 3+ ≥ 2 yr	≥2 yr	≥ 2 yr	≥2 yr	≥18 yr

Adapted from source: Ref. [5]
CGM continuous glucose monitor, *iCGM* integrative CGM, *isCGM* intermittently scanned CGM, *rtCGM* real time CGM

Guideline Recommendations and Clinical Evidence for CGM Use

Guideline Recommendations

The American Diabetes Association (ADA) Standards of Care (2024) strongly support the use of diabetes devices for all people with diabetes and notes that the type and selection of devices should be individualized based on the person's specific needs, preferences, and skill level, as well as the availability of devices [2]. The standards note that CGM use should be considered at the time of diagnosis in individuals that require insulin management, given the beneficial findings concluded above. This approach allows for close tracking of glucose levels with adjustments of insulin dosing and lifestyle modifications and removes the burden of frequent BGM. Based on ADA standards, the following grade evidence is noted [2]:

- Adults with diabetes on MDI or CSII: rtCGM (level A) or isCGM (level B)
- Adults with diabetes on basal insulin: rtCGM (level A) or isCGM (level B)
- Youth with type 1 diabetes (T1D) on MDI or CSII: rtCGM (level A) or isCGM (level E)
- Youth with type 2 diabetes (T2D): rtCGM or isCGM (level E)
- Pregnancy: when used as an adjunct to preprandial and post-prandial BGM (level B)
- Hospitalized patients using a personal CGM: continuation during hospitalization with confirmatory point-of-care (POC) glucose measurements (level B)

Similarly, the American Association of Clinical Endocrinology (AACE) guidelines (2021) on use of advanced technology provide recommendations in which CGM is strongly recommended for the following populations [6]:

- Persons with diabetes treated with intensive insulin therapy, defined as 3 or more administrations of insulin per day or the use of an insulin pump (grade A)
- Persons with complicated cases of hypoglycemia—frequent/severe hypoglycemia, nocturnal hypoglycemia, and hypoglycemia unawareness (grade A)
- Children and adolescents with T1D (grade A)
- Pregnant women with T1D, T2D, or gestational diabetes treated with intensive insulin therapy (grade A)
- Women with gestational diabetes not on insulin therapy and individuals with T2D who are treated with less intensive insulin therapy (grade B)

Of note, level/grade A is the strongest recommendation based on evidence from randomized controlled trials, whereas level/grade E is the weakest recommendation and is based on expert opinion.

The Endocrine Society Guidelines (2023) on management of individuals at high risk for hypoglycemia parallel the above, noting that CGM should be used rather than BGM in individuals with T1D on MDI and in patients with T2D on insulin and/or sulfonylureas [7]. Additionally, the guidelines recommend considering initiation of CGM in the inpatient setting for select patients in the hospital at high risk for hypoglycemia and that patients admitted with a CGM should be continued versus discontinued in the hospital setting. The guidelines note that inpatient use of CGM is not currently approved by the FDA but was granted emergency use authorization during the COVID pandemic. Therefore, BGM is still recommended for medication adjustments. The guidelines further recommend a hybrid approach where CGM findings are combined with "periodic POC blood glucose testing," which is consistent with the 2024 ADA Standards of Care recommendations [1, 7].

Data Interpretation

The CGM data are available as a standardized report called the *ambulatory glucose profile* (AGP), which includes the CGM key metrics, the AGP itself, and the daily tracings of CGM data for the past 14 days. The AGP is a visualization of data that contains the median and shaded areas representing the 25th to 75th percentile of data, with an additional shaded area representing the tenth to 90th percentile or the fifth to 95th percentile, depending on the reporting system. This approach is a way to quickly assess patterns, including glucose variability (GV), although this format works best for people with similar everyday routines [8].

Other key metrics included in the CGM reports are the *glucose management indicator (GMI)*, which reflects the CGM-estimated hemoglobin A1C, and *time in range* (TIR), which is the percentage of time an individual's glucose values are 70–180 mg/dL. The goal for most adults is to spend more than 70% TIR, which correlates to an estimated hemoglobin A1C value of less than 7%. The CGM key metrics are presented in Table 6.3, and the CGM goals are represented in Fig. 6.1. For older adults or those at higher risk of hypoglycemia and complications, the goal is to spend greater than 50% TIR at 70–180 mg/dL, while minimizing *time below range* (TBR) at less than 70 mg/dL to less than 1%. Pregnancy is the only period when the target range is modified to 63–140 mg/dL with a goal of at least 70% TIR for preexisting T1D in pregnancy. Because of a lack of evidence, there is no consensus for the recommended TIR for gestational diabetes or preexisting T2D in pregnancy [9].

Reviewing the data provides opportunities for the pharmacist to engage in discussions to empower the patient to achieve goal glucose targets. For optimal data interpretation, patients should be educated on the value of tracking food intake, exercise, and diabetes medication timing to understand how these factors influence glycemic management. These types of data can be tracked directly in mobile apps that are connected to diabetes technology devices [8].

Table 6.3 Standardized metrics for CGM data interpretation

Key metric	Measure
Number of days CGM is worn	14 days
Percentage of time CGM is active	Recommend >70% wear time over 14 days
Mean glucose	Average glucose over the wear period
Glucose management indicator	CGM version of estimated A1C
Glycemic variability (coefficient of variation)	Standard deviation/mean, stable ≤36%
TAR level 2	% readings and time >250 mg/dL
TAR level 1	% readings and time 181–250 mg/dL
TIR	% readings and time 70–180 mg/dL
TBR level 1	% readings and time 54–69 mg/dL
TBR level 2	% readings and time <54 mg/dL

Source: Ref. [9]
CGM continuous glucose monitoring, *TAR* time above range, *TBR* time below range, *TIR* time in range

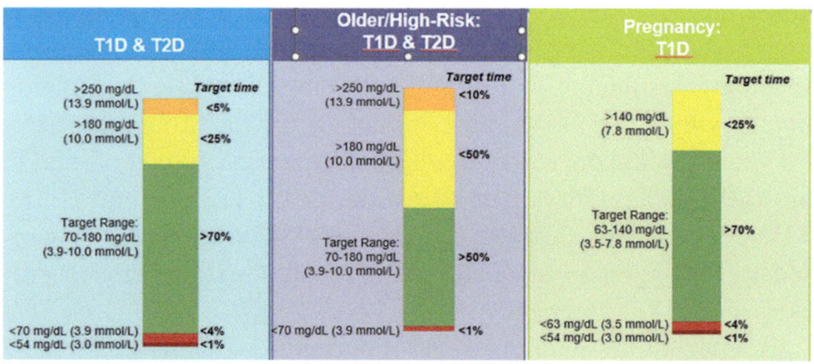

Fig. 6.1 Goals for time in range. *T1D* type 1 diabetes, *T2D* type 2 diabetes. (Adapted from source: Ref. 5)

The DATAA Model

The acronym *DATAA—download data, access safety, time in range, areas to improve, action plan*—can help with interpreting diabetes technology data and guiding patient interactions.

This model begins with obtaining or *downloading the data*. In this step, the glucose targets can be reviewed, and the pharmacist can ask the patient what is working well with diabetes self-management. The next step is to *assess safety*, which involves evaluating hypoglycemia symptoms and time spent below range. This step is important because hypoglycemia often leads to rebound hyperglycemia and more GV. Next, *time in range* is reviewed, which is evaluating the days or the times of day when the TIR is highest and replicating what is working well on those days. The next step includes *areas for improvement*, for which the time spent in hyperglycemia and possible causes are evaluated. All these data are used in the last step, which is to develop an *action plan* through shared decision-making with the patient. At each step, it is important to emphasize that this information is simply data and that numbers are not considered good or bad [10].

Education and Training

Pharmacists can play a role in educating and training on diabetes technology devices across many practice settings. For personal CGM, education and training can be performed in person or remotely given increased access to telehealth services since the COVID-19 pandemic. For CGM training, patients should be educated on the application of the sensor, wear time, warm-up period, differences between interstitial versus blood glucose, how often to scan or check sensor data, meaning of directional arrows, when to check glucose finger sticks, how to optimize alarms, interfering substances, and what to do if the sensor becomes detached from the body site.

When to Check the BGM

It is recommended to check blood glucose values using a traditional finger stick during the sensor warm-up period, when calibrations are needed (Medtronic, Eversense) or when symptoms do not match blood glucose values on the reader. Additionally, if a sensor falls off, the person with diabetes or caregiver should resume glucose monitoring with finger sticks if backup sensors are not available.

Lag Time

Given that CGM is measuring interstitial glucose values, a difference between CGM values and BGM values will be evident if checked at the same time. The capillary glucose must diffuse into the interstitial fluid. The lag time may range from 5 to 15 min. Therefore, the CGM values may be lower than the actual glucose values in the blood. The lag time varies after meals, during periods of exercise, and after administration of rapid-acting insulin.

Frequency of Checking/Scanning

With the isCGM, the Libre 14 day and Libre 2 sensors must be scanned every 8 h for the sensor to continuously monitor glucose levels every minute. If there is a delay in scanning the sensor, the data will be lost between scans. For rtCGM, the sensor does not need to be scanned; however, an important counseling point for patients would be on keeping their smart phone or reader/receiver nearby to hear alarms and for data transmission. For the Libre system, the reader needs to be within 20 feet, whereas the distance for Dexcom is 33 feet.

Optimizing Alerts

Alerts should be customized to the patient. Because of the potential for alert fatigue, alarms should be set to specific thresholds based on patient goals and/or current glucose levels. For example, if a patient tends to develop hypoglycemic symptoms with glucose levels in the range of 70 mg/dL, the alarm for low alert should be set to 75 mg/dL or 80 mg/dL to be given advanced notice of approaching low value. This method allows the patient time to treat before it becomes too low. Critical low alerts cannot be turned off. For hyperglycemia, clinicians can consider turning these alarms off for some patients or setting them only to alert when glucoses are very high. As time spent in range increases, the high alert settings can be lowered if the patient is aiming to achieve tight control.

Site Adhesiveness

Contact dermatitis—both irritant and allergic—has been reported with all devices that attach to the skin. In some cases, this dermatitis has been linked to the presence of isobornyl acrylate, which is a skin sensitizer and can cause an additional spreading allergic reaction. Patch testing can be performed to identify the cause of contact dermatitis in some cases. Identifying and eliminating tape allergens is important to ensure comfortable use of devices and to enhance patient adherence. Use of an implanted sensor may be helpful when avoiding skin reactions in patients who are sensitive to tape.

Rotating body sites is important between applications, as well as considering sleeping positions, exercise routines, and clothing. Sensors should be placed on clean dry skin, avoiding placement on broken or irritated skin. It may be necessary to shave areas to improve placement for some individuals. Patients should be counseled to avoid placement of CGM on wet skin immediately after a shower or bath. Also, to prevent sweating, unscented antiperspirant can be applied to the skin 10–15 min before insertion. Intranasal fluticasone applied before sensor application has also been shown to prevent skin irritation or itchiness [11].

Several products are available to aid in adhesiveness. Skin-Tac or Skin-Prep can be applied to the skin before sensor application to aid in adhesion. Other overlap products may be applied after sensor placement, such as Simpatch or Tegaderm. People with diabetes can be directed to the individual CGM websites for resources to improve adhesion.

If a sensor becomes detached from the body site and is lost, users should be instructed to contact the manufacturer for replacement. If a backup sensor is not quickly available, the patient should perform finger-stick testing until the sensor can be replaced.

Billing Opportunities for Pharmacists

Pharmacists can play a key role in educating patients and caregivers how to use CGM. Therefore, this involvement presents a billing opportunity for pharmacists as well. In Table 6.4 are the codes

Table 6.4 CGM billing codes

Code	Description	Who can bill
95249	Ambulatory CGM of interstitial fluid via subcutaneous catheter for minimum of 72 h with patient-provided equipment. Includes sensor placement, hook-up, calibration of monitor, patient training, and print-out of recording. This code is used once for the lifetime of the personal CGM device	Examples of staff who may perform this duty include MD/DO, PharmD, NP/PA, CDCES *other healthcare personnel may be able to perform this duty if within their scope of practice
95250	This code is used both for the placement of professional CGM and the downloading of the data. Multidisciplinary health-care providers can perform placement if it is within their scope of practice. This code should only be reported once per month per patient, although this may vary by payer	Examples of staff who may perform this duty include: MD/ DO, NP/PA, CDCES, RD, RN
95251	This code is used for interpretation of professional or personal CGM and does not require face-to-face visit. It cannot be billed more than once per month	Interpretation can be performed by MD/DO, or NP/PA. Pharmacists can DO this in many states with a collaborative practice agreement and co-signature of MD/DO or NP/ PA

Adapted from source: Refs [4, 5]
CDCES Certified Diabetes Care and Education Specialist, *CGM* continuous glucose monitor

associated with education and interpretation of CGM. Codes 95249 and 95250 can only be billed if there is a minimum of 72 h of glucose data available from CGM download. The codes 95250 and 95251 can also only be billed once per month. An E/M Code (Evaluation and Management) can be billed on the same day of either of these codes if a distinct and separate E/M service was medically necessary and provided over and above the Professional CGM service. In this case, the modifier -25 must be attached to the E/M code.

Insulin Pumps

Insulin pump therapy involves wearing a device designed to deliver insulin into subcutaneous tissue through a small cannula. Insulin pumps work best with rapid-acting insulin, although regular insulin can also be used. These pumps are designed to work with U-100 insulin. Of importance, a long-acting or basal insulin should never be used in a pump because the rapid-acting insulin serves as both the basal and the bolus insulin. The two categories of insulin pumps are *smart insulin pumps* and *wearable insulin pumps*, also called *patch pumps*. Smart insulin pumps also include sensor-augmented pump therapy and hybrid closed-loop technology [1].

Patch Pumps

Patch pumps are designed to be simple to use. These pumps are wearable devices that make it easier for the person with diabetes to administer insulin. Patch pumps administer insulin in 2-unit bolus increments. They do not contain integration with any glucose monitoring system, do not have a bolus calculator, and do not record data in a data management system. Two available products are currently marketed (Table 6.5). The V-Go offers three choices for background insulin: 20, 30, or 40 units, with up to 36 units/day of bolus insulin doses. The V-Go replaces both basal and bolus insulin, whereas Simplicity replaces bolus insulin only. Simplicity holds up to 200 units of bolus insulin and must be replaced every 3 days, whereas V-Go is replaced daily.

Smart Insulin Pumps

Smart insulin pumps include a background, 24-hour continuous infusion that replaces the need for long-acting insulin injections because rapid-acting or regular insulin formulation is continually being administered. Multiple basal rates can be programmed

Table 6.5 Comparison of patch pumps

Feature	V-Go	Simplicity
FDA approval	T2D	T1D, T2D
Model(s)	20 units 30 units 40 units	2 units
Maximum number of insulin units/reservoir	20–56 units 30–66 units 40–76 units	200 units
Minimum bolus increment (units)	2 units	2 units
Waterproof vs. resistant	IPX7 rating water resistant to a depth of 3′3″ for up to 30 min	IPX7 rating water resistant to a depth of 3′3″ for up to 30 min

Adapted from source: Refs [12, 13]
FDA Food and Drug Administration, *T1D* type 1 diabetes, *T2D* type 2 diabetes

throughout the day depending on the individual's insulin needs. For example, different basal pattern profiles can be set for sick days, workdays, and during exercise. Bolus calculators can recommend doses for meals and correct hyperglycemia based on a programmed individual insulin to carbohydrate ratio (ICR) and insulin sensitivity factor (ISF). This calculator also accounts for *active insulin* or *insulin on board*, which is defined as the amount of insulin still acting to lower glucose from a previous bolus. An *extended bolus feature* allows a portion of the bolus dose to be delivered immediately, with the remaining portion administered over time. This approach may be useful when consuming meals with high-fat or high-protein content, when the meal is consumed over a long period of time, or for people with gastroparesis. Multiple pumps are available on the market with different features, including ability to integrate with CGM or BGM, insulin reservoir volume, customization with insulin dosing, and the presence or absence of tubing. Devices with tubing can vary in terms of the material (steel vs. plastic cannula), insertion angle, cannula length, type of connection to tubing, and manual versus automatic insertion [14].

Hybrid Closed-Loop Pumps

The hybrid closed-loop (HCL) systems are the most advanced form of pump integration. The technology for HCL systems differs from LGS and PLGS technology because, in addition to insulin suspension to prevent hypoglycemia, HCL systems can also increase the basal infusion using an algorithm to reduce hyperglycemia. Some systems even deliver automated correction boluses, although they are based on current glucose levels. Of note, patients who use HCL technology are still required to count or estimate carbohydrates and bolus doses as needed for meals. A fully closed-loop system that automatically delivers mealtime bolus doses without the need to input carbohydrate loads is a goal for future technology. The available systems include Tandem T:Slim X2 and Mobi, which both utilize the Control IQ algorithm. There is the Medtronic 780, Beta Bionics iLet, and Omnipod 5. The newest approved device is the Sequel Med Tech Twiist, which will utilize the Tidepool Loop algorithm once available. The Omnipod 5 is a tubeless pump controlled from a smart phone or company-provided controller. Other insulin pumps have tubing that connects the infusion set to the pump. Certain settings can be adjusted in the automated mode for HCL systems, which will impact the algorithm. For example, the ICR can be adjusted in all systems. Only in the Control IQ system will modifying the basal rates have any effect on the HCL algorithm. The active insulin time can be adjusted with the Minimed 780G and Omnipod 5, but not with Control IQ. Some can do additional correction doses beyond the basal modulation (ex. 780G, Control IQ) [15]. The Beta Bionics iLet has only one setting that can be adjusted, which is the glucose target. Everything else is automatically calculated from the patient's weight and sensor glucose. The iLet is also the only pump that does not have a default manual mode, so a sensor must be connected to use.

Connected Pens

Connected insulin pens (CIP) and pen caps are synced to a mobile app that includes a dose calculator and/or dose tracker. The dose calculator is used to determine mealtime or correction insulin doses. Connected Pens use Bluetooth to provide alerts for upcoming and missed doses [16]. Three types of CIP and pen cap devices have FDA approval: InPen, which is a connected pen; Bigfoot Unity, which is a connected pen cap; and Lilly SmartTempo Button, which is a button that goes on top of Lilly Tempo pens.

Comparison of Types

The InPen is a reusable pen that works with compatible insulin cartridges. This device is approved for individuals aged 7 years and older, and younger individuals can use this device with caregiver assistance. The pen works with 3-mL lispro or aspart U-100 rapid-acting insulin cartridges. Doses may be delivered in one-half unit increments with a maximum of 30 units per injection. The InPen mobile app can connect to Guardian or Dexcom CGM. Doses of long-acting insulin are given with the traditional insulin pen, although they can be recorded in the mobile app. Reminders to take insulin can also be set together with alerts for insulin temperature extremes. The InPen does not require any charging or batteries, but the device itself needs to be changed every year. People with diabetes should be instructed on entry of ICR, ISF, target blood glucose, and insulin on board into the bolus calculator in the mobile app. Carbohydrate estimates or set meal doses are also options [17].

Connected Pen Cap

The Bigfoot Unity connected pen cap replaces the usual cap-on–compatible disposable insulin pens. This device has FDA approval for individuals aged 12 years and older. This system can record doses administered from both basal and bolus insulin by separate caps and is compatible with most long-acting and rapid-acting insulin pens. Pen caps are color-coded, with a black cap fitting basal insulin and a white cap fitting rapid-acting insulin. The white pen cap contains a reader that allows the users to scan their Libre 2 sensor to obtain a glucose value and trend arrow. When scanned before bolus administration, the sensor glucose reading is integrated into the bolus calculator to provide a dose recommendation based on programmed ICR, ISF, and target glucose. The pen caps require periodic charging. Correction doses will not be advised if insulin was given within the past 3 hours [18].

The Lilly Tempo Smart Button is used on Lilly Tempo pens which are disposable but require the specific Tempo type, which is different than the Lilly KwikPen. These are available as insulin glargine (Basaglar), insulin lispro (Humalog), and insulin lispro-aabc (Lyumjev). This is indicated for adults over 18 and works with the Tempo Smart mobile app. The app tracks doses of insulin and has additional features where you can take pictures of foods to estimate carbohydrate content. There is also diabetes education embedded within the app. The app also has a bolus calculator incorporating a carbohydrate ratio, correction factor, glucose target and insulin action time. There is also a basal titration feature when used with BGM; it can also pair with Dexcom G6 and G7 CGM. See Table 6.6 for calculations used for connected pens and insulin pumps.

Mobile Apps

All personal CGM devices allow for a smart device to be used in the CGM system, and many patients may opt to use their smart devices in place of a receiver or reader for either cost savings or convenience. An important educational point for patients starting with personal use CGM is to ensure they select "always allow" for all alerts when downloading the app; this can always be later changed in the smart device settings as warranted. Some patients may not have a compatible smart device and would therefore need to use a manufacturer-provided reader or receiver. One of the benefits to using smart devices is the ability to share data with family or friends as well as health-care providers. The Eversense Now, Dexcom Follow, and Freestyle LibreLink apps allow for up to 5, 10, and 20 people to track a user's glucose data and trends.

Table 6.6 Methods to calculate connected pen settings

Setting	Explanation/calculation	Considerations
TDD	Use 1 of the following: TDD of mealtime + long-acting insulin —OR— Weight-based dosing: Weight (kg) × 0.5 Weight (lb) × 0.23	If consistent hypoglycemia, use lower amount If consistent hyperglycemia, use higher amount Can also average the results of the two calculations
Insulin carbohydrate ratio	450 ÷ TDD	These are starting points and should be adjusted based on CGM or BGM readings
Insulin sensitivity factor (correction factor)	1700 ÷ TDD	These are starting points and should be adjusted based on CGM or BGM readings
Active insulin time or insulin on board	Usually set between 3–5 h Children, pregnancy: 3 h Older adults, impaired renal function: 5 h Most adults: 4 h	Based on duration of action of rapid-acting insulin
Maximum bolus	Maximum amount delivered at once; many systems have a maximum of 25 or 30 units	Safety precaution

Source: Refs [6, 16]
BGM blood glucose meter, *CGM* continuous glucose monitor, *TDD* total daily dose

The Jade Insulin Dose Calculator app can be synced with CGM devices and connect pens to aid in calculating and adjusting insulin doses. The app also helps with determining how many carbohydrates an individual will need to consume if experiencing hypoglycemia and how long to delay eating if experiencing significant hyperglycemia. Like alerts previously discussed with CGM, the app has available alerts for predicted hypoglycemia as well as reminders for mealtimes and insulin dosing. The Jade

Insulin Dose Calculator app can be synced to Dexcom and Freestyle Libre apps and is free for users.

The mySugr app is a glucose tracking platform which can help users monitor their glucose, meals, and medications. The app also provides "challenges" to help with glucose improvement and motivation as well as feedback on trends and an estimated A1C. The device is compatible with the Eversense app, LibreLink app, and Dexcom data. The basic version is free but advanced features (such as insulin dose calculations, sharing data with health-care providers, and e-coaching) are available at additional add-on or monthly fees.

Similar to the mySugr app, the Glooko app is a platform that helps with logging food, activity, and medications. The app also allows for sharing features with friends and family as well as health-care providers. In contrast to the two previously reviewed apps, Glooko syncs with multiple insulin pumps and can directly connect with many electronic health records, including EPIC. Glooko is compatible with Dexcom G6 and G7 and Eversense; unfortunately, direct input from Freestyle Libre apps is not available in the United States but can be accessed indirectly through AppleHealth. The app is free for users.

Finally, Tidepool Mobile is available and, like Glooko, providing opportunities for users to track glucose and log insulin use, food, and activity. Users can provide comments on different findings which can then be shared with health-care providers directly. Of note, the Tidepool Mobile app is different than the Tidepool Loop app which became the first FDA-approved app that integrates with insulin pumps and can be used to automatically adjust insulin delivery based on glucose readings. The Tidepool Mobile app is compatible with Dexcom G6 (through Apple Health, the online platform is available for Android users; G7 is only available for the online platform and not the app). Tidepool is compatible with other CGM devices (i.e., Freestyle Libre and Eversense), though only through the online platform and not the app. The app is free for users.

Downloadable connected pen reports allow the pharmacist to review items such as settings, bolus adherence, percent of daily insulin delivered as basal versus bolus, and CGM data, if integrated. The CGM reports may have this additional data if a person manually enters in doses and events. When using a mobile app, the data can be integrated directly with the clinic's account for 24-hour access to real-time updates by Bluetooth. For individuals using a reader, receiver, or insulin pump for the display without the use of a mobile app, the device must be downloaded into one of the respective platforms to view data. The data can be downloaded by the patient or health-care professional if they have the platform on their computer. Table 6.7 lists the different compatible data platforms and mobile apps for each type of connected pen or CGM.

Table 6.7 Data platforms and sources

System and website link	Associated mobile applications (apps)	Data sources
Glooko	Glooko	Dexcom G6, G7, InPen, T:Slim X2, Omnipod 5
Clarity	Dexcom G6, Dexcom G7, clarity, Dexcom follow	Dexcom G6, G7, InPen
LibreView	LibreLink, LibreLinkUp, libre 14 day, libre 2, libre 3	Libre 2, libre 3, libre 2+, libre 3+
CareLink	Guardian connect, CareLink	Medtronic insulin pumps, Guardian CGM
Tidepool	Tidepool Mobile	Dexcom G6, G7, InPen, tandem insulin pumps,
Tempo	TempSmart app	Tempo smart button, Dexcom G6, G7
Eversense Data Management System	Eversense	Eversense
InPen Insights Report	InPen	InPen, Dexcom G6, Guardian connect
Bigfoot Unity	Bigfoot Unity	Bigfoot Unity pen cap, libre 2
T:Connect/source	T:Connect	Tandem insulin pumps
Beta bionics user portal	Beta bionics smartphone app	iLet insulin pump

Role of the Pharmacist

Diabetes technology is an opportunity to help advance the care for individuals with diabetes to help with optimizing control and preventing long-term complications. Pharmacists should be at the front line to encourage use of diabetes technology and provide education for the health-care team and patients. People with diabetes vary in terms of their comfort level with technology, and some prefer in-person training and support; pharmacists are in an ideal position to help with both initiation of technology use as well as help develop more advanced skills and adjust therapies based on findings. Pharmacists should use the Pharmacists' Patient Care Process (PPCP) to collect subjective and objective information, assess individualized efficacy and safety of technology utilization, and plan/implement adjustments to medication results [19]. Additionally, pharmacists have the time and expertise to provide comfort and insight to individuals who are hesitant and address specific worries individual to each patient.

Prior research has demonstrated that individuals with more education and engagement regarding their diabetes and devices have better outcomes; ongoing as well as additional education and follow-up are needed both remotely and/or in person, specifically if outcomes are not being met. Pharmacists can help with interpreting data and, if practicing under a collaborative practice agreement, directly modify or initiate therapy as warranted. Pharmacists can also provide support for removing barriers to access, help with qualifying a patient for a device, and aid with cost concerns. As diabetes technology continues to expand and advance, it is critical that pharmacists advocate for initiating and continuing use of devices for patients with diabetes.

Conclusion

Diabetes technology is a growing area with new developments and advances in CGM and connected pens. Advanced diabetes technology can assist people with diabetes to achieve glycemic targets, improve quality of life, add greater convenience, potentially reduce burden of care, and offer a personalized approach to self-management safely and effectively. Furthermore, diabetes technology can improve the efficiency and effectiveness of clinical decision-making. Successful integration of these technologies into care requires knowledge about the functionality of devices in this rapidly changing field. This information will allow healthcare professionals to provide necessary education and training to persons accessing these treatments and to have the required expertise to interpret data and make appropriate treatment adjustments. Pharmacists can be integral in helping patients with diabetes to select the most optimal technology and educating them on use of technologies as well as interpretation of data to optimize the treatment plan.

References

1. American Diabetes Association Professional Practice Committee. 7. Diabetes technology: standards of Care in Diabetes—2024. Diabetes Care. 2024;47(Suppl. 1):S126–44.
2. Greenwood DA, Howell F, Scher L, et al. A framework for optimizing technology-enabled diabetes and cardiometabolic care and education: the role of the diabetes care and education specialist. Diabetes Educ. 2020;46:315–22.
3. MacLeod J, Scher L, Greenwood D, et al. Technology disparities and therapeutic inertia: a call to action for the diabetes care and education specialist. ADCES in Practice. 2021;9:34–41.
4. Association of Diabetes Care and Education Specialists (ADCES). In: American pharmacist association (APhA), APhA Foundation. Professional CGM implementation playbook. ADCES playbook series: implementing CGM into your practice. ADCES/AANP; 2020b. Available at www.diabeteseducator.org/docs/default-source/opencms_test/prof-cgm-playbook.pdf?sfvrsn=2.
5. Association of Diabetes Care and Education Specialists (ADCES). In: American Association of Nurse Practitioners (AANP). Personal CGM implementation playbook. ADCES playbook series: implementing CGM into your practice. ADCES/AANP; 2020a. Available at www.diabeteseducator.org/docs/default-source/practice/educator-tools/cgm-playbooks/apha-adces-personal-cgm-playbook_kbedits0921pdf5e8e8e42-8283-465e-ab8c-bd8399cc1eab.pdf?Status=Master&sfvrsn=8b8b9e58_5.

6. Grunberger G, Sherr J, Allende M, et al. American Association of Clinical Endocrinology clinical practice guideline: the use of advanced technology in the management of persons with diabetes mellitus. Endocr Pract. 2021;27:505–37.
7. McCall AL, Lieb DC, Gianchandani R, et al. Management of individuals with diabetes at high risk for hypoglycemia: an Endocrine Society clinical practice guidelines. J Clin Endocrinol Metab. 2023;108(3):529–62.
8. Schumacher C, Collier I, Isaacs D, et al. Use of continuous glucose monitoring to improve glycemic control: a clinician's guide. J Am Coll Clin Pharm. 2020;3:1333–43.
9. Battelino T, Danne T, Bergenstal RM, et al. Clinical targets for continuous glucose monitoring data interpretation: recommendations from the international consensus on time in range. Diabetes Care. 2019;42:1593–603.
10. Isaacs D, Cox C, Schwab K, et al. Technology integration: the role of the diabetes care and education specialist in practice. Diabetes Educ. 2020;46:323–34.
11. Messer LH, Berget C, Beatson C, a. Preserving skin integrity with chronic device use in diabetes. Diabetes Technol Ther. 2018;20:S254–64.
12. Mannkind Fill, Wear & go with V-go: using the V-go® wearable insulin delivery device. Instructions for patient use. Mannkind. 2022. Available at www.go-vgo.com.
13. CeQur Corporation. CeQur simplicity 3-day insulin patch user guide. CeQur Corporation; 2019. Available at https://myceqursimplicity.com/wp-content/uploads/User-Guide.pdf.
14. Zhou K, Isaacs D. Closed-loop artificial pancreas therapy for type 1 diabetes. Curr Cardiol Rep. 2022;24(9):1159–67.
15. Nallicheri A, Mahoney KM, Gutow HA, Bellini N, Isaacs D. Review of automated insulin delivery systems for type 1 diabetes and associated time in range outcomes. touchREV Endocrinol. 2022;18(1):27–34.
16. Warshaw H, Isaacs D, MacLeod J. The reference guide to integrate smart insulin pens into data-drive diabetes care and education services. Diabetes Educ. 2020;46(Suppl. 4):3S–20S.
17. InPen user guide: InPen-user-guide.pdf (medtronicdiabetes.com) Accessed 29 Sep 2024.
18. Bigfoot Unity. Bigfoot Unity Diabetes Management Program (bigfootbiomedical.com) Accessed 29 Sep 2024.
19. The Pharmacists' Patient Care Process. [Internet]. United States: Joint Commission of Pharmacy Practitioners. Available at: https//jcpp.net/patient-care-process/.

Special Populations

7

Jerry Wiles

Introduction

For diabetes management, pharmacists can address the unique challenges presented by special populations. The approach to care must be tailored to meet the specific needs of each person by considering factors such as age, presence of comorbidities, renal function, hepatic function, and educational level. Practical strategies can aid in understanding and applying practical information to clinical practice when caring for special populations, such as geriatrics, pediatrics, and other unique situations.

Considerations of Geriatric Population

Management of older adults with diabetes presents unique challenges due to numerous factors of aging that must be carefully considered when determining appropriate treatment. Distinguishing between older adults with type 1 (T1D) and type 2 diabetes (T2D) is important to guide management. Although most

J. Wiles (✉)
Pharmacy Department, AnMed, Anderson, SC, USA

© The Author(s), under exclusive license to Springer Nature Switzerland AG 2025

J. Clements (ed.), *The Pharmacist's Pocket Guide for Diabetes and Obesity*, https://doi.org/10.1007/978-3-031-88835-9_7

older adults with diabetes have T2D, improvements in medications and technology have allowed many people with T1D to live beyond the age of 65 [1]. It should also be noted that there are many problems common to the older adult and relevant to diabetes management, such as increased medication burden and impaired cognition. Older individuals are at increased risk for falling independent of diabetes, but this risk may be exacerbated by glucose-lowering medications, especially during hypoglycemic episodes. Predicted lifespan may also be taken into consideration when determining treatment and person-centered goals of therapy [1, 2]. Management of older adults with diabetes will differ from the treatment of otherwise healthy adults with diabetes. These considerations may affect goals, lifestyle recommendations, and drug therapy.

Treatment Goals

If an older adult's anticipated lifespan, cognitive function, and physical capabilities allow them to benefit from extended and intensive management of their diabetes, their treatment may resemble that of a non-geriatric adult with diabetes. Those with three or more coexisting chronic conditions may require less stringent goals. Coexisting conditions to consider include osteoarthritis, cancer, depression, emphysema, falls, heart failure, hypertension, myocardial infarction, stage 3 through 5 chronic kidney disease (CKD), and stroke [1].

For healthy, older adults characterized by minimal chronic conditions, and preserved cognitive and functional abilities, more stringent glycemic goals, such as A1C levels between 7.0% and 7.5%, are appropriate [1, 3]. Reasonable fasting glucose levels for this group would range from 80 to 130 mg/dL and a bedtime glucose goal of 80–180 mg/dL. However, individuals with multiple chronic conditions, cognitive impairment, or functional dependence should pursue less-stringent glycemic goals, aiming for an A1C level below 8.0%. For this group, a fasting glucose goal of 90–150 mg/dL and bedtime glucose goal of 100–180 mg/dL would be more appropriate due to treatment burden, elevated hypoglycemia and fall risk, and a more limited life expectancy. These tailored approaches account for the balance between glycemic control and potential risks associated with intensive treatment, recognizing the diverse health profiles and needs of older adults. Elevated risks of hypoglycemia requiring assistance have been associated with treatment protocols aimed at achieving A1C levels below 6.0%, particularly when involving complex drug regimens that heavily rely on insulin. This supports the tendency to relax, rather than intensify, A1C goals when dealing with medically complex older adults [1, 3].

Individualized care for older adults with diabetes may involve relaxing glycemic goals, particularly for those facing advanced diabetes complications, life-limiting comorbid illnesses, or substantial cognitive or functional impairments. Recommendations for deintensification of treatment goals are made, particularly to minimize the risk of hypoglycemia, provided it aligns with the individualized A1C target. While glycemic targets may be altered based on the individual's health status, it remains crucial to avoid hyperglycemia in all people with diabetes. Glycemic targets should prevent symptoms of hyperglycemia and hypoglycemia and acute complications of diabetes, such as impaired wound healing, dehydration, and hyperglycemic hyperosmolar syndrome [1]. The concept of reducing mortality and time to benefit is pertinent, guiding the understanding that those with advanced complications may have reduced capacity to reap the advantages of intensive glycemic control. Therefore, older adults with advanced diabetes complications have a diminished likelihood of benefiting from reducing the risk of microvascular complications through intensive glycemic control [4]. Additionally, they are more susceptible to serious adverse effects, such as hypoglycemia, emphasizing the need for a careful balance in therapeutic approaches [5].

Screening for Complications

Screening for diabetes complications is essential in the care of older adults. Special consideration should be given to complications with the potential to result in reduced cognitive and/or physical function. Emphasis should be placed on complications that may manifest over short periods and have a significant impact on physical function, including issues related to vision and lower extremities [6]. It is also recommended to conduct screenings for the early detection of cognitive impairment or individuals with dementia for aged 65 or older with their first visit, with subsequent annual assessments or as frequently as deemed appropriate [1]. This targeted screening strategy acknowledges the unique health challenges faced by older adults with diabetes and underscores the importance of early detection to mitigate the impact of complications on overall function and well-being.

Treatment of Comorbidities

In the management of older adults with diabetes, goals often extend beyond glycemic control due to the prevalence of comorbidities in this population. Evidence supports the significance of treating hypertension in older adults, emphasizing individualized target levels for optimal outcomes [7]. However, the effects of intensive glycemic and blood pressure control on reducing brain function decline remain inconclusive [8]. While the evidence for lipid-lowering therapy and aspirin use is inconclusive, their potential benefits for primary and secondary prevention are applicable to older adults whose life expectancies align with or surpass the durations studied in clinical trials [9]. Notably, studies on statins, with trial durations ranging from 2 to 6 years, suggest a time to benefit of 2.5 years [10]. Managing other risk factors for comorbid conditions should be individualized, considering the anticipated time frame for beneficial effects.

A reasonable blood pressure goal for healthy older adults with diabetes and minimal additional chronic conditions is <130/80 mmHg. This is also appropriate for individuals with multiple chronic conditions, cognitive impairment, or functional dependence who still have an intermediate life expectancy. Older adults with more medically complex treatment, poor health, and a limited life expectancy could benefit from a more relaxed goal of <140/90 mmHg [1].

Some older adults have lived with a diabetes diagnosis for many years, experiencing a range of complications or none, due to effective management. Others are diagnosed with either new-onset diabetes, without serious complications, or potentially years of undiagnosed diabetes, which may have led to extensive complications. This variability is further compounded by the presence of underlying chronic conditions, and limitations in cognitive or physical functioning, as well as frailty among some individuals [1]. This diverse spectrum of diabetes in older adults leads to many individualized treatment goals.

Continuous Glucose Monitoring

Continuous glucose monitoring (CGM) emerges as a crucial component for older adults with T1D, as well as insulin-dependent T2D, offering enhanced control and risk reduction of hypoglycemia [1]. Notably, it has been shown that CGM results in a reduction in time spent with hypoglycemia compared to standard blood glucose monitoring [11, 12]. Observational data from studies support the use of routine CGM and insulin pump in older adults with long-standing T1D, correlating with fewer hypoglycemic events, hyperglycemic excursions, and lower A1C concentrations [13, 14]. The evidence base, primarily rooted in T1D, is expanding to show clinical benefits for people with T2D using insulin [15]. CGM has also shown a positive impact in adults over 60 years of age with either T1D or T2D using multiple daily injections, associating its use with improved A1C, and reduced glycemic variability [16].

As the role of CGM continues to evolve, older adults with physical or cognitive limitations, who require blood glucose monitoring, represent a population where CGM may play an increasing role. The availability of accurate CGM devices communicating with insulin pumps through Bluetooth has facilitated the development of advanced insulin-delivery algorithms, including predictive low-glucose suspend and hybrid closed-loop algorithms. New developments in this type of technology show promise for improving glycemic outcomes [1].

Polypharmacy

Older adults with diabetes are prone to polypharmacy and heightened vulnerability to medication side effects and interactions. Individuals over 80 years of age, using insulin or a sulfonylurea medication, face an increased risk of hypoglycemia in comparison to those aged 65–70 years. Comprehensive care often necessitates an escalation in prescribed medications as diabetes and its complications advance over time. This means the decision to introduce new medications, whether diabetes-related or otherwise, for older adults should be approached with careful consideration, weighing the potential benefits against the associated risks [2]. For otherwise healthy older adults with diabetes, deprescribing or deintensification may be warranted if they experience severe or recurrent hypoglycemia, wide glucose excursions or if cognitive or functional status begin to decline due to acute illness. For more medically complex older adults with multiple coexisting illnesses or mild-to-moderate cognitive impairment, treatment simplification may be warranted in the same situations as healthy older adults, as well as if there is a significant change in social circumstances such that they are unable to manage the complexity of the regimen. For older adults in long-term care facility, with end-stage chronic illness, or significant cognitive/physical impairments, they may simplify their regimen to fewer daily injections and finger sticks. Regimens can also be simplified if they eat inconsistent meals. For end-of-life care, the regimen can be deintensified if there is any pain or discomfort caused by their medications, medications with no clear benefits for comfort or symptom improvement may be removed, or if there is significant caregiver stress. For individuals who live in the community but have a short-term rehab stay, their regimen may have become more complicated while hospitalized before their stay. It is reasonable to simplify their regimen to restart their home regimen prior to hospitalization if simplification is needed [1].

Hypoglycemia Risk

Older adults with diabetes face an elevated risk of hypoglycemia due to numerous factors, including insulin deficiency necessitating insulin therapy and progressive renal insufficiency [17]. Given the higher risk of hypoglycemia in older adults compared to younger individuals, routine visits should prioritize the identification and management of episodes of hypoglycemia [1]. To proactively address future risks, validated risk calculators, such as the Kaiser Hypoglycemia Model, can be employed to stratify older adults based on their susceptibility to hypoglycemic events [18]. Factors contributing to hypoglycemia in this population include certain behaviors, such as skipping meals or inadvertently repeating medication doses [19]. Acknowledging these challenges is a recommended approach for mitigating the risk of hypoglycemia, as deintensification would align with individualized A1C targets [1]. This strategy aims to balance effective diabetes management while minimizing the potential for hypoglycemic events in geriatric individuals.

Cognitive, Physical, and Functional Status

Managing diabetes in older adults presents challenges when cognitive impairment is a factor, hindering individuals from performing complex self-care tasks [1]. Screening tools, such as the Mini-Mental State Examination, help identify those needing neuropsychological evaluation, crucial for early detection of mild cognitive impairment or dementia in adults aged 65 and older [20, 21]. Assessing treatment knowledge and self-management skills is essential at treatment onset, with regular reassessments recommended when changing treatment plans or when there is evidence of declining functional abilities [6, 22]. Struggling with adherence to rigorous blood glucose monitoring and insulin regimens is common in older adults. Therefore, it would be essential to establish individualized glycemic targets when accounting for chronic conditions, functional status, and cognitive function [19]. Beyond medical considerations, impaired social functioning poses a risk to the quality of life and may lead to functional dependency [23]. Evaluating living situations and involving social support networks in decision-making processes, including adult children and caretakers, is vital for comprehensive diabetes care in older people [1].

End-of-Life and Advanced Disease States

In end-of-life care for older adults with diabetes, the focus is avoiding hypoglycemia and symptomatic hyperglycemia while alleviating the burdens of glycemic management. As organ failure progresses, deintensification or discontinuation of several agents for T2D is often necessary, though there is no consensus on the management of T1D in this context [24, 25]. Palliative care discussions in older adults with diabetes should address the goals and intensity of care, with a shift away from strict glucose and blood pressure control [1]. Simplification of regimens, deintensification of therapy, and potential withdrawal may be considered, aligning with the overarching goals of preserving comfort, preventing distressing symptoms, and maintaining quality of life and dignity [26].

Management strategies vary during end-of-life for those within different advanced disease categories. For those who are stable, continuation of the previous regimen is advised. In individuals with organ failure, preventing hypoglycemia is paramount, with careful attention to hydration. For those approaching the end of life, discontinuation of all medications may be reasonable for T2D with limited oral intake. However, in T1D, a small amount of basal insulin may be considered to maintain glucose levels and prevent acute hyperglycemic complications [24]. These tailored approaches aim to optimize care while respecting individual needs and circumstances.

Lifestyle Management

Lifestyle management requires a holistic approach emphasizing optimal nutrition and protein intake is paramount. Older adults with diabetes should be encouraged to exercise regularly. Aerobic activity, weight-bearing exercises, and resistance training are recommended for all older adults, who can safely engage in these activities. For those with T2D, where overweight/obesity coexists with the capacity for safe exercise, an intensive lifestyle intervention becomes crucial. This intervention, centered on dietary modifications, physical activity, and achieving modest weight loss (typically 5–7%), holds potential benefits for enhancing quality of life, maintaining mobility and physical functioning, and effectively managing cardiometabolic risk factors [1].

Diabetes in aging individuals is often associated with reduced muscle strength, poor muscle quality, and accelerated loss of muscle mass, contributing to conditions such as sarcopenia and osteopenia [27, 28]. In the management of frailty in diabetes, an integrated strategy involving optimal nutrition with adequate protein intake should be coupled with a comprehensive exercise program. This type of program aims to mitigate sedentary behavior, prevent mobility disability, and reduce frailty in older adults [29, 30]. Intensive lifestyle interventions in non-frail older adults, designed to reduce weight, have been shown to improve quality of life, reduce A1C, and reduce need for medications [31].

Financial Considerations

In the domain of drug therapy for T2D, a comprehensive approach involves addressing cost considerations, overtreatment concerns, and the choice of medications based on individualized risk profiles. The considerations for older adults with diabetes extend beyond medical factors to encompass economic and practical facets. Cost implications and insurance coverage rules should be factored into the development of treatment plans to mitigate potential barriers to adherence [1]. Given that older adults often contend with multiple medications and fixed incomes, understanding and addressing these cost-related challenges become integral to minimizing the risk of cost-related barriers to adherence [32, 33].

Pharmacological Treatment

The recommendation for the simplification of complex treatment plans, particularly regarding insulin, aims to not only reduce the risk of hypoglycemia but also address polypharmacy concerns, lessening the overall burden of the disease, provided it aligns with the individualized A1C target. It is crucial to recognize that intensive glycemic control, especially with regimens involving insulin and sulfonylureas, may be identified as overtreatment in older adults with complex medical conditions. This practice is unfortunately common in clinical settings, emphasizing the need for a tailored approach. Additionally, the risk of hypoglycemia in older adults necessitates a preference for medication classes with a minimal risk of such events. Overtreatment, a common issue in this demographic, should be actively avoided [1]. Deintensification of non-insulin diabetes medications may involve lowering doses or discontinuing the medication entirely, if the person continues to meet glycemic targets [34].

Metformin emerges as the first-line agent for older adults with T2D, with safety considerations for renal function, and cautious use in those with impaired hepatic function or decompensated heart failure [1, 35]. Thiazolidinediones are suggested with caution, especially in individuals on insulin therapy and those with or at risk of heart failure. Insulin secretagogues (e.g., sulfonylureas) warrant careful use due to their association with hypoglycemia, with preference given to shorter-acting options [1].

Dipeptidyl peptidase-4 inhibitors (DPP-4i) can be considered due to few side effects and minimal risk of hypoglycemia, though cost may pose a barrier for some older adults. Additionally, DPP-4i may require renal dose adjustments, except for linagliptin; sitagliptin and linagliptin have a neutral effect on major cardiovascular outcomes. Glucagon-like peptide-1 (GLP-1) receptor agonists offer cardiovascular benefits across age groups, and while injectable, they may be associated with gastrointestinal side effects. Sodium-glucose cotransporter-2 inhibitors (SGLT-2i), administered orally, present convenient options, particularly for those with cardiovascular and kidney concerns.

Insulin plays a crucial role in managing glycemic control for older adults with T1D and T2D. In the aging population, complexities associated with diabetes, cognitive impairment, and functional limitations can pose challenges in administering insulin. Basal insulin is recommended for older adults with T1D, even when meal ingestion is challenging, to prevent diabetes-related ketoacidosis. The administration of insulin may become more difficult as complications arise and simplifying the insulin plan based on an individual's self-management abilities has been demonstrated to reduce hypoglycemia and disease-related distress without compromising glycemic outcomes [1]. Once-daily basal insulin injection therapy, associated with minimal side effects, emerges as a reasonable option for many older adults [36]. Long-acting insulin analogs are favored over NPH insulin due to a lower risk of hypoglycemia. However, the complexity of multiple daily insulin injections may be challenging for older individuals with advanced complications or limited functional status. Therefore, a tailored approach to insulin regimen simplification is advocated to align with individualized glycemic targets and minimize the burden of diabetes in the geriatric population [1].

For older adults with T1D, the use of advanced insulin delivery devices, such as automated insulin-delivery systems and connected pens, is recommended to mitigate the risk of hypoglycemia. The choice of insulin therapy requires good visual, motor skills, and cognitive ability either from the individual or their caregiver [1]. Recent advancements in hybrid closed-loop insulin delivery strategies show potential benefits for older individuals with long-standing T1D. These strategies have demonstrated significant improvements in time spent in the desired glucose range, accompanied by notable reductions in hypoglycemia [37, 38]. However, it is emphasized that the adoption of such advanced technologies should be subject to periodic reassessment, especially for those experiencing declining cognitive or functional status [1].

Deintensification is an important component of therapy for older adults with diabetes since this age group may acquire comorbidities over time that potentially reduce life expectancy, cognitive ability, or physical ability to maintain their current diabetes regimen. Non-insulin diabetes medications may require doses to be reduced or medications to be discontinued to make a regimen more manageable for people if glycemic targets are maintained. Healthy individuals and those with multiple chronic illnesses that remain in the community may require deintensification if there is polypharmacy, hypoglycemia, or glycemic variability. Those in Skilled Nursing Facilities for short-term rehab may require deintensification in acute illness/condition resulting in temporary cognitive decline, sudden weight loss, or temporary physical decline. Individuals in long-term care facilities or that are nearing end of life may require the removal of medications that show no clear benefit and do not aid in comfort. Strategies for simplifying insulin regimens include switching basal doses to the morning instead of bedtime, eliminating rapid or short-acting insulin doses that are near bedtime, and attempting to remove or reduce prandial doses. If prandial doses are greater than 10 units, consider reducing the dose by 50% and adding an oral agent. If prandial doses are less than 10 units, consider discontinuing prandial doses altogether.

Pediatric Considerations

Management of pediatric people with diabetes presents unique challenges due to several factors that are unique to childhood. T1D is the predominant form of diabetes among the pediatric population, and recent data suggest its significant presence in cases diagnosed during adulthood [39, 40]. The rates of T2D diagnosis continue to increase in the pediatric population [41]. Problems that are common to children with diabetes include barriers to the comprehension of self-management, coordination of medical and nutritional care with family and school, and transition from childhood to adulthood.

Managing diabetes in children and adolescents necessitates a specialized approach, considering various distinctive aspects. Health-care professionals must be attuned to the evolving insulin sensitivity linked to physical growth and sexual maturation, self-care capabilities, and supervision required in childcare and school settings. Neurological susceptibility to hypoglycemia and hyperglycemia in young children, coupled with potential adverse neurocognitive effects of diabetic ketoacidosis (DKA), further underscores the need for specialized care [42, 43].

Tailored nutrition therapy is crucial for pediatric diabetes management, recognizing the unique challenges faced by children and adolescents with T1D and their families [41]. A comprehensive approach extends beyond medical settings to encompass the school environment. Students diagnosed with T1D or T2D must receive support for utilizing advanced diabetes technologies, such as continuous glucose monitors, insulin pumps, connected insulin pens, and automated insulin-delivery systems, as prescribed by their diabetes care team. Given that a substantial portion of a youth's day is spent in school or day care, educating and training school personnel becomes imperative. This training ensures that the child's individualized diabetes medical management plan is adhered to facilitating optimal diabetes management and safe participation in all school-sponsored activities [44]. The collaborative efforts of health-care providers, families, and educational institutions are pivotal in addressing the unique concerns of pediatric people with both T1D and T2D.

Diabetes Self-Management

Ensuring comprehensive care for youth diagnosed with T1D is paramount, extending beyond the individual to encompass their parents or caregivers for those aged below 18 years. Culturally sensitive and developmentally appropriate diabetes self-management education and support, in alignment with national standards, should be initiated at the time of diagnosis and maintained as an ongoing practice. This personalized approach recognizes the evolving needs of young people and their families [41].

Moreover, an integral facet of pediatric diabetes care involves the assessment of educational requirements and skills of day-care workers, school nurses, and other school personnel responsible for the child's care and supervision. Providing targeted training to these individuals is essential, ensuring they are equipped to navigate the unique challenges posed by diabetes in a school or day-care setting [44–46]. This collaborative effort strives to create an environment where pediatric youth receive holistic and tailored support, fostering their well-being and successful diabetes management throughout their formative years.

Nutrition Therapy

For youth diagnosed with T1D, individualized medical nutrition therapy stands as a crucial pillar within the overarching treatment framework. The monitoring of carbohydrate intake, facilitated by approaches such as carbohydrate counting or experiential-based estimation, emerges as a pivotal strategy for optimizing glycemic management. A cornerstone of this approach involves the provision of comprehensive nutrition education at the time of diagnosis and complemented by annual updates, preferably by an experienced registered dietitian nutritionist [41]. This ongoing nutritional guidance serves to assess caloric and nutritional intake relative to weight status and cardiovascular disease risk factors, providing a foundation for informed macronutrient choices [41]. Notably, adherence to recommended nutrition plans has been correlated with improved glycemic outcomes in the youth with T1D [47]. This concerted focus on individualized nutrition equips young people with the tools to navigate their dietary choices effectively, contributing to enhanced glycemic control and overall well-being.

Transitioning into Adulthood

As children and adolescents age with T1D or T2D, there is a discernible shift in the responsibility and oversight of diabetes management from parents and caregivers to the young individuals themselves throughout their formative years. This transition becomes particularly noteworthy during the pivotal phase of emerging adulthood, marking a shift from pediatric to adult health-care professionals. However, the transfer of care often unfolds abruptly as older teens traverse this developmental stage [48]. The ensuing transition period from pediatric to adult care introduces a susceptibility to fragmentation in health-care delivery, potentially compromising the quality, cost, and overall outcomes of health care [49]. Notably, documented evidence indicates a concerning trend of worsening diabetes health outcomes during this transitional phase into adult care and early adulthood [50]. Recognizing and addressing the unique challenges posed by this transitional period is crucial for sustaining optimal diabetes management and ensuring positive health outcomes as individuals navigate the complexities of adulthood.

Screening for Comorbidities/Complications

A proactive approach to mental health considerations is paramount for comprehensive care among the pediatric population. At the time of diagnosis and throughout routine follow-up care, diligent screening for psychosocial issues and family stresses is essential, recognizing their potential impact on diabetes management. Appropriate referrals to trained mental health professionals can be offered, preferably those with experience in childhood diabetes, who should be regarded as integral members of the pediatric diabetes multidisciplinary team. Moreover, judicious employment of age-appropriate standardized tools is recommended for screening youth with T2D for diabetes distress, depressive symptoms, and broader mental/behavioral health concerns. Special attention should be given to symptoms of depression and disordered eating, with timely referrals to qualified mental health professionals, when indicated [41].

Beyond mental health considerations, a comprehensive screening approach extends to the identification and management of additional autoimmune conditions associated with T1D. This involves vigilant monitoring for symptoms and the early assessment of conditions such as thyroid disease and celiac disease. Additionally, screening and appropriate management protocols should be implemented for common comorbidities associated with T2D, including hypertension, dyslipidemia, nonalcoholic fatty liver disease, obstructive sleep apnea, polycystic ovary syndrome, and cardiovascular disease [41].

The importance of long-term follow-up is underscored by data revealing that a significant proportion of individuals diagnosed with T2D during youth developed microvascular complications by young adulthood [51]. Notably, retinopathy commonly manifests after the onset of puberty and 5–10 years into the duration of T1D [52]. To address the potential impact on neuropathy, an annual comprehensive foot exam is recommended, encompassing various aspects such as inspection, palpation of pulses, and assessments of proprioception, vibration, and monofilament sensation [53]. Consistent foot inspection during each visit serves an educational purpose, emphasizing the importance of ongoing foot care for youth with diabetes [41].

Glucose Monitoring

Effective blood glucose monitoring is crucial for the comprehensive management of pediatric diabetes, and its approach should be tailored to the individual's needs, preferences, and treatment plans. Youth with T2D on multiple daily injections or insulin pumps, who possess the capability to safely use the device either independently or with caregiver assistance, should be offered real-time CGM or intermittently scanned CGM [41]. The choice of monitoring device should align with the individual and family's circumstances, preferences, and needs. While data on CGM in youth with T2D are limited, it may be considered for those requiring frequent blood glucose monitoring [54].

Real-time or intermittently scanned CGM should be considered for those on multiple daily injections or insulin pump therapy, capable of safely using the device [41]. For youth with T1D, who are not using a CGM device, a robust blood glucose monitoring routine is essential, involving multiple daily checks (up to 6–10 times/day) using blood glucose meters. This includes checks before meals and snacks, at bedtime, and as needed for safety during specific activities like physical exertion or driving or in the presence of hypoglycemia symptoms.

Treatment Goals

Glycemic status evaluation, with an A1C target of <7%, is recommended every 3 months for most children and adolescents with T2D. However, more stringent A1C targets (<6.5%) might be appropriate for selected individuals, especially those with a short duration of diabetes, lesser degrees of beta-cell dysfunction, or significant weight improvement through lifestyle or metformin-only treatment. More stringent A1C targets can be achieved without significant hypoglycemia or other adverse effects. Conversely, less stringent A1C goals (e.g., 7.5%) may be considered in situations where there is an increased risk of hypoglycemia or hypoglycemia unawareness, a lack of access to advanced insulin technologies, or limitations in regular blood glucose monitoring. For youth on insulin, A1C targets should be personalized, considering the low rates of hypoglycemia observed in youth-onset T2D. In situations where glycemic control may be affected by non-glycemic factors, even more lenient A1C goals may be appropriate. Individuals with specific circumstances, such as a history of severe hypoglycemia, limited life expectancy, or a greater risk of treatment-related harms compared to benefits, may warrant even less stringent A1C goals [41].

In conjunction with A1C assessment, metrics derived from CGM over the most recent 14 days, or longer for youth with increased glycemic variability, should be integrated. These metrics, including time in range (70–180 mg/dL), time below target (<70 and <54 mg/dL), and time above target (>180 and >250 mg/dL), offer valuable insights into glycemic control and should be utilized whenever possible to enhance the precision of diabetes management [41].

Lifestyle Management

Lifestyle management is integral to the comprehensive care of pediatric people with diabetes, emphasizing physical activity and nutrition. For youth with T1D, T2D, or prediabetes, engaging in 60 min of daily moderate-to-vigorous aerobic activity, including resistance and flexibility training, is recommended [41, 55]. CGM and meticulous glucose monitoring before, during, and after exercise play crucial roles in preventing, detecting, and managing hypoglycemia and hyperglycemia associated with physical activity. Education for both youth and parents/caregivers on glycemic targets and management strategies tailored to the type and intensity of planned physical activities is paramount [41].

Preventing hypoglycemia during and after exercise involves strategic adjustments to insulin dosages, carbohydrate intake, and leveraging technologies. Intense activity should be postponed in the presence of marked hyperglycemia or ketosis [56]. Reducing basal rates or adjusting long-acting insulin doses by approximately 20% following exercise could potentially mitigate the risk of delayed exercise-induced hypoglycemia [57]. Hybrid closed-loop systems and "exercise mode" can enhance safety during exercise, optimizing time in the target glucose range [58]. Blood glucose targets prior to exercise should be individualized, and additional carbohydrate intake may be necessary depending on activity duration and intensity. To prevent hypoglycemia during low-to-moderate-intensity aerobic activities lasting 30–60 min, and in situations where the youth is fasting, it is advisable to consume 10–15 g of carbohydrates. Following insulin boluses, characterized by relative hyperinsulinemia, incorporate 0.5–1.0 grams of carbohydrates per kilogram of body weight per hour of exercise. This aligns with the carbohydrate needs recommended for optimizing performance in athletes without T1D [41].

Psychosocial Considerations

Health-care professionals should address various social determinants of health, including food security, housing stability, financial barriers, and social/community support, incorporating this information into treatment decisions. Furthermore, screening for psychosocial aspects such as social adjustment, school performance, and mental health distress is essential, with timely referrals to qualified professionals when indicated. Adolescents should be provided time alone with their health-care professionals to foster open communication. For those with T1D, screening for disordered eating is initiated between 10 and 12 years of age. Lastly, a chronic care model is recommended for youth with T2D, integrating developmentally and culturally appropriate lifestyle programs aimed at achieving a 7–10% decrease in excess weight, alongside a focus on healthy eating patterns [41].

Choosing Pharmacologic Treatment

The initial treatment approach for pediatric persons with obesity and diabetes must be adapted to the uncertainty often present in the early stages, where the distinction between diabetes types may not be immediately clear. In cases of overlapping symptoms and potential ketoacidosis, the priority is to address hyperglycemia and associated metabolic imbalances, irrespective of the definitive diabetes type. Treatment adjustments can be made once metabolic compensation is established, considering additional information such as islet autoantibody results [59].

For individuals presenting with an A1C less than 8.5% without acidosis or ketosis, initiating treatment with metformin is recommended, titrating up to 2000 mg per day as tolerated [60]. In cases where the A1C is ≥8.5%, with or without ketosis, metformin should be initiated along with a long-acting insulin regimen (0.5 u/kg/day), titrating every 2–3 days based on blood glucose monitoring. Management of acidosis, DKA, or hyperosmolar hyperglycemic nonketotic state (HHNS) takes precedence in people with these complications. Intravenous insulin is administered until acidosis resolves, followed by subcutaneous insulin as if T1D is responsible, pending testing for pancreatic autoantibodies [41].

After initiating treatment, pancreatic autoantibody testing should be collected. If the results are negative, metformin can be continued or started, and insulin (if already initiated) can be titrated based on glucose values. If the results are positive, metformin should be discontinued (if started), and multiple daily injection (MDI) insulin or pump therapy for T1D is initiated. In cases where A1C targets are not met with metformin alone for T2D, the consideration of a glucagon-like peptide-1 (GLP-1) receptor agonist approved for youth, such as liraglutide and exenatide, may be appropriate. If insulin is necessary, starting with a long-acting insulin is recommended, with the option to add prandial insulin if needed [41].

Other Considerations

Renal Impairment

The interplay between diabetes and renal function requires a nuanced approach to care. The renin–angiotensin system (RAS) inhibitors have emerged as pivotal agents in slowing kidney disease progression, particularly in individuals with diabetes, hypertension, and albuminuria. CKD is classified based on the cause of dysfunction, estimated glomerular filtration rate (eGFR), and albuminuria. In these people, titration to the maximum tolerated dose is important. Close monitoring of serum potassium and serum creatinine levels within 2–4 weeks of initiation or dose adjustment is imperative to ensure optimal therapeutic outcomes [61].

Cautionary advice discourages the combination therapy involving both ACE inhibitors (ACEis) and angiotensin receptor blockers (ARBs) in those with diabetes and CKD due to potential harm. Additionally, mineralocorticoid receptor antagonists, such as spironolactone and eplerenone, have demonstrated effectiveness in managing resistant hypertension. Finerenone, a selective nonsteroidal mineralocorticoid receptor antagonist, shows benefit in reducing risks associated with CKD progression and cardiovascular events among those with CKD and T2D on RAS blockade [61].

Monitoring remains important with an individualized target ranging from <6.5% to 8.0%. The A1C is maintained down to an eGFR of 30 mL/min/1.73 m^2, below which considerations for erythrocyte lifespan alterations must be acknowledged. CGM can serve as an addition or alternative unaffected by CKD, offering crucial insights for those with discordant A1C levels or clinical symptoms [61].

Beyond glycemic control, dietary and lifestyle interventions assume significance. Protein intake is recommended at 0.8 g protein/kg/day, while sodium intake should be limited to <2 g/day. Physical activity, often lacking in those with diabetes and CKD, is endorsed, with a cumulative duration of at least 150 min per week recommended to enhance overall well-being [61].

In the management of T2D and CKD, SGLT-2i takes precedence as the preferred first-line pharmacologic therapy. The initiation of SGLT-2i is recommended for individuals with an eGFR of at least 20 mL/min/1.73 m^2. The benefits of SGLT-2i extend beyond glycemic control, emphasizing their role in organ protection, particularly for the heart and kidneys, in those with CKD. Clinical trials have demonstrated cardiovascular and kidney advantages across various eGFR categories, with consistent benefits observed in different albuminuria statuses, including normal albumin excretion. As a second-line drug class for glucose lowering in T2D and CKD, GLP-1 receptor agonists demonstrate potential kidney-related benefits, specifically liraglutide and semaglutide. The cardiovascular benefits of GLP-1 receptor agonists persist across various eGFR categories. Additionally, the potential advantages of weight loss associated with GLP-1 RAs are highlighted, recognizing the importance of weight management in certain CKD scenarios, such as pre-kidney transplantation [62]. Metformin is also appropriate to use with an eGFR ≥30 mL/min/1.73 m^2. Dosing should be reduced to a maximum of 500 mg twice daily when eGFR is between 45 and 30 mL/min/1.73 m^2 [61]. Structured self-management education programs and team-based, integrated care models are advocated to empower individuals and comprehensively address the multifaceted challenges posed by diabetes and renal impairment. In navigating this complex terrain, a person-centered and evidence-based approach is paramount for optimizing outcomes and enhancing the quality of life for individuals with diabetes and CKD [61].

For those requiring dialysis, metformin and SGLT-2i should be stopped as soon as a person requires dialysis. A range of options is still available to those on dialysis. Medication classes to choose from include GLP-1 receptor agonists, DPP-4i, sulfonylureas, alpha-glucosidase inhibitors, thiazolidinediones, and insulin. Although GLP-1 receptor agonists are preferred due to their additional benefits, these other drug classes may be considered if GLP-1 receptor agonists cannot be used due to contraindication or factors such as cost [61].

Hepatic Impairment

Hepatic impairment is a decline in the functionality of the liver, which plays a critical role in the homeostasis of blood glucose. Diagnosing and treating diabetes with hepatic impairment presents a unique set of challenges, demanding a careful balance between glycemic control and the limitations imposed by liver disease. Fasting plasma glucose, while a simple and cost-effective diagnostic tool, faces hurdles in widespread adoption due to prolonged fasting requirements and stringent processing needs. Stress, acute illness, and alcohol consumption can further impact glucose accuracy. Controversies surrounding the optimal fasting plasma glucose threshold for diagnosing diabetes in individuals with chronic liver disease or end-stage liver disease underscore the complexity of this issue [63].

The oral glucose tolerance test is encumbered by prolonged fasting, test complexity, and limited reproducibility. However, it remains crucial, especially for detecting gestational diabetes and cystic fibrosis-related diabetes. A1C offers an advantage in its ease of use and absence of fasting requirements, making it valuable for assessing long-term glycemic control. Nevertheless, its reliability in advanced liver diseases is questionable due to factors such as erythrocyte turnover abnormalities, which are common in chronic liver disease and end-stage liver disease [63]. Nontraditional glycemic markers, such as glycated albumin, fructosamine, and serum 1,5-anhydroglucitol, provide alternatives. Glycated albumin and fructosamine reflect glycemic control over shorter durations, but their accuracy is compromised by liver disease-related variations in protein metabolism. Serum 1,5-anhydroglucitol, although sensitive in assessing glycemic control, may be influenced by liver disease and dietary intake [63].

While the American Diabetes Association recommends an A1C goal of <7% for the general population, the impact of glycemic control on the natural history of chronic liver disease remains inadequately explored. Moreover, antihyperglycemic therapy choices should consider the potential benefits and risks in the context of liver disease [63].

In the context of managing diabetes in people with hepatic impairment, various antidiabetic medications exhibit distinct advantages and limitations. Metformin stands out with its favorable safety profile, cardioprotective effects, and improvements in insulin resistance, aminotransferases, and liver morphology, particularly in nonalcoholic fatty liver disease. Its continued use after cirrhosis diagnosis contributes to increased overall median survival. However, a rare risk of metformin-associated lactic acidosis should be considered [63].

Pioglitazone, another therapeutic option, proves beneficial in improving aminotransferases and liver histology in nonalcoholic steatohepatitis, with a minimal risk of hypoglycemia and inhibitory effects on hepatocellular carcinoma development. Long-term safety concerns and the potential for weight gain are notable drawbacks. Alpha-glucosidase inhibitors demonstrate positive outcomes by reducing postprandial hyperglycemia, glycemic variation, and serum ammonia levels while enhancing intellectual function. However, their use may lead to flatulence and diarrhea [63].

GLP-1 receptor agonists offer benefits such as weight loss, low hypoglycemia risk, and improvements in insulin sensitivity and hepatic outcomes in nonalcoholic fatty liver disease and steatohepatitis, but their efficacy in advanced cirrhosis remains less explored. DPP-4i show promise in improving hepatic steatosis and inflammation. On the downside, uncertainties surround their impact on heart failure exacerbation and their use in advanced cirrhosis [63].

SGLT-2i induce weight loss, pose a low hypoglycemic risk, and improve hepatic outcomes in nonalcoholic fatty liver disease and steatohepatitis; yet, concerns about infections and limited experience in advanced cirrhosis warrant caution. Conversely, sulfonylureas and meglitinides present heightened risks of hypoglycemia, extensive hepatic metabolism, and ineffectiveness under certain hepatic conditions [63].

Insulin, while effective for glycemic control, necessitates careful use due to the associated high risk of hypoglycemia, weight gain, and potential exacerbation of underlying insulin resistance with an increased risk of malignancy. Managing diabetes with hepatic impairment demands a tailored and vigilant approach. Consideration of hepatic function, glycemic markers, and therapeutic nuances is paramount to optimize care and improve outcomes in this complex population [63].

Visual Impairment

Diabetes, irrespective of its type, poses an elevated risk of vision loss due to the relentless progression of the disease, often manifesting as retinopathy. For individuals grappling with diabetes, safeguarding vision becomes a paramount concern. A proactive approach to eye care is essential, involving annual dilated eye exams to detect potential issues at their earliest, most manageable stages. Tight control of blood sugar levels is crucial, as persistently elevated levels not only compromise blood vessels in the eyes but can also distort lens shape, leading to blurred vision. Additionally, maintaining blood pressure and cholesterol within target ranges emerges not only as a safeguard against systemic complications but as a vital strategy to mitigate the risk of eye diseases. Lifestyle modifications, such as smoking cessation and regular physical activity, further fortify the defense against diabetes-related vision impairments [64].

The visually impaired face unique challenges in adhering to monitoring and treatment measures. Insulin pens are preferred over syringes. When a person with visual impairment requires the use of insulin pens, it is important that they be counseled on the increments of insulin units that are dialed with each rotation. Pens with a more audible clicking noise during each adjustment of units are preferable in this population. Blood glucose monitors should have large, high-contrast screens with sufficient backlighting to allow for ease of reading under low visibility conditions such as dim lighting. CGM devices encounter a barrier in the absence of vocalized information [65]. Encouragingly, a preliminary study suggests that integrating CGM with voice-enabled technology, such as Siri, significantly reduces the incidence of severe hypoglycemia over a 12-month period for this specific group [66]. Despite this setback, a range of diabetes-specific devices tailored for those with low vision offer solutions. Audio glucometers that vocalize glucose readings, lancets with user-friendly drum mechanisms, and CGM devices equipped with audio alerts for critical glucose levels cater to the needs of visually impaired individuals. These tailored technologies illuminate a path toward comprehensive care, enhancing both glycemic control and the preservation of precious eyesight [67].

Low Literacy

Low health literacy and numeracy pose significant challenges in managing diabetes, affecting approximately one in three adult Americans. These limitations are linked to adverse health outcomes, particularly in the realm of chronic diseases. In the context of diabetes, individuals with low health literacy encounter difficulties comprehending their condition, engaging in self-care activities, and achieving optimal glycemic control. Similarly, those with low numeracy skills exhibit lower disease knowledge, reduced participation in self-care, lower self-efficacy in managing diabetes, higher body weight, and modest associations with poor glycemic control [68].

To address the communication barriers associated with low health literacy, health-care providers can employ various strategies. First, avoiding ambiguous phrases that might have dual interpretations is crucial. For instance, explaining nuanced statements like, “Insulin may prevent your diabetes from getting worse,” ensures that people understand the uncertainty in such language. Some individuals could interpret the word “may” to mean that there is no conclusive evidence showing that insulin is effective, while the word “will” would better convey the intended meaning. Additionally, providers should write out acronyms and introduce new terms explicitly to enhance comprehension. For example, using “Body Mass Index (BMI)” or “Blood Pressure (BP)” instead of their respective acronyms aids in clarity [68].

Using common words in their typical contexts and being mindful of potential cultural differences in interpreting language are essential considerations. Providers should recognize that what may be plain language for one cultural group might not be clear to another. Cultural sensitivity becomes even more critical when dealing with diverse racial and ethnic backgrounds and generational cultures. Furthermore, encouraging open-ended questions is a valuable practice to gauge understanding. People may be hesitant to admit difficulty comprehending information, so asking, “What questions do you have?” provides an opportunity for clarification [68].

The teach-back method is a powerful tool in ensuring comprehension. Instead of simply asking if someone understands, they are prompted to explain or demonstrate what they have been told. This method minimizes the likelihood of responses with a generic “yes” when they may not comprehend the information [68]. To support both individuals with diabetes and providers in diabetes education, tools like the Diabetes Literacy and Numeracy Education Toolkit offer interactive guidance. This comprehensive resource facilitates cooperative learning between special populations with diabetes and health-care providers, enhancing diabetes education and encouraging optimal self-care activities [69]. Additionally, the American College of Physicians Foundation Living with Diabetes Guide addresses key topics, including diet, physical activity, blood glucose monitoring, medication adherence, and insulin use, contributing to improved diabetes education and self-care for individuals with low health literacy [68].

Diabetes in Pregnancy

Preconception

Preconception counseling is an essential component of diabetes care for individuals of reproductive age, starting at puberty and continuing throughout adulthood. Family planning discussions, including the use of effective contraception, are recommended until an individual's treatment plan and glycemic control are optimized for pregnancy, ideally achieving A1C <6.5% [70]. Achieving near-normal glucose levels before conception has been shown to reduce the risk of stillbirth, spontaneous abortion, congenital anomalies, and other complications [71]. Elevated A1C levels during the first 10 weeks of pregnancy are associated with an increased risk of diabetic embryopathy, emphasizing the importance of glycemic optimization prior to conception. Preconception counseling should educate individuals about the risks of unplanned pregnancies and the benefits of pregnancy planning, including the use of long-acting, reversible contraception. Prior to conception, attention should also be given to avoiding harmful drugs, such as ACEi, ARBs, and statins since these medications may be commonly prescribed to people with diabetes. By providing comprehensive preconception education, health-care providers can help individuals with diabetes make informed decisions to optimize maternal and fetal outcomes while minimizing the occurrence of complications [70].

Treatment Goals

In both gestational diabetes mellitus and preexisting diabetes during pregnancy, monitoring of fasting and postprandial blood glucose levels is crucial to achieving optimal glucose control. Recommended targets are fasting plasma glucose <95 mg/dL and either 1-h postprandial glucose <140 mg/dL or 2-h postprandial glucose <120 mg/dL. Some individuals with preexisting diabetes may need to check blood glucose levels preprandially. Due to increased red blood cell turnover during pregnancy, A1C levels tend to be slightly lower, with an ideal target of <6% if achievable without significant hypoglycemia; however, this target may be relaxed to <7% if necessary to avoid hypoglycemia [70, 72]. CGM, when used alongside traditional blood glucose monitoring, can aid in achieving glycemic targets during pregnancy, potentially reducing complications such as macrosomia and neonatal hypoglycemia. While CGM metrics can complement traditional monitoring, they should not replace blood glucose monitoring entirely. Estimated A1C and glucose management indicator calculations commonly used outside of pregnancy should not be relied upon during pregnancy [70].

Lifestyle Management

Lifestyle interventions, including medical nutrition therapy, physical activity, and weight management, are critical aspects of diabetes management during pregnancy. Medical nutrition therapy involves developing an individualized nutrition plan in collaboration with a registered dietitian nutritionist. This plan should ensure adequate calorie intake to support fetal and maternal health, achieve glycemic goals, and promote appropriate weight gain during pregnancy. While there is no specific recommendation for calorie intake in GDM, dietary plans should align with dietary reference intake guidance, emphasizing a minimum of 175 g of carbohydrates, 71 g of protein, and 28 g of fiber daily [73]. Nutrition counseling in pregnancy should emphasize a balanced intake of macronutrients, including nutrient-dense foods such as fruits, vegetables, legumes, whole grains, and healthy fats containing n-3 fatty acids [74]. Carbohydrate intake, comprising about 35% of a 2000-calorie diet, significantly impacts glucose levels, with higher quality carbohydrates leading to better glycemic control. Physical activity also plays a crucial role, with evidence showing improved glucose control and reduced insulin requirements with exercise interventions. Various types and durations of exercise, including aerobic and resistance exercises for 20–50 min per day, 2–7 days per week at moderate intensity, have demonstrated efficacy in improving glycemic outcomes [70].

Pharmacologic Treatment

Pharmacologic management of gestational diabetes mellitus relies on insulin as the primary treatment. While metformin and glyburide have shown efficacy in reducing glucose levels, they are not recommended as first-line treatments due to concerns about their ability to cross the placenta and limited long-term safety data for offspring [75]. Sulfonylureas, including glyburide, have been associated with increased neonatal hypoglycemia and other adverse outcomes, while metformin, although associated with a lower risk of neonatal hypoglycemia and maternal weight gain compared to insulin, has raised concerns about its impact on offspring health, including increased risk of childhood obesity [70, 76]. For individuals unable to use insulin safely or effectively due to various factors, oral agents may be considered after discussing the known risks, but caution is advised, especially regarding metformin use in pregnant individuals with hypertension, preeclampsia, or those at risk for intrauterine growth restriction. Insulin remains the recommended therapy for gestational diabetes, as well as T1D and T2D during pregnancy, with both multiple daily injections and continuous subcutaneous insulin infusion being viable delivery strategies, neither of which has shown superiority over the other during pregnancy [70].

In pregnancy, blood pressure tends to be lower than in non-pregnant individuals. It has been demonstrated that a blood pressure threshold of 140/90 mm Hg reduces adverse pregnancy outcomes without negatively impacting fetal growth. Data supports a target blood pressure range of 110–135/85 mmHg to minimize maternal hypertension and fetal growth impairment [77]. It is crucial to avoid ACEi and ARBs during pregnancy due to potential fetal complications, though first-trimester exposure may not be associated with congenital malformations. Safe antihypertensive options during pregnancy include methyldopa, nifedipine, labetalol, diltiazem, clonidine, and prazosin, while chronic diuretic use and statins should generally be avoided [70].

Conclusion

Pharmacists play a pivotal role in the comprehensive management of diabetes in special populations, serving as indispensable members of the health-care team. As drug experts, they provide essential guidance on dosing, contraindications, and unique benefits of drugs in intersecting comorbidities, ensuring safe and effective medication therapy for individuals. Pharmacists also serve as educators, empowering people with the knowledge and tools they need to manage their condition effectively with medication as well as lifestyle management. In geriatric and pediatric diabetes care, pharmacists offer specialized support to those with diabetes and their caregivers, while also collaborating with other health-care providers to address the unique needs of these populations. In the settings of renal and hepatic impairment, pharmacists are excellent resources regarding the nuances of drug therapy required in these conditions. Pharmacists can offer insights on diabetes care to those with visual and educational limitations and provide tools to help them succeed in their diabetes management. Pregnant women can benefit from the pharmacist's knowledge regarding safe and effective diabetes care for the mother and her developing child. Overall, pharmacists' expertise and advocacy contribute significantly to optimizing therapeutic outcomes and improving the quality of life for individuals living with diabetes.

References

1. ElSayed NA, and Professional Practice Committee on behalf of the American Diabetes Association. 13. Older Adults. Standards of care in diabetes – 2023. Diabetes Care. 2023;46(Suppl. 1):S216–29.
2. Laiteerapong N, Huang ES. Diabetes in older adults. In: Cowie CC, Casagrande SS, Menke A, et al., editors. Diabetes in America. 3rd ed. Bethesda: National Institute of Diabetes and Digestive and Kidney Diseases; 2018.
3. Duckworth W, Abraira C, Moritz T, et al. VADT investigators. Glucose control and vascular complications in veterans with type 2 diabetes. N Engl J Med. 2009;360:129–39.

4. Huang ES, Zhang Q, Gandra N, Chin MH, Meltzer DO. The effect of comorbid illness and functional status on the expected benefits of intensive glucose control in older patients with type 2 diabetes: a decision analysis. Ann Intern Med. 2008;149:11–9.
5. Huang ES, Laiteerapong N, Liu JY, et al. Rates of complications and mortality in older patients with diabetes mellitus: the diabetes and aging study. JAMA Intern Med. 2014;174:251–8.
6. Kirkman MS, Briscoe VJ, Clark N, et al. Diabetes in older adults. Diabetes Care. 2012;35:2650–64.
7. de Boer IH, Bangalore S, Benetos A, et al. Diabetes and hypertension: a position statement by the American Diabetes Association. Diabetes Care. 2017;40:1273–84.
8. Launer LJ, Miller ME, Williamson JD, et al. Effects of intensive glucose lowering on brain structure and function in people with type 2 diabetes (ACCORD MIND): a randomised open-label substudy. Lancet Neurol. 2011;10:969–77.
9. Gencer B, Marston NA, Im K, et al. Efficacy and safety of lowering LDL cholesterol in older patients: a systematic review and meta-analysis of randomised controlled trials. Lancet. 2020;396:1637–43.
10. Yourman LC, Cenzer IS, Boscardin WJ, et al. Evaluation of time to benefit of statins for the primary prevention of cardiovascular events in adults aged 50 to 75 years: a meta-analysis. JAMA Intern Med. 2021;181:179–85.
11. Carlson AL, Kanapka LG, Miller KM, et al. Hypoglycemia and glycemic control in older adults with type 1 diabetes: baseline results from the WISDM Study. J Diabetes Sci Technol. 2021;15:582–92.
12. Pratley RE, Kanapka LG, Rickels MR, et al. Effect of continuous glucose monitoring on hypoglycemia in older adults with type 1 diabetes: a randomized clinical trial. JAMA. 2020;323:2397–406.
13. Miller KM, Kanapka LG, Rickels MR, et al. Benefit of continuous glucose monitoring in reducing hypoglycemia is sustained through 12 months of use among older adults with type 1 diabetes. Diabetes Technol Ther. 2022;24:424–34.
14. Gubitosi-Klug RA, Braffett BH, Bebu I, et al. Continuous glucose monitoring in adults with type 1 diabetes with 35 years duration from the DCCT/EDIC Study. Diabetes Care. 2022;45:659–65.
15. Karter AJ, Parker MM, Moffet HH, Gilliam LK, Dlott R. Association of real-time continuous glucose monitoring with glycemic control and acute metabolic events among patients with insulin-treated diabetes. JAMA. 2021;325:2273–84.
16. Ruedy KJ, Parkin CG, Riddlesworth TD, DIAMOND Study Group. Continuous glucose monitoring in older adults with type 1 and type 2 diabetes using multiple daily injections of insulin: Results from the DIAMOND trial. J Diabetes Sci Technol. 2017;11:1138–46.

17. Lee AK, Lee CJ, Huang ES, Sharrett AR, Coresh J, Selvin E. Risk factors for severe hypoglycemia in black and white adults with diabetes: the atherosclerosis risk in communities (ARIC) study. Diabetes Care. 2017;40:1661–7.
18. Karter AJ, Warton EM, Lipska KJ, et al. Development and validation of a tool to identify patients with type 2 diabetes at high risk of hypoglycemia-related emergency department or hospital use. JAMA Intern Med. 2017;177:1461–70.
19. Centers for Disease Control and Prevention. National Diabetes Statistics Report, 2020: Estimates of Diabetes and its Burden in the United States. Accessed 26 Nov 2023.
20. Folstein MF, Folstein SE, McHugh PR. "Mini-mental state". A practical method for grading the cognitive state of patients for the clinician. J Psychiatr Res. 1975;12:189–98.
21. Moreno G, Mangione CM, Kimbro L, American Geriatrics Society Expert Panel on Care of Older Adults with Diabetes Mellitus. Guidelines abstracted from the American geriatrics society guidelines for improving the care of older adults with diabetes mellitus: 2013 update. J Am Geriatr Soc. 2013(61):2020–6.
22. American Psychological Association. Guidelines for the Evaluation of Dementia and Age-Related Cognitive Change, 2021. Accessed 26 Nov 2023.
23. Laiteerapong N, Karter AJ, Liu JY, et al. Correlates of quality of life in older adults with diabetes: the diabetes and aging study. Diabetes Care. 2011;34:1749–53.
24. Sinclair A, Dunning T, Colagiuri S. IDF global guideline for managing older people with type 2 diabetes. International Diabetes Federation; 2013
25. Angelo M, Ruchalski C, Sproge BJ. An approach to diabetes mellitus in hospice and palliative medicine. J Palliat Med. 2011;14:83–7.
26. Kutner JS, Blatchford PJ, Taylor DH Jr, et al. Safety and benefit of discontinuing statin therapy in the setting of advanced, life-limiting illness: a randomized clinical trial. JAMA Intern Med. 2015;175:691–700.
27. Park SW, Goodpaster BH, Strotmeyer ES, et al. Decreased muscle strength and quality in older adults with type 2 diabetes: the health, aging, and body composition study. Diabetes. 2006;55:1813–8.
28. Park SW, Goodpaster BH, Strotmeyer ES, et al. Accelerated loss of skeletal muscle strength in older adults with type 2 diabetes: the health, aging, and body composition study. Diabetes Care. 2007;30:1507–12.
29. Pahor M, Guralnik JM, Ambrosius WT, et al. Effect of structured physical activity on prevention of major mobility disability in older adults: The LIFE study randomized clinical trial. JAMA. 2014;311:2387–96.
30. Gill TM, Baker DI, Gottschalk M, et al. A program to prevent functional decline in physically frail, older adult persons who live at home. N Engl J Med. 2002;347:1068–74.

31. Wing RR, Bolin P, Brancati FL, et al. Cardiovascular effects of intensive lifestyle intervention in type 2 diabetes. N Engl J Med. 2013;369:145–54.
32. Zhang JX, Bhaumik D, Huang ES, Meltzer DO. Change in insurance status and cost-related medication non-adherence among older U.S. adults with diabetes from 2010 to 2014. J Health Med Econ. 2018(4):7.
33. Patel MR, Resnicow K, Lang I, Kraus K, Heisler M. Solutions to address diabetes-related financial burden and cost-related nonadherence: results from a pilot study. Health Educ Behav. 2018;45:101–11.
34. Seidu S, Kunutsor SK, Topsever P, et al. Deintensification in older patients with type 2 diabetes: a systematic review of approaches, rates and outcomes. Diabetes Obes Metab. 2019;21:1668–79.
35. Inzucchi SE, Lipska KJ, Mayo H, Bailey CJ, McGuire DK. Metformin in patients with type 2 diabetes and kidney disease: a systematic review. JAMA. 2014;312:2668–75.
36. Bradley MC, Chillarige Y, Lee H, et al. Severe hypoglycemia risk with long-acting insulin analogs vs neutral protamine Hagedorn insulin. JAMA Intern Med. 2021;181:598–607.
37. McAuley SA, Trawley S, Vogrin S, et al. Closed-loop insulin delivery versus sensor-augmented pump therapy in older adults with type 1 diabetes (ORACL): a randomized, crossover trial. Diabetes Care. 2022;45:381–90.
38. Boughton CK, Hartnell S, Thabit H, et al. Hybrid closed-loop glucose control compared with sensor augmented pump therapy in older adults with type 1 diabetes: an open-label multicentre, multinational, randomised, crossover study. Lancet Healthy Longev. 2022;3:e135–42.
39. Lawrence JM, Divers J, Isom S, et al. Trends in prevalence of type 1 and type 2 diabetes in children and adolescents in the US, 2001-2017. JAMA. 2021;326:717–27.
40. Thomas NJ, Jones SE, Weedon MN, et al. Frequency and phenotype of type 1 diabetes in the first six decades of life: a cross-sectional, genetically stratified survival analysis from UK Biobank. Lancet Diabetes Endocrinol. 2018;6:122–9.
41. ElSayed NA, and Professional Practice Committee. 14. Children and adolescents: standards of care in diabetes – 2023. Diabetes Care. 2023;46(Suppl. 1):S230–53.
42. Barnea-Goraly N, Raman M, Mazaika P, et al. Alterations in white matter structure in young children with type 1 diabetes. Diabetes Care. 2014;37:332–40.
43. Cameron FJ, Scratch SE, Nadebaum C, et al. Neurological consequences of diabetic ketoacidosis at initial presentation of type 1 diabetes in a prospective cohort study of children. Diabetes Care. 2014;37:1554–62.
44. Jackson CC, Albanese-O'Neill A, Butler KL, et al. Diabetes care in the school setting: a position statement of the American Diabetes Association. Diabetes Care. 2015;38:1958–63.

45. Driscoll KA, Volkening LK, Haro H, et al. Are children with type 1 diabetes safe at school? Examining parent perceptions. Pediatr Diabetes. 2015;16(8):613–20.
46. Siminerio LM, Albanese-O'Neill A, Chiang JL, et al. Care of young children with diabetes in the child care setting: a position statement of the American Diabetes Association. Diabetes Care. 2014;37:2834–42.
47. Mehta SN, Volkening LK, Anderson BJ, et al. Dietary behaviors predict glycemic control in youth with type 1 diabetes. Diabetes Care. 2008;31:1318–20.
48. Arnett JJ. Emerging adulthood. A theory of development from the late teens through the twenties. Am Psychol. 2000;55:469–80.
49. Mays JA, Jackson KL, Derby TA, et al. An evaluation of recurrent diabetic ketoacidosis, fragmentation of care, and mortality across Chicago, Illinois. Diabetes Care. 2016;39:1671–6.
50. Lotstein DS, Seid M, Klingensmith G, et al. Transition from pediatric to adult care for youth diagnosed with type 1 diabetes in adolescence. Pediatrics. 2013;131:e1062–70.
51. Bjornstad P, Drews KL, Caprio S, et al. Long-term complications in youth-onset type 2 diabetes. N Engl J Med. 2021;385:416–26.
52. Cho YH, Craig ME, Hing S, et al. Microvascular complications assessment in adolescents with 2- to 5-yr duration of type 1 diabetes from 1990 to 2006. Pediatr Diabetes. 2011;12:682–9.
53. Pop-Busui R, Boulton AJM, Feldman EL, et al. Diabetic neuropathy: A position statement by the American Diabetes Association. Diabetes Care. 2017;40:136–54.
54. Chan CL. Use of continuous glucose monitoring in youth-onset type 2 diabetes. Curr Diab Rep. 2017;17:66.
55. U.S. Department of Health and Human Services. Physical activity guidelines for Americans, 2nd ed., 2018. Accessed 26 Nov 2023.
56. Tsalikian E, Kollman C, Tamborlane WB, et al. Prevention of hypoglycemia during exercise in children with type 1 diabetes by suspending basal insulin. Diabetes Care. 2006;29:2200–4.
57. Taplin CE, Cobry E, Messer L, et al. Preventing post-exercise nocturnal hypoglycemia in children with type 1 diabetes. J Pediatr. 2010;157:784–8.e1.
58. Eckstein ML, Weilguni B, Tauschmann M, et al. Time in range for closed-loop systems versus standard of care during physical exercise in people with type 1 diabetes: a systematic review and meta-analysis. J Clin Med. 2021;10:2445.
59. Pinhas-Hamiel O, Dolan LM, Zeitler PS. Diabetic ketoacidosis among obese African-American adolescents with NIDDM. Diabetes Care. 1997;20:484–6.
60. Zeitler P, Hirst K, Pyle L, et al. A clinical trial to maintain glycemic control in youth with type 2 diabetes. N Engl J Med. 2012;366:2247–56.

61. Navaneethan SD, Zoungas S, Caramori ML, et al. Diabetes management in chronic kidney disease: synopsis of the 2020 KDIGO clinical practice guideline. Ann Intern Med. 2021 Mar;174(3):385–94.
62. Navaneethan SD, Zoungas S, Caramori ML, et al. Diabetes management in chronic kidney disease: synopsis of the KDIGO 2022 clinical practice guideline update. Ann Intern Med. 2023 Mar;176(3):381–7.
63. Chung W, Promrat K, Wands J. Clinical implications, diagnosis, and management of diabetes in patients with chronic liver diseases. World J Hepatol. 2020;12(9):533–57.
64. Centers for Disease Control and Prevention. Diabetes and vision loss. Accessed 28 Nov 2023.
65. Heinemann L, Drossel D, Freckmann G, Kulzer B. Usability of medical devices for patients with diabetes who are visually impaired or blind. J Diabetes Sci Technol. 2016;10(6):1382–7.
66. Akturk HK, Snell-Bergeon JK, Shah VN. Continuous glucose monitor with Siri integration improves glycemic control in legally blind patients with diabetes. Diabetes Technol Ther. 2021 Jan;23(1):81–3.
67. Living with Low Vision. American Diabetes Association. diabetes.org. 2023. Available from: https://diabetes.org/health-wellness/eye-health/living-low-vision#:~:text=There%20are%20also%20a%20variety
68. Osborn CY, Cavanaugh K, Kripalani S. Strategies to address low health literacy and numeracy in diabetes. Clin Diabetes. 2010;28(4):171–5.
69. Wolff K, Cavanaugh K, Malone R, et al. The Diabetes Literacy and Numeracy Education Toolkit (DLNET): materials to facilitate diabetes education and management in patients with low literacy and numeracy skills. Diabetes Educ. 2009;35:233–44.
70. ElSayed NA, and Professional Practice Committee. 15. Management of diabetes in pregnancy: standards of care in diabetes – 2023. Diabetes Care. 2023;46(Suppl 1):S254–66.
71. Nielsen GL, Møller M, Sørensen HT, et al. HbA1c in early diabetic pregnancy and pregnancy outcomes: a Danish population-based cohort study of 573 pregnancies in women with type 1 diabetes. Diabetes Care. 2006;29(12):2612–6.
72. Nielsen LR, Ekbom P, Damm P, et al. HbA1c levels are significantly lower in early and late pregnancy. Diabetes Care. 2004;27(5):1200–1.
73. Institute of Medicine. Dietary Reference Intakes: The Essential Guide to Nutrient Requirements. Washington: The National Academies Press; 2006. p. 1344.
74. Marshall NE, Abrams B, Barbour LA, et al. The importance of nutrition in pregnancy and lactation: lifelong consequences. Am J Obstet Gynecol. 2022 May;226(5):607–32.
75. Committee on Practice Bulletins—Obstetrics. ACOG Practice Bulletin No. 190: gestational diabetes mellitus. Obstet Gynecol. 2018;131:e49–64.

76. Hanem LGE, Stridsklev S, Júlíusson PB, et al. Metformin use in PCOS pregnancies increases the risk of offspring overweight at 4 years of age: follow-up of two RCTs. J Clin Endocrinol Metab. 2018;103:1612–21.
77. Tita AT, Szychowski JM, Boggess K, et al. Chronic hypertension and pregnancy (CHAP) trial consortium. Treatment for mild chronic hypertension during pregnancy. N Engl J Med. 2022;386:1781–92.

Diabetes: Monitoring and Follow-Up

8

Christopher R. Downey

Introduction

Pharmacists' extensive training and drug knowledge ensure the safety and well-being of individuals with diabetes and populations throughout drug treatment, both retrospectively and prospectively [1].

Pharmacists are specifically trained in monitoring drug therapy. They can track the effectiveness of medications, identify any adverse reactions or therapeutic problems that may arise, and provide early and effective intervention if needed. Pharmacists can collaborate with other health-care professionals to adjust in real-time to treatment plans, ensuring safe and effective medication use.

Patient self-monitoring is also a necessary aspect of diabetes management because it enables individuals to manage their blood glucose levels, which is vital for preventing the short-term and long-term complications associated with diabetes. Regular monitoring provides valuable feedback on how different factors such

C. R. Downey (✉)
Pharmacy Department, New Horizon Family Health Services, Inc, Greenville, SC, USA

ITS Pharmacy Systems, Prisma Health, Greenville, SC, USA
e-mail: cdowney@newhorizonfhs.org; Christopher.Downey5@PrismaHealth.org

© The Author(s), under exclusive license to Springer Nature Switzerland AG 2025

J. Clements (ed.), *The Pharmacist's Pocket Guide for Diabetes and Obesity*, https://doi.org/10.1007/978-3-031-88835-9_8

as dietary intake, physical activity, and medication affect blood glucose levels. This information empowers individuals to make informed decisions about their lifestyle and treatment options.

Another critical aspect of monitoring in diabetes management is the early detection of hypo- or hyperglycemic episodes. These conditions, if not addressed promptly, can lead to severe health emergencies such as hypoglycemia, requiring the assistance of another person, diabetes-related ketoacidosis, or hyperosmolar hyperglycemic state. Regular monitoring identifies episodes early, allowing for quick intervention, which can be lifesaving.

Monitoring for safety and efficacy in diabetes management extends beyond tracking blood glucose levels. It encompasses a range of other vital parameters that contribute to overall health and well-being in people with diabetes [2].

In addition, pharmacist follow-up is an indispensable component of diabetes management, serving as a bridge between initial treatment decisions and long-term health outcomes. Through follow-up, pharmacists and health-care professionals assess the evolution of diabetes over time, addressing any emerging challenges and adjusting treatment strategies to align with the changing health statuses of people with diabetes.

Monitoring

This section is structured into five key sections, each addressing elements of diabetes management from both the individual and provider/pharmacist perspectives. The first section, "Patient Safety Self-Monitoring," focuses on techniques and tools individuals can use to monitor their own health safely. The second section, "Patient Efficacy Self-Monitoring," focuses on how individuals can effectively assess the impact of self-care routines on their diabetes management. In the third section, "Provider Safety Monitoring," the emphasis shifts to how health-care providers and pharmacists can monitor and ensure the safety of people with diabetes. The fourth section "Provider Efficacy Monitoring" discusses methods providers and pharmacists use to evaluate the effectiveness of treatment and care plans. Lastly, the fifth section, "Provider Monitoring Frequency," provides a quick reference and structured approach to monitoring frequencies. Each section combines practical advice with detailed insights to support comprehensive diabetes care and management.

Patient Safety Self-Monitoring

Blood Glucose Self-Monitoring

Fingerstick Blood Glucose Safety Monitoring

Capillary blood glucose monitoring allows for a quick measurement of blood glucose levels at any time. This is particularly beneficial in detecting and managing episodes of hyper- and hypoglycemia. People with diabetes should be properly trained on how to correctly check blood glucose using an at-home blood glucose monitor, how to correct hypoglycemia using "The Rule of 15," and what warrants immediate medical attention. Refer to Table 8.1 for the definitions of hypoglycemia.

Important "The Rule of 15"

If blood glucose is less than 70 mg/dL, consume 15 g of carbohydrates. Wait 15 min and recheck blood glucose. If blood glucose is not above 70 mg/dL, REPEAT. Once the blood glucose level is above 70 mg/dL, the individual should eat a snack or meal containing balanced carbohydrates, fats, and proteins. A patient or bystander should seek medical attention if the blood glucose level continues to drop below 54 mg/dL, the individual becomes unconscious, or requires the usage of glucagon [2].

Table 8.1 Classification of hypoglycemia

Level 1	Glucose <70 mg/dL and ≥54 mg/dL
Level 2	Glucose <54 mg/dL
Level 3	A severe event characterized by altered mental and/or physical status requiring assistance for treatment of hypoglycemia

Adapted from source: Ref. [2]

When medications are being adjusted or titrated, self-testing blood glucose levels can also be effective at keeping people with diabetes safe and aware of improvement from medications. Self-testing also serves as a benchmark for atypical symptoms or symptoms inconsistent with normal glucose levels. Similarly, on sick days, when illness can unpredictably affect blood glucose levels, more frequent glucose testing is advisable. Illnesses, especially those involving fever, infection, or changes in diet and fluid intake, can cause fluctuations in blood glucose levels. During such times, testing helps in making timely decisions about medication adjustments, dietary changes, or the need for medical intervention [2].

CGM Self-Safety Monitoring

CGMs can play a beneficial role for a person with diabetes in self-safety monitoring by providing real-time glucose level tracking. In situations where blood glucose levels rise rapidly, CGMs can send immediate alerts to people warning them of potential hyperglycemia. Similarly, for rapidly falling glucose levels, the CGM alerts the user to the risk of hypoglycemia [3]. For more information regarding CGMs, see the section Diabetes Technology.

Fingerstick Versus CGM Self-Safety Monitoring

While CGMs provide the most data, there is still a place for fingerstick blood glucose monitoring. Financial burden and strain on resources are common barriers. At the time of this publishing, CGMs can range anywhere from $100 to $300 per month for sensors among cash-paying individuals [4]. If a one-time reader is included, start-up costs could well exceed those monthly estimates. Regarding coverage, many insurance plans place restrictions on payments for CGMs and often reserve payment for type 1 diabetes (T1D), type 2 diabetes (T2D) on insulin, or history of hypoglycemia unawareness [5]. Also, fingerstick blood glucose is more accurate than the CGM, especially in times of quick glycemic changes. CGMs can lag causing occasional inappropriate decision-making [6].

Important

Instruct people with diabetes to always check a fingerstick blood glucose if they feel different than the reading shown by their CGM.

Ketone Self-Monitoring

Monitoring urine ketones can be situationally beneficial for people with diabetes, especially those with T1D and ketosis-prone diabetes, in the early detection and prevention of diabetic ketoacidosis (DKA). In a state of no insulin production, the body is unable to use glucose for energy. In response, the body starts to break down fats that lead to the production of serum ketones, specifically, the final products of aceto-acetate and beta-hydroxybutyrate. Because these ketone bodies have a low pKa, they can cause the blood to become more acidic, leading to metabolic acidosis. The body is initially able to compensate but is easily overwhelmed. These ketone bodies are freely filtered into the urine and can be detected with at-home urine ketone test strips. Early detection of ketones in urine may indicate the need to seek early intervention before the progression to DKA [7].

Important

DKA is more common in T1D where there is a complete lack of insulin production. The amount of insulin produced in T2D is usually enough to suppress ketogenesis, however, DKA can still be present in T2D.

Self-Foot Exam

People with diabetes should practice daily foot care and foot examinations. A daily visual inspection of the feet should be performed by the person to check for cuts, sores, swelling, blisters, and toenail abnormalities. Any of the aforementioned warrants an evaluation by a qualified health-care professional. Any injuries, infections, or significant changes should also warrant a prompt visit to a health-care provider, especially a podiatrist [2].

Patient Efficacy Self-Monitoring

Fingerstick Glucose Efficacy Monitoring

People with diabetes may be prescribed a blood glucose testing regimen specific to their medication regimen. Based on practice experience, noninsulin-dependent people with T2D are usually prescribed testing once daily but may also test 3 times per week or not at all. People using insulins may be prescribed once daily up to 4 times daily and as needed. The "basal plus" regimens add one, two, or three doses of short-acting insulin before meals (basal plus one, basal plus two, basal plus three) to manage the rise in blood glucose after eating. The "basal-bolus plus correctional" regimen includes a basal dose, premeal bolus doses for carbohydrate coverage, and additional correctional doses as needed to adjust for blood glucose variations. Blood glucose testing frequencies vary with each regimen's complexity; basal alone might require testing 2–4 times a day, while more intensive regimens like basal-bolus plus correction could necessitate testing 4–10 times daily, depending on meal patterns, physical activity, and individual glucose targets.

Despite the commonality of prescribed self-testing regimens in people with diabetes, there has been no high-quality evidence that suggests blood glucose efficacy monitoring leads to an improvement in glycemic control [2]. Glucose monitoring should be reserved for safety monitoring, and de-prescribing intensive regimens for efficacy may save on additional resources. As a general statement, providers may review self-efficacy monitoring among people with diabetes to make tailored treatment decisions.

CGM Efficacy Monitoring

For people with diabetes, CGMs can provide additional insights into understanding how various factors, such as food, exercise, alcohol, sleep, and stress, impact their daily blood glucose levels. This continuous and detailed feedback empowers people with diabetes to make more informed and personalized decisions about their lifestyle and diabetes management, leading to better glycemic control and overall health [2]. Additional information regarding CGMs can be found in the technology section.

Home A1C Testing

At-home A1C tests offer people with diabetes a convenient means to track their diabetes management progress over time, allowing for frequent monitoring without the need for clinical visits. However, it is important to understand that the accuracy of at-home tests may not be fully validated against standard laboratory methods [8]. This means that while they can be a useful tool for ongoing self-monitoring, the results should be interpreted with caution and supplemented with periodic, professional medical evaluations to ensure comprehensive diabetes management.

Provider Safety Monitoring

Laboratory Monitoring

Tables 8.2, 8.3, 8.4, 8.5, and 8.6 highlight laboratory tests or panels that are routinely monitored to ensure patient safety. This is not an exhaustive list but includes the most common laboratory tests and their significance in diabetes monitoring. Table 8.7 presents common equations used in clinical practice, based on laboratory tests, to accurately determine an individual's clinical status.

Important

If a person with diabetes presents acutely with high glucose, then the presence of an anion gap should be screened. Anion gaps are typically caused by acid-base shifts which is a classic presentation of DKA. Anion gaps can be calculated using formula Eq. (8.2) within Table 8.7, which calculates the difference of the sum of common serum cations and the sum of common serum anions. A true gap never exists because serum is always neutral but rather the calculation exposes variations in the specified ions [32].

Table 8.2 Basic/complete metabolic panel

Obtain:

Initially—Everyone [2]

2 weeks—After initiating or adjusting ACEi, ARB, MRA (renal function/potassium) [9]

4 weeks—After initiating nonsteroidal MRA (potassium) [10]

1–3 months—Stage G5 CKD (renal function) [2]

3–5 months—stage G4 CKD, any renal impairment and metformin or insulin use (renal function) [2], for first year of acarbose (transaminases) [11], TZD [12]

6–12 months—Stage G3 CKD (renal function) [2]

Yearly—Everyone [2]

Yearly + as needed—Therapies including SGLT-2i) [13, 14], GLP-1 receptor agonist [15, 16], DPP-4i (renal function, no renal monitoring for linagliptin) [17, 18], SU (renal function, LFTs) [19], TZD (LFTs, electrolytes) [20], acarbose (renal function) [11], bromocriptine (renal and hepatic function) [21], GABA analogs (renal function) [22], SNRIs (renal and hepatic function), TCAs (renal and hepatic function) [23]

PRN—Therapies including statins if signs and symptoms of hepatic disease (LFTs) [24]

Analyte	**Ref. range** [25]	**Units**	**Acute care considerations**	**Chronic care considerations**
Sodium (Na+)	136–145	mmol/L	Sodium can appear falsely low in the presence of high blood glucose. People presenting in DKA or HHS may have a pseudo-hyponatremia. It is important to mathematically correct sodium lab values in these cases. See Eq. (8.1) [26].	

Potassium (K+)	3.5–5.0	mmol/L	Close monitoring of potassium should occur in the acute care setting especially with the use of insulin to rapidly correct blood glucose. Insulin can shift potassium intracellularly through the stimulation of sodium-potassium transporters causing serum potassium levels to drop [27].	Potassium is important when monitoring medications used to reduce risk in diabetes such as ACEi and ARBs. Diabetes is often a comorbid condition with hypertension and heart disease. It is important to keep in mind the additive effects of potassium-sparing drugs and monitor potassium routinely [2]
Chloride (Cl-)	98–106	mmol/L	Pseudo-hyperchloremia can occur caused by hypertriglyceridemia but is dependent on the assay method [28]	
Bicarbonate (CO3-)	2–28	mmol/L	Bicarbonate is not routinely monitored closely but may drop as a result of DKA. Due to the lack of evidence of administering sodium bicarbonate in DKA, using serum bicarbonate to determine if sodium bicarbonate should be administered is not recommended [29]	

(continued)

Table 8.2 (continued)

Glucose	70–100 (normal)	mg/dL	Hypoglycemia is a significant risk, presenting immediate dangers such as confusion, loss of consciousness, seizures, and in severe cases, even death Hyperglycemic conditions, such as HHS and DKA, also pose significant immediate risks In HHS, glucose levels may exceed 1000 mg/dL, though they often fall below 800 mg/dL In DKA, glucose levels typically range from 350 to 500 mg/dL [2] Target glucose of 140–180 mg/dL for hospitalized people with diabetes may be appropriate [2]	Chronic hypoglycemia can lead to long-term complications, including neurological damage and impaired cognitive function [2]

Blood urea nitrogen (BUN)	8–20	mg/dL	People with diabetes are at higher risk for AKI. AKI can be defined as any of the following: Increase in SCr by ≥0.3 mg/dL within 48 hours; or Increase in SCr to ≥1.5 times baseline, which is known or presumed to have occurred within the prior 7 days Or Urine volume <0.5 mL/kg/h for 6 h [2]	Monitoring kidney function is important due to the high risk of diabetic nephropathy. Regular assessment of kidney function, through BUN, SCr, eGFR, and urine albumin-to-creatinine ratio allows for early detection of kidney damage [2]
Serum creatinine (SCr)	Men: 0.7–1.2 Women: 0.5–1.0	mg/dL		
Estimated glomerular filtration rate (eGFR)	>59	mL/min/1.73 m^2		
Albumin	3.5–5.4	g/dL	Albumin is not directly related to diabetes monitoring, but abnormal levels should be taken into consideration to calculate other corrected lab values [30]	

(continued)

Table 8.2 (continued)

Alkaline phosphatase (ALP)	36–150	IU/L		Elevations of LFTs, particularly in the setting of T2D, can be associated with NAFLD. This condition often manifests as elevated levels of AST and ALT. However, the presence of NAFLD should be confirmed through additional testing or imaging Monitoring liver function tests is also important due to the mechanism of action of many glucose-lowering agents. Since glucagon stimulates glucose production in the liver, it is often targeted by these drugs to maintain lower glucose levels. It is worth mentioning that some glucose-lowering medications may occasionally lead to liver inflammation [2, 15, 31]
Aspartate transaminase (AST)	<35	IU/L		
Alanine transaminase (ALT)	<45	IU/L		

Adapted from sources: Refs. [2, 10–31]

ACE angiotensin-converting enzyme inhibitor(s), *AKI* acute kidney injury, *ARB* angiotensin II receptor blocker(s), *CKD* chronic kidney disease, *DPP-4i* dipeptidyl peptidase-4 inhibitor(s), *GLP-1* glucagon-like peptide-1, *GABA* gamma-aminobutyric acid, *HHS* hyperosmolar hyperglycemic state, *LFTs* liver function tests, *MRA* mineralocorticoid receptor antagonist(s), *NAFLD* nonalcoholic fatty liver disease, *PRN* as needed, *SGLT-2i* sodium glucose co-transportor-2 inhibitor(s), *SNRIs* serotonin norepinephrine reupdate inhibitor(s), *SU* sulfonylurea(s), *TCAs* tricyclic antidepressant(s), *TZD* thiazolidinedione(s), *T2D* type 2 diabetes

Table 8.3 Complete blood count

Obtain: Initially—Everyone [2] Yearly—Everyone, especially if taking metformin PRN—Neuropathy reported while taking metformin [33]				
Analyte	**Ref. range** [25]	**Units**	**Acute care considerations**	**Chronic care considerations**
Hemoglobin (Hgb)	Males: 14–17 Females: 12–16	g/dL	In cases of severe anemia necessitating blood transfusion, A1C can be artificially lowered.	Mild anemias rarely affect diagnostic tests such as A1C, however moderate to severe anemias can artificially elevate it [34]
Mean cell volume (MCV)	80–100	fL		MCV can be used as a secondary marker to screen for B12 deficiencies specifically caused by metformin

Adapted from sources: Refs. [25, 33, 34]

Important

LDL is often reported as a calculated number using the Friedewald equation as seen in Eq. (8.4). Because the equation considers TGs, hypertriglyceridemia can falsely lower LDL. An LDL-direct measurement can be performed where the actual LDL is measured rather than calculated if the provider desires. Keep in mind, that LDL is not part of the ASCVD 10-year risk score [36, 38].

CGM Safety Monitoring

CGM Remote Monitoring

CGMs also offer the ability for remote monitoring of people with diabetes. This allows providers to routinely check on people with diabetes and have real-time information regarding their glucose

Table 8.4 Iron and B12 testing

Obtain: Initially—Everyone 1–3 months—Stage G5 CKD 3–5 months—Stage G4 CKD 6–12 months—Stage G3 CKD Yearly—Therapies including metformin PRN—Neuropathy reported and taking metformin [2]				
Analyte	**Ref. range** [25]	**Units**	**Acute care considerations**	**Chronic care considerations**
Iron	Males: 50–150 females: 35–145	mg/dL		Both iron and iron saturation can be affected by anemia of CKD [35]
Iron saturation	20–50	%		
B12	200–800	pg/mL		As mentioned previously, metformin can cause B12 deficiency with long-term use

Adapted from sources: Refs. [2, 25, 35]
CKD chronic kidney disease, *PRN* as needed

control. This is extremely beneficial, especially in times of medication changes and titrations. For more information on CGMs, see the section Diabetes Technology.

Professional CGM Office Monitoring

Professional CGM office monitors are also another product available to monitor patient safety. When a patient's drug coverage does not include an at-home CGM, a provider's office can supply a sensor as a medical device without the need to use drug benefits. Some devices are blinded to the person, but the advantage is that the device does not require a minimum number of scans per time period. This method is not without its barriers. Coverage under medical insurance is often payer-dependent and requires a second visit at the end of the sensor's life to collect the data [39].

Table 8.5 Urinalysis

Obtain: PRN				
Analyte	**Ref. range** [25]	**Units**	**Acute care considerations**	**Chronic care considerations**
Glucose	Negative	mg/dL	The presence of glucose in the urine can be an indicator of uncontrolled diabetes. In times of hyperglycemia, glucose transporters become saturated in the proximal tubule leading to the presence of glucose in the urine. Glucose presence in the urine can also indicate SGLT-2i use due to the mechanism of action of the drug. Typically the higher the average blood glucose, the higher the amount of glucose filtered into the urine attributed to the SGLT-2i [2, 13, 14]	
Ketones	Negative	mg/dL	Moderate-to-high levels of ketones indicate need for urgent/emergent action as it can be an indicator of DKA [2]	Ketone bodies are freely filtered into the urine and may be present in trace amounts in controlled and moderately uncontrolled people with diabetes [2]
Obtain: Initially—Everyone Yearly—Everyone [2]				

(continued)

Table 8.5 (continued)

Analyte	Ref. range [25]	Units	Acute care considerations	Chronic care considerations
Microalbumin	Negative/trace	mg/mL		Microvascular damage of the kidneys causes the leakage of protein into the urine. Regular testing for albuminuria helps identify diabetes-related kidney dysfunction. The UACR is an even more accurate assessment and is the preferred test. In highly concentrated urine, there will be slightly increased albuminuria but also more creatinine present. The UACR accounts for variations in urine concentration [2]
Urine albumin-to-creatinine ratio (UACR)	Normal: 0–29 Moderately increased: 30–300 Severely increased: >300 [2]	mg/g creatinine		

Adapted from sources: Refs. [2, 25]
SGLT-2i sodium glucose cotransporter-2 inhibitor(s)

Table 8.6 Lipid panel

Analyte	Ref. range [25]	Units	Acute care considerations	Chronic care considerations
Obtain: Initially—Everyone, especially when initiating colesevelam for glucose control 1–3 months—After initiating statins, ezetimibe, and PCSK9-i (efficacy only) Yearly—Everyone [2]				
Total cholesterol (TC)	150–199	mg/dL		While there is no guideline recommended targets for diabetes, total cholesterol, and HDL are used in estimating ASCVD risk [36]
High-density lipoprotein (HDL)	≥ 40	mg/dL		
Fasting triglycerides (TG)	Normal: <150 Borderline: 150–199 High: 200–499 Very high: ≥500	mg/dL	People with diabetes with fasting TGs ≥ 500 mg/dL and especially ≥1000 mg/dL, are at high risk of pancreatitis [2]	Pharmacotherapy should be considered to reduce risk of pancreatitis [2] Colesevelam should not be used if TG >500 mg/dL or history of severe hypertriglyceridemia [37]
Low-density lipoprotein (LDL)	≤130	mg/dL		Goal of <70 mg/dL is appropriate if aged 40–75 years at higher cardiovascular risk [2]

ASCVD atherosclerotic cardiovascular disease, *PCSK9-i* proprotein convertase subtilisin/kexin type 9 inhibitor(s)

Table 8.7 Equations to consider [25, 32, 38]

$Na_{corrected} = Na_{measured} + [(Glucose - 100) \times 0.016]$	(8.1)
$\text{Anion Gap} = (Na^+ + K^+) - (Cl^- + HCO_3^-)$	(8.2)
$AG_{corrected} = AG_{observed} + 0.25(\text{albumin}_{normal} - \text{albumin}_{measured})$	(8.3)
$LDL = TC - \left(\frac{TG}{5} + HDL\right)$	(8.4)

Provider Efficacy Monitoring

This section emphasizes health-care providers' role in diabetes management through strategic blood glucose monitoring, including the essential A1C test for long-term control and the nuanced use of daily glucose measurements. Providers guide the timing of A1C tests, adhere to a minimum 3-month interval, and utilize fasting, preprandial, and postprandial glucose tests to adjust treatment plans effectively. Additionally, fructosamine testing offers an alternative in specific cases, enhancing the tailored approach to patient care. All these tests can be used independently or in conjunction to measure efficacy and help guide treatment decisions.

Glycated Hemoglobin A1C (A1C) Testing

A1C reflects long-term glycemic exposure, representing the average glucose concentration over the preceding 8–12 weeks. This test is critical for predicting the risk of microvascular complications in diabetes, with its value strongly correlating with retinopathy and other complications. Importantly, lowering A1C concentrations significantly reduces the rate of progression of these complications [2].

Important
Do not check A1C earlier than every 3 months due to the cellular turnover rate of erythrocytes.

Capillary Fingerstick and Serum Blood Glucose Monitoring

Fasting Blood Glucose

Fasting blood glucose is not only an accepted criterion for diagnosing diabetes but also a useful tool for monitoring general diabetes safety and control. Its advantages include ease of use, widespread availability and access, and low cost. However, it requires an individual to fast for at least 8 hours and is subject to large biological variability, diurnal variation, and instability of lab samples. Factors such as stress, acute illness, and sample handling can alter glucose concentrations. Additionally, there is no standardization of glucose testing across different laboratories, and glucose concentration can vary depending on the sample's source (venous, capillary, or arterial blood) [40, 41].

Preprandial Blood Glucose

Preprandial blood glucose testing is another method for assessing the efficacy of drug treatments, specifically insulin. However, drugs such as thiazolidinediones, DPP-4i, GLP-1 receptor agonists, and meglitinides can lower postprandial glucose levels, thereby affecting the following meal's preprandial blood glucose [15, 18, 30].

Important

Preprandial and fasting blood glucose share the same goal of 80–130 mg/dL [2].

Postprandial Blood Glucose Monitoring

Postprandial monitoring is yet another way to monitor the effectiveness of dietary changes and prescribed medications. While there is no set preference to measure pre- versus postprandial blood glucose, postprandial measurements can provide insight for people who have controlled fasting and preprandial who are still not otherwise at goal when looking A1C.

Important

A goal of <180 mg/dL for people living with diabetes is appropriate. Peak postprandial blood glucose is around 1–2 h after a meal, and this is when the measurement should be taken. In addition, provider monitoring of these values is dependent on accurate patient reporting [2].

Relationship of Average Blood Glucose and A1C

$$\text{eAG} = (28.7 \times \text{A1c}) - 46.7 \tag{8.5}$$

To estimate average blood glucose (eAg) Eq. (8.5) can be used. This equation can be a helpful tool when explaining the A1C test results to people with diabetes or prediabetes. People who self-monitor often have an idea of “good” and “bad” numbers. This describes their A1C result in a relatable fashion [42].

Fructosamine Monitoring

Fructosamine reflects glycemic control over a shorter period (1–3 weeks) compared to A1C. It provides an index of longer-term control than glucose levels, especially in people with abnormal hemoglobin and in T1D. Fructosamine is found in the plasma and is a result of proteins being glycated (i.e., derivatives of the nonenzymatic reaction product of glucose and albumin).

Fructosamine testing is used in health-care settings but is not a standard of care. It is considered superior in people with abnormal hemoglobin, where A1C testing may be unreliable due to interference. The published reference interval for healthy subjects is 205–285 μmol/L, and in people not meeting treatment goals it ranges from 228 to 563 μmol/L with a mean of 396 μmol/L [43].

Summary

In summary, while blood glucose testing provides immediate insights into current glucose levels, fructosamine and A1C tests offer a broader view of glucose control over longer periods. The choice of test depends on individual’s specific health conditions, the presence of abnormal hemoglobin, and the need for short-term versus long-term glucose monitoring. Understanding the limitations and variations inherent in each test is important for effective diabetes management.

Monitoring Frequency

Table 8.8 is a comprehensive list outlining a structured approach to monitoring and managing people with diabetes or prediabetes, emphasizing the importance of regular assessments to optimize treatment outcomes and prevent complications.

Follow-Up

The Importance of Follow-Up in Diabetes Management

Diabetes is a chronic disease that even when well managed requires continuous monitoring. For this reason, follow-up is crucial in the management of diabetes. People with T1D should have their glucose control along with medication safety assessed regularly. Times of growth, hormonal changes, and illness can all affect glucose control. Among people with T2D, the disease can further progress even if initially well controlled. Treatment plans and goals can change the longer the individual has diabetes. Regular follow-up allows for continued education and can help each individual with diabetes to better understand their condition.

Comorbidity Follow-up

Cardiovascular

Cardiovascular comorbidities are often present in diabetes. One of the prioritized goals of diabetes is preventing and reducing morbidity and mortality from cardiovascular complications. More information on the management complications can be found in the chapter Management of Complications [2].

Retinopathy

Diabetes can lead to microvascular complications that affect vision. Regular screenings are important for early detection and

Table 8.8 Monitoring frequencies

Every follow-up regardless of timing	Hypoglycemia frequency, causes, timing, and patient hypoglycemic awareness Weight Body mass index Blood pressure Skin examination by a medical provider Physical activity Medication compliance
Every 3 months	A1C in people with diabetes who are not meeting treatment goals
Every 6 months	A1C in people with diabetes who are meeting glycemic target Kidney function if eGFR drops below 60 mL/min
Annually assess	Development of diabetes in people with diabetes with prediabetes Eating patterns and weight Familiarity with carbohydrate counting Physical activity Alcohol and substance use Medication compliance Medication intolerance or adverse effects Complementary medicine use (B12, statins, BP meds) Vaccine status CGM results and glucose data Insulin pump settings and use Social drivers of health (food insecurity, housing, transportation, financial security, community safety) Height, weight, body mass index Blood pressure Funduscopic eye examination (refer as needed) Comprehensive foot examinations Depression, anxiety, and disordered eating screening A1C Lipids CMP Specifically, potassium levels with people with diabetes on ACEi, ARB, MRA, and diuretics Liver function test Serum creatinine and eGFR UACR or microalbumin if UACR is not possible TSH (T1D) CBC Vitamin B12 (metformin use) Assess the need for diabetes self-management education and support

Adapted from source: Ref. [2]

ACEi angiotensin-converting enzyme inhibitor(s), *ARB* angiotensin II receptor blocker(s), *CBC* complete blood count, *CGM* continuous glucose monitoring, *CMP* comprehensive metabolic panel, *eGFR* estimated glomerular filtration rate, *MRA* mineralocorticoid receptor antagonist(s), *TSH* thyroid stimulating hormone, *UACR* urinary albumin-to-creatinine ratio management, which can prevent progression to more severe outcomes such as loss of vision. More information on the management complications can be found in the chapter Management of Complications [2].

Neuropathy Monitoring

Diabetes can affect the nervous system, leading to diabetic neuropathy, which often presents as numbness, tingling, or pain in the extremities. Regular neurological exams, including comprehensive foot exams, are important. More information on the management complications can be found in the chapter Management of Complications [2].

Foot Health

Foot complications are common in diabetes due to poor circulation and nerve damage. Regular foot exams are critical for early detection of problems such as ulcers, infections, and deformities. More information on the management complications can be found in the chapter Management of Complications [2].

Pharmacotherapy Follow-up

Tables 8.9 and 8.10 outline suggested considerations for follow-up with glucose-lowering drugs, while Table 8.11 summarizes follow-up for other medications prescribed for people with diabetes.

Methods of Follow-Up

Effective monitoring is essential in diabetes management, and each type of medical follow-up contributes uniquely to this goal. In-office visits are foundational, providing detailed physical assessments and immediate medical interventions, crucial for accurate and timely monitoring of a patient's condition. In-pharmacy visits offer supplementary monitoring opportunities, especially useful for checking medication compliance and basic

Table 8.9 Glucose lowering drugs

Drug class	Drug	Considerations during follow-up
Biguanide	Metformin [31]	Development of peripheral neuropathy due to vitamin B12 deficiency GI adverse effect Risk factors for lactic acidosis such as concurrent alcohol abuse, kidney dysfunction, dehydration, increased age
Dipeptidyl peptidase 4 inhibitors (DPP-4i)	Alogliptin [44] Linagliptin [17] Saxagliptin [45] Sitagliptin [18]	Comorbid heart failure or signs and symptoms of heart failure (saxagliptin and alogliptin) Skin eruptions Signs and symptoms of pancreatitis
Glucagon-like peptide-1 (GLP-1) receptor agonists	Dulaglutide [16] Exenatide [46] Liraglutide [47] Lixisenatide [48] Semaglutide [15]	Body weight Signs and symptoms of pancreatitis BP, HR Signs and symptoms of gallbladder disease Monitoring for worsening of diabetic retinopathy if present Monitoring for psychiatric changes (new or worsening depression or anxiety)
GLP-1 and glucose-dependent insulinotropic polypeptide (GIP) receptor agonist	Tirzepatide [49]	Back up contraception should be used whenever initiating or changing dose for 4 weeks

(continued)

Table 8.9 (continued)

Drug class	Drug	Considerations during follow-up
Insulin	Regular NPH Glargine Lispro Aspart Glulisine degludec Premixed insulins	Awareness of symptoms of hypoglycemia and hyperglycemia [2]
Sodium glucose transporter type 2 inhibitors (SGLT2i)	Bexagliflozin [50] Canagliflozin [51] Dapagliflozin [13] Empagliflozin [14] Ertugliflozin [52]	Signs/symptoms of diabetic foot infection, genital mycotic infections, UTI Risk of ketoacidosis, particularly euglycemic presentation
Sulfonylureas [19]	Glipizide Glimepiride Glyburide	Weight gain Occurrence of hypoglycemia
Thiazolidinedione [20]	Pioglitazone	Watch for signs of heart failure, especially after starting treatment or increasing doses Regular liver function tests before and during treatment, with more frequent monitoring in liver disease Monitoring for signs of fluid retention like edema or weight gain

BP blood pressure, *GI* gastrointestinal, *HR* heart rate, *UTI* urinary tract infection

Table 8.10 Other glucose lowering drugs

Drug class	Drug	Considerations during follow-up
Alpha-glucosidase inhibitor	Acarbose [11]	Worsening GI symptoms
Meglitinide analogs	Repaglinide Nateglinide	Check for drug-drug interactions (numerous)
Dopamine agonist	Bromocriptine [21]	BP and heart rate
Bile acid sequestrant	Colesevelam [37]	Signs and symptoms of pancreatitis (secondary to hypertriglyceridemia)

BP blood pressure, *GI* gastrointestinal

Table 8.11 Non-glucose lowering drugs

Drug class	Drug	Considerations during follow-up
2-Azetidinone	Ezetimibe [53]	Lipid panel
ACEi/ARB	Numerous	Blood pressure Potassium and serum creatinine Signs of bradykinin buildup (dry cough) [2]
Fibrates	Fenofibrate [54] Gemfibrozil [55]	Lipid panel Renal function *gemfibrozil
GABA analogs	Gabapentin [56] Pregabalin [57]	Renal function Behavioral changes Alertness/symptoms of respiratory depression especially with respiratory disease Overuse
Nonsteroidal mineralocorticoid receptor antagonist	Finerenone [10]	Signs and symptoms of hyperkalemia Serum creatinine eGFR
PCSK-9 inhibitors	Alirocumab [58] Evolocumab [59]	Lipid panel Injection site reactions

(continued)

Table 8.11 (continued)

Drug class	Drug	Considerations during follow-up
Serotonin-norepinephrine reuptake inhibitors (SNRI) [23]	Duloxetine Venlafaxine	BP (venlafaxine) US boxed warning for suicidal thoughts and behavior Discontinuation symptoms (venlafaxine)
Statins [24]	Numerous	Lipid panel LFTs as needed CPK Signs and symptoms of myopathies/rhabdomyolysis
Tricyclic antidepressants (TCA) [23]	Amitriptyline Nortriptyline	Heart rate BP Signs and symptoms of serotonin syndrome especially when combined with SSRIs or SNRIs

ACEi angiotensin-converting enzyme inhibitor(s), *ARB* angiotensin II receptor blocker(s), BP blood pressure, *CPK* creatinine phosphokinase, *eGFR* estimated glomerular filtration rate, *GABA* gamma-aminobutyric acid, *LFTs* liver function tests, *PCSK-9* proprotein convertase subtilisin/kexin type 9, *SSRIs* selective serotonin reuptake inhibitors

health parameters, although they have limitations in scope and depth. Remote follow-ups, through telemedicine and other digital communications, extend monitoring capabilities to those who might otherwise face barriers to regular health-care access, enabling frequent health status updates and education on disease management. Each mode of follow-up plays a critical role in creating a comprehensive monitoring strategy that accommodates the diverse needs and circumstances of individuals with diabetes.

In-Office Visits

In-office visits allow for comprehensive physical exams and immediate access to medical resources. These types of visits offer the ability to measure objective information, such as vital signs and point-of-care testing. Being face-to-face with people with diabetes facilitates mutual trust and understanding with the health-care team. If needed immediate intervention or referral to urgent or emergent care can take place.

While in-office visits are the standard for follow-up, there are also barriers to care that should be considered. Often, office visits can be time-consuming. Most offices set a goal cycle time of 1 h from the time of check-in until the time of check-out. This does not include any other auxiliary services, such as laboratory tests or visiting in-house pharmacies, if available. Office hours are typically during standard business hours so working individuals must make arrangements to miss work. For some populations, missing work also means not getting paid for time away from work. Upfront costs of office visits can also be difficult for individuals to understand and may cause avoidance of appointments, even if insured.

While office visits may be the preferred method for providers, often it is the least preferred for people with diabetes, especially those in underserved communities.

In-Pharmacy Visits

Pharmacy visits offer flexibility for people with diabetes, usually at a lower cost than office visits. Pharmacies are often open for extended hours for more days during the week. They play an important role in assessing medication compliance and providing education about the importance of their prescriptions. While pharmacies offer convenience, some barriers prevent pharmacists from billing for their services. Additionally, pharmacists are limited to performing basic health monitoring, such as blood pressure checks and some point-of-care tests. They often lack access to electronic health records, which restricts their ability to provide comprehensive drug monitoring. In addition, to start, stop, or change medications, pharmacists require oversight from a medical provider and must establish collaborative practice agreements. Due to the high volume of prescription production, larger retail chain and mail-order pharmacies are often unable to allow pharmacists to practice to their full potential. While there are both pros and cons to pharmacy follow-ups (visits), in the community setting, pharmacists should always provide retrospective reviews and monitoring.

Remote Medical Follow-up (Telemedicine, Telephone, and EMR Messaging)

Remote medical follow-up allows for the most convenient healthcare provided, which may be beneficial to those limited by work, cost, location, and mobility. Individuals would not have to pay for indirect medical costs such as transportation. Remote medical care may also provide benefits to those who are immunocompromised and limit their exposure to pathogens. Again, like all non-office visit follow-ups, physical exams are limited. There may be technology barriers for some people with diabetes, especially those in remote locations where internet and phone service may not be available. Lacking face-to-face interaction can also introduce miscommunication and misunderstandings. Nuances such as body language and facial expressions can be missed. Telemedicine and telephone encounters are instantaneous, but electronic medical record (EMR) messaging is dependent on provider and staff availability. Urgent and emergent matters should not be communicated through EMR messages and SMS texting services. Lastly, HIPAA compliance can be more challenging to ensure confidentiality within a digital environment. While convenience is the biggest advantage of remote follow-up, many disadvantages limit its usage.

Conclusion

In conclusion, monitoring and follow-up in diabetes management are crucial components that ensure the effectiveness and safety of treatment regimens. Pharmacists, with their extensive training in drug therapy and patient care, are pivotal in this process. They provide thorough monitoring that detects any therapeutic issues or side effects early, allowing for timely interventions that can prevent serious complications. Furthermore, regular follow-up by pharmacists ensures continuous assessment and adjustment of treatment plans as a patient's condition evolves. This proactive approach not only helps in maintaining optimal blood glucose levels but also supports overall health and well-being, underscoring the indispensable role of pharmacists in enhancing the quality of care for individuals with diabetes.

References

1. Hughes JD, Wibowo Y, Sunderland B, Hoti K. The role of the pharmacist in the management of type 2 diabetes: current insights and future directions. Integr Pharm Res Pract. 2017;6:15–27.
2. American Diabetes Association. Standards of care in diabetes – 2024. Diabetes Care. 2024;47(Suupl. 1):S1–S322.
3. FreeStyle Libre, 2022. Available: https://freestyleserver.com/Payloads/IFU/2022/q2/ART46090-003_rev-A.pdf. Accessed 28 Apr 2024.
4. Silva L. How Much Does A Continuous Glucose Monitor Cost? 31 October 2023. Available: https://www.forbes.com/health/conditions/diabetes/continuous-glucose-monitor-cost/. Accessed 28 Apr 2024.
5. American Diabetes Association. FAQs on CGM Coverage Criteria Changes in Medicare, 2023. Available: https://diabetes.org/advocacy/cgm-continuous-glucose-monitors/faqs-medicare-coverage#:~:text=Medicare%20now%20allows%20people%20to,day%20to%20access%20a%20CGM. Accessed 28 Apr 2024.
6. Basu A, Dube S, Veettil S, et al. Time lag of glucose from intravascular to interstitial compartment in type 1 diabetes. J Diabetes Sci Technol. 2015;9(1):63–8.
7. Kitabchi AE, Umpierrez GE, Miles JM, Fisher JN. Hyperglycemic crises in adult patients with diabetes. Diabetes Care. 2009;32(7):1335–43.
8. Jacobsen LM, Bocchino LE, Lum JW, et al. Accuracy of three commercial home-use hemoglobin A1c tests. Diabetes Technol Ther. 2002;24(11):789–96.
9. Momoniat T, Ilyas D, Bhandari S. ACE inhibitors and ARBs: managing potassium and renal function. Cleve Clin J Med. 2019;86(9):601–7.
10. Kerendia (finerinone) [Package insert], Wippany: Bayer HealthCare Pharmaceuticals Inc., 2021.
11. Precose (acarbose) [package insert], Wayne, NJ: Bayer HealthCare Pharmaceuticals Inc., 2011.
12. Actos (pioglitazone HCl) [package insert], Lincolnshire, IL: Takeda Pharmaceuticals America, Inc., 1999.
13. Farxiga (dapagliflozin) [package insert], Wilmington, DE: AstraZeneca Pharmaceuticals, 2014.
14. Jardiance (empagliflozin) [package insert], Ingelheim: Boehringer Ingelheim, 2014.
15. Ozempic (semaglutide) [package insert], Bagsvaerd, Denmark: Novo Nordisk, 2017.
16. Trulicity (dulaglutide) [package insert], Indianapolis, IN: Eli Lilly and Company, 2014.
17. Tradjenta (linagliptin) [package insert], Ridgefield, CT: Boehringer Ingelheim Pharmaceuticals, Inc., 2011.
18. Januvua (sitagliptin) [package insert], Rahway, NJ: Merck Sharp & Dohme LLC, 2006.

19. Costello RA, Nicolas S, Shivkumar A. Sulfonylureas. Treasure Island: StatPearls Publishing; 2024.
20. Eggleton JS, Jialal I. Thiazolidinediones. Treasure Island: StatPearls Publishing; 2024.
21. Cycloset (bromocriptine) [package insert], Tiverton, RI: VeroScience, LLC, 1978.
22. Burns ML, Kinge E, Opdal MS, Johannessen SI, Landmark SJ. Therapeutic drug monitoring of gabapentin in various indications. Acta Neurol Scand. 2019;139(5):446–54.
23. Fiaturi N, Greenblatt DJ. Therapeutic drug monitoring of antidepressants. In: Macaluso M, Preskorn S, editors. aNtidepressants. Handbook of experimental pharmacology. Springer; 2018. p. 115–33.
24. Sizar O, Khare S, Jamil RT, Talati R. Statin medications. Treasure Island: StatPearls; 2024.
25. Padilla O, Abadie J. Normal laboratory values. Merck Manual: Professional Version, 2021. Available: https://www.merckmanuals.com/professional/resources/normal-laboratory-values/normal-laboratory-values. Accessed 15 May 2024.
26. Katz MA. Hyperglycemia-induced hyponatremia – calculation of expected serum sodium depression. N Engl J Med. 1973;289(16):843–4.
27. Li T, Vijayan A. Insulin for the treatment of hyperkalemia: a double-edged sword? Clin Kidney J. 2014;7(3):239–41.
28. Nagami G. Hyperchloremia – why and how. Nefrología (English Edition). 2016;36(4):347–53.
29. Chua HR, Schneider A, Bellomo R. Bicarbonate in diabetic ketoacidosis – a systematic review. Ann Intensive Care. 2011;1(1):23.
30. Payne RB, Little AJ, Williams RB, Milner JR. Interpretation of serum calcium in patients with abnormal serum proteins. Br Med J. 1973;15(4):643–6.
31. Glucophage (metformin) [package insert], Princeton, NJ: Bristol-Myers Squibb Company, Rev 2017.
32. Oh MS, Carroll HJ. The anion gap. N Engl J Med. 1977;297(15):814.
33. Pan QI, Luo J, Guo L. The relationship between diabetic peripheral neuropathy and metformin treatment in type 2 diabetes mellitus. Diabetes. 2022;71(1):467.
34. Christy AL, Manjrekar PA, Babu RP, Hegde A, Rukmini MS. Influence of iron deficiency anemia on hemoglobin A1c levels in diabetic individuals with controlled plasma glucose levels. Iran Biomed J. 2014;18(2):88–93.
35. Shaikh H, Hashmi MF, Aeddula NR. Anemia of chronic renal disease. Treasure Island: StatPearls; 2023.
36. Goff DC, Lloyd-Jones DM, Bennett G, et al. 2013 ACC/AHA guideline on the assessment of cardiovascular risk: a report of the American College of Cardiology/American Heart Association task force on practice guidelines. Circulation. 2013;129:S49–73.
37. WelChol (colesevelam hydrochloride) [package insert], Parsippany, NJ: Daiichi Sankyo, Inc., 2000.

38. Krishnaveni P, Gowda VMN. Assessing the validity of Friedewald's formula and Anandraja's formula for serum LDLcholesterol calculation. J Clin Diagn Res. 2015;9(12):BC01–4.
39. FreeStyle Libre, Compare CGM systems, Abbott, Available: https://www.freestyleprovider.abbott/us-en/compare-cgms.html. Accessed 15 May 2024.
40. Odegard PS, Beach JR. Blood glucose monitoring: a practical guide for use in the office and clinic setting. Diabetes Spectr. 2008;21(2):100–11.
41. Hellman R. Glycemic variability in the use of point-of-care glucose meters. Diabetes Spectr. 2012;25(3):135–40.
42. American Diabetes Association. eAG/A1C Conversion Calculator. Available: https://professional.diabetes.org/glucose_calc. Accessed 15 May 2024.
43. Labcorp. Fructosamine; 2021. Available: https://www.labcorp.com/tests/100800/fructosamine. Accessed 15 May 2024.
44. Nesina (alogliptin) [package insert], Deerfield, IL: Takeda Pharmaceuticals America, Inc, 2013.
45. Onglyza (saxagliptin) [package insert], Princeton, NJ: Bristol-Myers Squibb Company, 2009.
46. Byetta (exenatide) [package insert], San Diego, CA: Amylin Pharmaceuticals, Inc., 2005.
47. Victoza (liraglutide) [package insert], Bagsvaerd, Denmark: Novo Nordisk, 2010.
48. Adlyxin (lixisenatide) [package insert], Bridgewater, NJ: Sanofi-Aventis US LLC, 2016.
49. Mounjaro (tirzepatide) [package insert], Indianapolis, IN: Lilly USA, LLC; 2022.
50. Brenzavvy (bexagliflozin) [package insert], Marlborough, MA: TheracosBio, LLC, 2023.
51. Invokana (canagliflozin) [package insert], Titusville, NJ: Janssen Pharmaceuticals, Inc., 2013.
52. Steglatro (ertugliflozin) [package insert], Whitehouse Station, NJ: Merck & Co., Inc. 2017.
53. Zetia (ezetimibe) [package insert], Jersey City, NJ: Organon & Co, 2002.
54. Tricor (fenofibrate) [package insert], North Chicago, IL: AbbVie, 1993.
55. Lopid (gemfibrozil) [package insert], Kirkland, Quebec: Warner-Lambert Company, 2009.
56. Neurontin (gabapentin) [package insert], New York, NY: Parke-Davis, 1993.
57. Lyrica (pregabalin) [package insert], New York, NY: Parke-Davis, 2004.
58. Praluent (alirocumab) [package insert], Tarrytown, NY: Regeneron Pharmaceuticals, Inc., 2015.
59. Repatha (evolocumab) [package insert], Thousand Oaks, CA: Amgen Inc., 2015.

Population-Based Care

9

Elizabeth G. Schlosser

Introduction

Population health is a term that has been utilized with various definitions for many years, but its usage within the United States and specifically within pharmacy, has greatly expanded in recent decades due to health-care reform [1]. The Affordable Care Act (ACA) and the Triple Aim framework of the Institute for Healthcare Improvement (IHI) brought population health to the forefront of providing higher quality care. Initiatives and payment models created in response to the ACA have focused on providing quality care and developing ways to continue to improve care. The IHI Triple Aim framework includes population health as a direct contributor to optimizing health for individuals [1, 2]. In these contexts, the most common definition of population health is "the health outcomes of a group of individuals, including the distribution of such outcomes within the group" [3, 4]. While this can be applied broadly, at times it can be difficult to understand or

E. G. Schlosser (✉)
Department of Pharmacy Practice and Administrative Sciences, University of Cincinnati James L. Winkle College of Pharmacy, Cincinnati, OH, USA
e-mail: Elizabeth.schlosser@uc.edu

© The Author(s), under exclusive license to Springer Nature Switzerland AG 2025

J. Clements (ed.), *The Pharmacist's Pocket Guide for Diabetes and Obesity*, https://doi.org/10.1007/978-3-031-88835-9_9

translate into direct action. Table 9.1 provides definitions for some commonly used terminology in population health.

Many health-care organizations are now participating in alternative payment models that financially reward organizations meeting certain quality standards or metrics. Many types of alternate payment models exist, but they can all be classified as value-based agreements, and include quality metrics to determine payment. Metrics or measures are developed and validated through rigorous processes and eventually incorporated into value-based contracts between health-care organizations and payors. There are many sets of metrics available, but commonly utilized ones include Healthcare Effectiveness Data and Information Set (HEDIS) measures, Centers for Medicare and Medicaid Services (CMS) 5-star measures, and CMS Hospital Readmissions Reduction Program, among others [5]. Pharmacists can be instrumental in these organizations by providing services that specifi-

Table 9.1 Population health terminology

Term	Definition
Population health	The health outcomes of a group of individuals, including the distribution of such outcomes within the group
Population health management	Programs targeted to a defined population that use a variety of individual, organizational, and societal interventions to improve health outcomes
Population health improvement	The enhancement of the health of all individuals in a population, with a greater emphasis on factors and influences unrelated to health care
Public health	This science-based, evidence-backed field strives to give everyone a safe place to live, learn, work and play
Care gap or gap in care	Gap between optimal patient care and care a patient receives
Payor	The entity that pays for services rendered by a health-care provider. (i.e., commercial insurance company, government program, employer, etc.)
Accountable care organization	Groups of doctors, hospitals, and other health-care providers who come together to give coordinated high-quality care to the Medicare patients they serve

Sources: Refs. [3–9]

cally address these measures. This chapter combines these definitions, frameworks, and recommendations into practical applications for pharmacist-provided population health management services for people living with diabetes.

Developing a Diabetes Population Health Management Service

Identify Organizational Priorities and Quality Metrics Related to Diabetes Management

The first step in developing a pharmacist-led diabetes population health management service is to examine the organization's priorities. Determination of what priorities currently exist within the organization related to the health of people living with diabetes, and how pharmacy services can align with those priorities should be made. The organization may be striving to meet goals related to diabetes medication adherence, hemoglobin A1C (A1C), diabetes complications, etc., and population health pharmacists can collaborate to reach these goals. Additionally, organizations may already be participating in alternative payment models such as ACOs and a pharmacist or pharmacy team can assist with meeting quality measures tied to value-based reimbursement [5].

Quality metrics or measures may originate from several sources and be incorporated into population health initiatives. As mentioned above, commonly used tools include HEDIS or CMS Stars Measures, examples of which are shown in Table 9.2. It is important to note that while measures within value-based contracts are based on these national standards, there may be differences in how the measure is specifically calculated for each contract or organization. It is also possible that the measure itself may be the same as the national measure, but the way it is incorporated into each value-based contract will vary. For example, two contracts may include medication adherence for diabetes medications, but one may offer a greater financial incentive for meeting a high rating on the measure. For this reason, an optimally successful population health program will align with measures and incentives specific to the organization [5].

Table 9.2 Nationally recognized quality metrics related to diabetes

HEDIS measures 2023		
Measure	Code	Description
A1C control for patients with diabetes	HBD	Percentage of members 18–75 years of age with T1D and T2D whose A1C was at the following levels: A1C control (<8.0%) A1C poor control (>9.0%)
Blood pressure control for patients with diabetes	BPD	Percentage of members 18–75 years of age with T1D and T2D whose blood pressure was controlled (<140/90 mmHg)
Eye exam for patients with diabetes	EED	Percentage of members 18–75 years of age with T1D and T2D who had a retinal eye exam
Kidney health evaluation for patients with diabetes	KED	Percentage of members 18–75 years of age with T1D and T2D who received a kidney evaluation using eGFR AND uACR
Statin therapy for patients with diabetes	SPD	Percentage of members 40–75 years of age with diabetes without ASCVD who met the following criteria. Received statin therapy—Members who were dispensed at least one statin medication of any intensity during the measurement year Statin adherence 80%—Members who remained on a statin medication of any intensity for at least 80% of the treatment period
CMS star measures		
Diabetes care—Eye exam	C09	Percentage of members with diabetes who had an eye exam to check for damage from diabetes during the year
Diabetes care—Kidney disease monitoring	C10	Percentage of members with diabetes who had a kidney function test during the year

(continued)

Table 9.2 (continued)

HEDIS measures 2023		
Measure	Code	Description
Diabetes care—Blood sugar controlled	C11	Percentage of members with diabetes who had an A1C lab test during the year that showed their average blood sugar is under control
Medication adherence for diabetes medications	D08	Percentage of members with a prescription for diabetes medication who fill their prescription often enough to cover 80% or more of the time they are supposed to be taking the medication

Sources: Refs. [10, 11]

A1C hemoglobin A1C, *ASCVD*, atherosclerotic heart disease, *CMS* Centers for medicare and medicaid services, *HEDIS* healthcare effectiveness data and information set, *eGFR* estimated glomerular filtration rate, *T1D* type 1 diabetes, *T2D* type 2 diabetes, and *uACR* urine albumin-creatinine ratio

Example

EGS Physicians is an accountable care organization (ACO) that has entered into multiple value-based contracts with several payors including Medicare, Medicaid, and commercial contracts. The organization has examined data that showed only 50% of people living with diabetes who have primary care physicians within the organization have an A1C <7.0%, and 30% have an A1C >8.0%. Several of the value-based contracts include a diabetes control measure and the organization would like to increase percentage of people living with diabetes with an A1C <7.0–60% and decrease the percent of those with an A1C above 8.0–20%.

Identify Patient Population

Once organizational goals are elucidated and aligned with the proposed population health program, the patient population must be selected. Quality measures may also guide the patient selection, as the population should reflect those currently being measured. In the case of people living with diabetes, it should be considered whether to include all people with diabetes in the program. Below are considerations to determine the patient population:

- Should people with type 1 diabetes (T1D) and type 2 diabetes (T2D) be included? Should classification be grouped together or separated and approached differently?
- Should an emphasis be placed on patients within certain value-based contracts (i.e., Medicare, Medicaid, commercial)? There may be special incentives under certain contracts or organizational goals related to certain payors that could influence who should be prioritized. The population may also be predetermined by the payor.
- How many patients can be included with the current available resources? It may not be practical to try to include too many patients that cannot be accommodated by current resources.
- What data is available that is accurate, and timely? If data is not available consistently for the chosen population, it will be impossible to make substantial improvements.

Risk stratification is also important depending on the size of the population. Resources are limited and must be allocated to the most impactable patients in the population. Two strategies exist for determining which patients to intervene with first: the patients who are closest to meeting the quality measure, and those who are at highest risk and furthest from meeting the measure. Both strategies have merit, and depending on current goals, each may be appropriate. It may make sense to target patients whose diabetes is severely uncontrolled and who may be at high risk of hospitalization to reduce health resource utilization, but this may also require significant time and resources to make the desired impact. It could also make sense to target patients who are close to the goal A1C and may need minimal support to meet the measure. This second group would be considered "low hanging fruit" meaning small interventions may make a big impact in meeting the measure. Additionally, many risk calculators exist and organizations may develop internal calculators to determine who may be at highest risk for negative outcomes [1, 5].

Example

EGS Physicians identifies 10,000 patients who are seen for primary care within the organization who are living with diabetes and have an A1C >7.0%. Of those, 6000 have an A1C >8.0% and 2000 have an A1C >9.0%. Additionally, XYZ Insurance Group contract data indicates that EGS is at three stars for diabetes control and may be eligible for a $20,000 shared savings bonus if the organization achieves four stars for the year or $30,000 if the organization reaches five stars. XYZ Insurance Group also sends a weekly report of members who are not currently meeting the diabetes control measure. For these reasons, EGS decides to allocate population health resources for XYZ contract patients with an A1C >8.0%. This leads to a panel of approximately 4500 patients.

Define Roles and Responsibilities of Population Health Team

The nature of population health programs requires collaborative teams to address various barriers to quality care. Members of the population health team can include nurses, medical assistants, care coordinators, physicians, dietitians, Certified Diabetes Care and Education Specialists (CDCES), nurse practitioners, physician assistants, and, of course, pharmacists. It is important to define the role of each of these members of the population health team prior to beginning services to avoid unintentional overlap. Each member of the team should be functioning optimally and at the top of their license to provide the best patient care. Table 9.3 provides examples of complementary health professionals and how their services could coordinate with pharmacist services [5].

Table 9.3 Potential population health team members

Professional	Complementary role to pharmacist-led services
Nurses	Assist in management of quality dashboards Provide diabetes education to identified patients or groups of patients Provide telehealth diabetes monitoring Review continuous glucose monitor data and communicate to physicians or pharmacists
Dieticians	Provide identified patients with diet-related education Develop suggested meal plans for identified patients.
Medical assistants	Schedule and room for pharmacist appointments Gather data related to diabetes control for evaluation by pharmacists Triage questions to physicians, pharmacists, or other members of the team
Physicians	Refer to pharmacist diabetes management services Collaborate to manage diabetes care with pharmacists and the rest of the population health team Place necessary referrals
CDCES	Provide specialized diabetes education to patient panel Educate on diabetes devices Follow-up with patients and relay information to physicians and/or pharmacists
Health informaticists	Obtain data related to population health measures Collate data into actionable information Develop quality dashboards for frontline staff usage
Payor contacts	Provide data related to population health measures at regular intervals Serve as a liaison between the organization and payor to answer questions, share strategies for addressing measures, update on status of measure achievement, etc
Pharmacy technicians	Collect data for pharmacist evaluation Outreach to patients who are not meeting quality measures Schedule patients for pharmacist visits

Source: Refs. [1, 5]
CDCES certified diabetes care and education specialist

Example

EGS Physicians has allocated 0.5 pharmacist full time equivalent (FTE), 1 medical assistant FTE, 0.25 dietician FTE, and 0.5 CDCES FTE to the population health management of the 4500 people living with diabetes identified above. It is decided that medical assistants will be responsible for scheduling appointments and triaging questions/phone calls for all members of the population health team. Pharmacists will enter into a collaborative practice agreement (CPA) with primary care physicians who provide care to the patient panel. This CPA will allow the pharmacists to order, adjust, and discontinue diabetes medications. They will also be able to order laboratory tests related to diabetes management and continuous glucose monitors. The dietician on the team will provide weekly group educational sessions and individual educational sessions by appointment related to diet for people living with diabetes. Finally, the CDCES will provide initial diabetes education for all patients enrolled in the population health management program in group or individual settings and via video visit.

Develop Diabetes Population Health Workflows

Once a patients and a population health team has been identified, workflows should be established. Workflows will differ by organization and will depend on what team members are available. Figure 9.1 displays a generic workflow for a population health pharmacist.

Population health interventions begin with data mining. Obtaining and verifying data to have accurate lists of patients who are not currently meeting quality measures is of the utmost importance. In population health, interventions are only as effective as data allows. Data may be obtained from a variety of sources including electronic health records, insurance companies, pharmacy fill history, etc. Individuals whose care is not currently

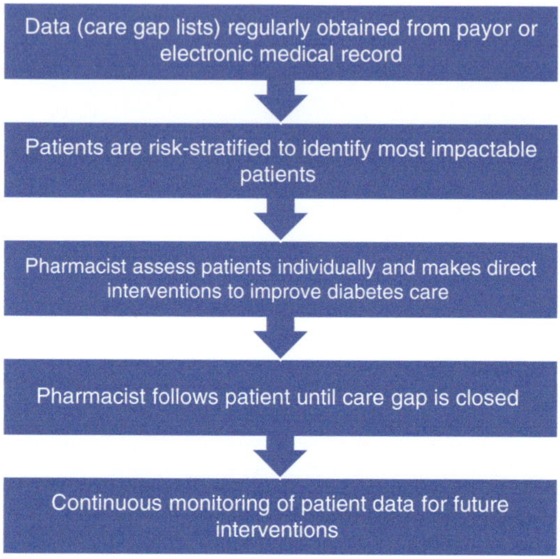

Fig. 9.1 Example population health pharmacist workflow

meeting the quality measure are referred to as "care gaps." Once accurate and timely care gap data is obtained, a pharmacist will risk stratify individuals to determine the most impactful interventions, and act upon them. For people living with diabetes, the most impactable individuals may be those with the highest A1C or who have had complications of diabetes [5].

After stratifying patients based on risk, the pharmacist will utilize patient specific data within the medical chart to assess what interventions can be made to help close the care gap. These interventions vary greatly but may include placing a referral for medication management with a pharmacist under a CPA, investigating medication adherence barriers, and providing or referring for education. The most important part is assessing the patient and connecting them to appropriate quality care [5].

Example

EGS Physicians obtains care gap lists weekly from XYZ Insurance Company that shows patients who currently have an A1C >8.0% on the patient panel. A pharmacist receives this list and determines which patients are highest risk and most impactable. An automatic referral is placed for patients to be seen by the pharmacist under the collaborative practice agreement with a primary care physician. Once the referral is placed, the medical assistant calls to set up a telehealth visit with the pharmacist and patient. The pharmacist conducts the visit with a patient to assess and adjust their diabetes medication regimen, place additional referrals as necessary, and monitor outcomes long term. The patient is referred for diabetes education with the CDCES. A continuous glucose monitor is ordered, and education is provided by the pharmacist. The pharmacist follows the patient until their A1C is <8.0% and remains stable for 6 months. XYZ Insurance Company continues to send care gap reports each week with updated data.

Financial Sustainability

When considering any intervention, costs must be considered. New services come at a cost to the organization and for the practice to be sustainable, it must at least be cost neutral, if not profitable. Direct or "incident-to" billing for pharmacist services may be an option to improve financial sustainability, though there are many caveats per state regulations. Pharmacists may also have provider status in some states, which improves billing options. If providing pharmacist services in a hospital facility, facility fees may also be billed. Other options for financial justification include improved performance on value-based contracts, though it is a complicated process to show direct impact of pharmacist services, considering that the many other members of the population health management team are also impacting performance. Revenue could also be generated through downstream services, like increased laboratory tests or referrals to other professionals who are also able to bill for services. Overall, the most important attribute that will encourage sustainability of the practice is diversification of revenue streams or justification of services. Reliance on one aspect of financial justification will not be sufficient as revenue streams have the potential to change quickly [12].

Continuous Monitoring

Continuous monitoring of performance is necessary to ensure consistent improvement of quality performance over time. One way that many organizations have addressed continuous monitoring is through patient dashboards. Dashboards can provide real-time data that can be continuously evaluated for potential changes and need for interventions. They pose an ideal solution, but not all health systems are equipped to develop them. Other strategies include frequent data mining to obtain up-to-date, though not real-time, data. Employing the assistance of health informaticists may also be beneficial in this data mining and continuous monitoring phase [5, 12].

It is also important to continue to evaluate what measures are being tracked as part of continuous monitoring. Yearly evaluation may be prudent to validate that measures are still relevant to practice and organizational goals. In addition to patient outcome quality metrics, other outcomes such as patient and provider satisfaction with pharmacist and population health services can be useful. Gaining perspectives from these groups may enable process improvements [5, 12].

Other Considerations

When thinking about population health services by pharmacists it is also important to consider involving pharmacy technicians, students, and residents. Advanced pharmacy technician roles are emerging in many areas, especially population health. Models have been described within the Veterans Administration for pharmacy technicians to address medication adherence and refer to pharmacists for intervention [13]. Technicians are also being employed in emerging areas of ambulatory care that may affect population health, including responding to medication refill requests [14, 15]. Pharmacy learners are also great resources to incorporate into population health processes. Each level of learner may be able to assist with different diabetes-related quality measures and collaboration may provide opportunity for layered learning [16].

It is also important to ensure that all population health initiatives for people living with diabetes account for a pharmacoequity perspective. Pharmacoequity was defined by Dr. Utibe Essien in 2021 as "ensuring that all individuals regardless of race and ethnicity, socioeconomic status, or availability of resources, have access to the highest quality medication required to manage their health needs" [17]. This is especially important for people living with diabetes because the newest and most effective diabetes medications lack equitable access due to the high cost of new diabetes medications, inadequate insurance coverage, drug shortages, etc. [18]. Population health initiatives should consider these barriers to optimal care and attempt to mitigate them.

Conclusion

Population health is a key piece of the puzzle to improve the quality of health care provided to people living with diabetes. Pharmacists, pharmacy technicians, and student pharmacists are important members of the health-care team and are well positioned to develop and implement population health initiatives. People living with diabetes can benefit from these initiatives through continuous monitoring and improvement in the quality of care provided.

References

1. Pearson TL, et al. Population health: the diabetes educator's evolving role. Diabetes Educ. 2019;45(4):333–48.
2. IHI. Triple Aim and Population Health; 2023.; Available from: https://www.ihi.org/improvement-areas/triple-aim-population-health
3. Kindig DA, Asada Y, Booske B. A population health framework for setting national and state health goals. JAMA. 2008;299(17):2081–3.
4. Kindig D, Stoddart G. What is population health? Am J Public Health. 2003;93(3):380–3.
5. Saito E et al. FAQ: Getting started with population health management, A.S.o.H.S. Pharmacists, Editor; 2021, American Society of Health System Pharmacists: ASHP.org.
6. Swarthout M, Bishop MA. Population health management: review of concepts and definitions. Am J Health Syst Pharm. 2017;74(18):1405–11.
7. APHA.org. What is public health? 2023
8. CMS.gov. Accountable Care Organizations (ACOs): general information; 2023
9. AMA. Payor Contracting 101; 2021, American Medical Association: ama-assn.org
10. NCQA. HEDIS MY 2023 measures and descriptions; 2023, NCQA: NCQA.org
11. CMS. 2023 medicare-medicaid plan performance data technical notes, C.f.M.a.M. Services, Editor; 2023, CMS: CMS.gov
12. Kliethermes MA, Brown TR. Building a successful ambulatory care practice: a complete guide for pharmacists. American Society of Health-System Pharmacists; 2012.
13. Will S et al. Utilization of PACT Clinical Pharmacy Technician (CPhT) in Population Health Management; 2022. Available from: https://marketplace.va.gov/innovations/utilization-of-pact-clinical-pharmacy-technician-cpht-in-population-health-management
14. Schlosser EG, et al. Implementation of a protocol-driven pharmacy technician refill process at a large physician network. J Am Pharm Assoc. 2003;60(6):e341–8.
15. Schlosser EG, et al. Assessment of pharmacy technician job satisfaction and duties in ambulatory care pharmacy settings: a mixed-methods analysis. Am J Health Syst Pharm. 2023;80(3):137–47.
16. ASHP, N.P.F.R.A.A.G. Residency guide: recommendations for practice and engagement in a layered learning model as a resident; 2019
17. Essien UR, Dusetzina SB, Gellad WF. A policy prescription for reducing health disparities – achieving Pharmacoequity. JAMA. 2021;326(18): 1793–4.
18. Taylor SI. The high cost of diabetes drugs: disparate impact on the most vulnerable patients. Diabetes Care. 2020;43(10):2330–2.

Part III

Obesity Section: Clinical Assessment Chapter

10

Sarah A. Kain

Purpose

The purpose of this chapter is to provide an evidence-based, person-centered guide on the clinical assessment of overweight and obesity. There are multiple modalities for assessment, each having its own advantages and disadvantages in terms of accessibility, feasibility, classification, and risk stratification. As a rapidly evolving and focused area of medicine, it is important to have an outline of the steps of care necessary to have a strong practitioner-patient relationship and improve the experience of health care and well-being of every life touched.

Comprehensive History

There are numerous considerations and areas of care to review and assess in the initial encounter for obesity or overweight (refer to Table 10.1) [1]. Following the initial steps to the 5 A's frame-

S. A. Kain (✉)
Ambulatory Care Pharmacy Department, Community Health Network, Indianapolis, IN, USA
e-mail: skain@ecommunity.com

© The Author(s), under exclusive license to Springer Nature Switzerland AG 2025

J. Clements (ed.), *The Pharmacist's Pocket Guide for Diabetes and Obesity*, https://doi.org/10.1007/978-3-031-88835-9_10

Table 10.1 Initial assessment considerations

Adults	Children and adolescents
Willingness and motivation to change lifestyle	
Any presenting symptoms	
Underlying causes of overweight or obesity	
Family history of overweight or obesity and comorbidities	
Risk factors assessed using lipid profile (preferably done when fasting), blood pressure measurement, and A1C measurement	
Lifestyle (diet and physical activity)	
Psychosocial distress, such as low self-esteem, teasing, and bullying	
Environmental, social, and family factors that may contribute to overweight or obesity, and the success of treatment	
Medical problems and medications	
The role of family and care workers in supporting individuals with varying learning abilities to make lifestyle changes	
Comorbidities (e.g., type 2 diabetes (T2D), hypertension, cardiovascular disease, osteoarthritis, dyslipidemia, sleep apnea)	Comorbidities (e.g., type 2 diabetes (T2D), hypertension, hyperinsulinemia, dyslipidemia, psychosocial dysfunction, exacerbation of conditions, such as asthma)
Psychological problems	Growth and pubertal status
The potential of weight loss to improve health	
Eating behaviors	

Source: Ref. [1]

work is an approach to seek permission, gather information, and assess each individual [2]. This person-centered comprehensive review can be used to aid clinical judgment and investigate comorbidities and other factors, taking into account the individual, the timing of the assessment, the degree of overweight or obesity, and the results of previous assessments.

In each evaluation, determining patient readiness and willingness for weight loss is an essential component to care. It is important to first seek permission to collaborate and discuss overweight or obesity using a person-centered approach. If that encounter is not the right time for the individual, let them know you are ready to support and talk about this part of their health when they are. If permission is given, assess the individual's motivation and support, priorities and health beliefs, cultural dimensions, stressful life events, psychiatric status, time availability or constraints, and appropriateness of goals and expectations to help establish the likelihood of lifestyle change [2]. Providers must also assess factors affecting adherence and patient disposition to pursue and trial various treatment modalities.

Asking the individual to complete a lifestyle events-body weight graph or self-reflection of life events in relation to weight can help review the behavioral and biopsychosocial determinants of weight gain [3]. Insight into predisposing genetic factors can be obtained by taking a family history. Similarly, it is important to ascertain whether the patient was overweight as a child or adolescent because early onset of obesity is a predictor of severe obesity in adulthood.

Before counseling advisement is initiated, dietary habits, physical activity, psychological health, and psychiatric history should be evaluated [3]. A confidential psychosocial assessment that includes questions about eating behaviors, body image, and mood should be routinely conducted, especially in adolescents and young adults, to assess for disordered eating, including but not limited to, anorexia nervosa, binge eating disorder, bulimia nervosa, avoidant/restrictive food intake disorder, pica, rumination, other specified feeding and eating disorders (OSFED), and unspecified feeding and eating disorders (UFED) [4]. Some examples of screening tools include SSHADESS and HEEADSSS, and these tools should be utilized in combination with the rest of the clinical assessment to help determine whether an eating disorder is present or not. The occurrence of a major depressive episode, eating disorder, or other serious psychological condition indicates an immediate referral to an age-appropriate mental health provider for further assessment and treatment [3]. Social determinants of health (SDOH) burden are associated with a higher prevalence of obesity. Therefore, prioritizing the use of SDOH screening questions and tools at each visit, such as Health Leads Social Needs Screening Toolkit, Protocol for Responding to and Assessing Patients' Assets, Risks, and Experiences (PRAPARE), or American Academy of Family Physicians (AAFP) Social Needs Screening Tool is imperative [5].

Comorbidities, medications, and bariatric surgery history require assessment due to their implications in future treatment considerations and risk assessment. Obesity is a chronic relapsing disease in which multiple modalities of treatment are utilized across the age span, including lifestyle counseling, pharmacotherapy, and surgery.

Physical Examination

Vital signs, including heart rate, blood pressure, height, and weight, should be measured at baseline and at each visit. The objective assessment of risk status resulting from overweight or obesity is based on multiple factors including the adult patient's age, body mass index (BMI) (Table 10.2), duration of time spent in a BMI category, waist circumference (WC), body fat location and percentage, muscle mass quality or quantity, gender, ethnicity, medically significant familial-determined mortality effectors, presence of disordered eating, and existence of comorbid conditions [3, 6]. BMI and WC provide a better assessment of total body fat than weight alone and are independent predictors of obesity-related disease risk [3]. Some literature suggests BMI definitions of overweight 23–27.4 kg/m^2 and obesity 27.5 kg/m^2 and above for people with a South Asian, Chinese, Asian, Middle Eastern, Black African, or African-Caribbean family background due to central adiposity and cardiometabolic risk occurring at a lower BMI in these populations [1, 7–9]. Additionally, for people in these groups, obesity classes II and III are usually identified by

Table 10.2 BMI classifications in adults

Classification	BMI range (kg/m^2)
Normal	18.5–24.9
Overweight	25–29.9
Obesity	≥30
Class I	30.0–34.9
Class II	35.0–39.9
Class III	≥40

reducing the thresholds by 2.5 kg/m^2 [1]. In many instances and groups, the use of height and weight alone for calculation of BMI, as a surrogate measure of body fat, can lead to an incorrect estimation of risk. Individuals who are pregnant, have a unique body habitus, are weightlifters with increased muscle mass, or are older adults with reduced lean body mass may be misclassified if solely using the BMI categories listed below. The American Medical Association supports the removal of BMI as a standard measure in medicine due to its inaccuracy in measuring body fat in multiple groups, especially with a BMI less than 35 kg/m^2, and recognizes culturally diverse and varied presentations across racial and ethnic groups, sexes, and age spans [6].

Additionally, it is important to assess for sarcopenia, especially in adults 50 years and older, due to its implications in the setting of weight loss therapy. Sarcopenia may be assessed using the strength, assistance with walking, rising from a chair, climbing stairs, and falls (SARC-F) questionnaire, handgrip test, and chair stand test [10]. Muscle mass quantity or quality may be further evaluated using MRI, CT, dual-energy x-ray absorptiometry (DXA), or bioimpedance. Although the use of MRI or CT are considered the gold standards for accurate lean muscle mass measurement, these present challenges with access, cost, requirement of a highly trained healthcare provider, and overall practicality. Therefore, DXA and bioelectrical impedance analysis (BIA) are more widely utilized due to greater convenience, lower cost, and availability [10].

Further, there is a standardized method for people to measure the waist and calculate the waist-to-height ratio (Table 10.3) [1]. The waist-to-height ratio can be classified into varying degrees of central adiposity and used for people with a BMI under 35 kg/m^2 of both sexes and all ethnicities, including adults with high muscle mass, children, and adolescents (Table 10.4) [1]. Additionally, waist-to-hip ratio may be a better measurement than WC alone in predicting disease risk. To calculate the waist-to-hip ratio, a measuring tape is used to measure WC (Table 10.3) and hip circumference at its widest part [6]. Abdominal obesity is defined by the World Health Organization (WHO) as having a waist-to-hip ratio above 0.90 for males and above 0.85 for females [6, 11]. WC

Table 10.3 How to measure WC

Measure: Find the bottom of the ribs and the top of the hips Wrap a tape measure around the waist midway between these points (just above the belly button) and breathe out naturally before taking the measurement
Calculate: Measure waist circumference and height in the same units (centimeters or inches) Divide the waist measurement by height measurement

Source: Refs. [1, 6]

Table 10.4 Defined degrees of central adiposity based on waist-to-height ratio

Central adiposity	Waist-to-height ratio	Health risks
Healthy	0.4–0.49	
Increased	0.5–0.59	↑
High	0.6 or more	↑↑

Source: Ref. [1]

should be a standard component and vital sign of each clinical encounter, as it is associated with improved ability to predict health outcomes including mortality compared to BMI [12]. The combination of BMI and WC identifies a high-risk obesity phenotype better than either measure alone [12].

Metabolic syndrome is the co-occurrence of metabolic risk factors for both T2D and cardiovascular disease (CVD), which is defined as the presence of any three of the five criteria per the National Cholesterol Education Program (NCEP) ATP III and International Diabetes Federation (IDF) (Table 10.5) [13]. Although central adiposity with an elevated WC may be a factor in the pathophysiology of metabolic syndrome, it is not a requirement for diagnosis.

When talking to a person about the waist-to-height ratio, explain the goal of maintaining a WC half of the height. Some known health risks associated with higher levels of central adiposity include T2D, hypertension, and CVD [1]. In addition to BMI, the risk of overweight and obesity is independently associated

Table 10.5 Metabolic syndrome clinical criteria

Parameters	NCEP ATP3 2005	IDF 2009
Obesity	White of European origin, sub-Saharan African, eastern Mediterranean, and middle eastern populations: Waist ≥102 cm (men) or ≥88 cm (women) South Asian, Chinese, Japanese, and south and central American populations: Waist ≥90 cm (men) or ≥80 cm (women)	Waist ≥94 cm (men) or ≥ 80 cm (women)
Hypertension	≥130/85 mmHg or drug treatment for hypertension	≥130/85 mmHg or drug treatment for hypertension
Glucose	Fasting glucose ≥5.6 mmol/L (100 mg/dL) or drug treatment for elevated blood glucose	Fasting glucose ≥5.6 mmol/L (100 mg/dL) or diagnosed diabetes
High-density lipoprotein (HDL) cholesterol	<1.0 mmol/L (40 mg/dL) (men); <1.3 mmol/L (50 mg/dL) (women) or drug treatment for low HDL cholesterol (fibrate or niacin)	<1.0 mmol/L (40 mg/dL) (men); <1.3 mmol/L (50 mg/dL) (women) or drug treatment for low HDL cholesterol
Triglycerides	≥1.7 mmol/L (150 mg/dL) or drug treatment for elevated triglycerides (fibrate or niacin)	≥1.7 mmol/L (150 mg/dL) or drug treatment for high triglycerides

Source: Ref. [13]

with central adiposity and fitness level [3]. People with larger WCs have elevated obesity-related health risks compared with those with healthy WCs and within similar BMI categories. Determination of fitness level is another modifier of assessing risk associated with BMI. Cardiorespiratory fitness has been shown to be an important predictor of all-cause mortality independent of BMI and body composition [3].

For adults with BMI of 40 kg/m^2 or more, or between 35 and 39.9 kg/m^2 with a significant health condition that could be improved if weight lost, consider bariatric surgery [1]. Beyond the

Table 10.6 Assessment considerations for bariatric surgery

Medical needs and existing comorbidities
Nutritional status (e.g., dietary intake, eating habits and behaviors)
Any psychological needs that, if addressed, would help ensure surgery is suitable and support adherence to postoperative care requirements
Previous attempts to manage weight, and any past response to a weight management intervention
Any factors that may affect response after surgery (e.g., language barriers, learning abilities and neurodevelopmental conditions, factors related to health inequities)
Whether any individual arrangements need to be made before the day of the surgery (e.g., if need additional dietary or psychological support, or support to manage existing or new comorbidities)
Fitness for anesthesia and surgery

necessary long-term follow-up needed for bariatric surgery, there are many considerations that should be assessed initially for bariatric surgery (Table 10.6) [1].

In children and adolescents, BMI charts adjusted for age and sex may be used as a practical estimate of overweight and obesity. As above, interpret BMI with caution, because it is not a direct measure of central adiposity. The WHO growth and BMI charts can be used to plot and classify BMI percentile and z-scores [14]. The childhood and puberty close monitoring (CPCM) form can also be used for continued BMI monitoring in children aged 2 and over, especially in instances where puberty is either premature or delayed [1]. There are explicit growth charts to refer to for children and young people with specific health conditions, including Down syndrome, Turner Syndrome, Marfan Syndrome, Cornelia de Lange Syndrome, Williams Syndrome, Prader Willi Syndrome, and achondroplasia [15–23]. Consider using waist-to-height ratio in children aged 5 and older to assess and predict health risks associated with central adiposity (refer to Tables 10.3 and 10.4). In children and adolescents, the degree of overweight or obesity is classified in BMI centiles (Table 10.7) [24]. Use clinical judgment when interpreting BMI, irrespective of BMI percentile, because a child or young person may nevertheless have central adiposity warranting care [1].

Table 10.7 BMI classification in children and adolescents

Classification	BMI range
Underweight	<5th percentile
Healthy weight	5th percentile to <85th percentile
Overweight	85th percentile to <95th percentile
Obesity	≥95th percentile
Severe obesity	120% of the 95th percentile or greater OR ≥35 kg/m^2

Laboratory and Clinical Markers

No single laboratory test or diagnostic evaluation is indicated for all patients with overweight or obesity. The specific evaluation performed should be based on the presenting symptoms, risk factors, index of suspicion, and screening guidelines appropriate for the patient. Current literature suggests, at a minimum, completing a fasting glucose, hemoglobin A1c, and fasting lipid profile in adults with overweight or obesity [1, 3, 25]. Specific lipid markers with known risk include elevated triglyceride concentration, a low HDL cholesterol concentration, a high ratio of triglycerides to HDL cholesterol, or a combination of an enlarged waist and elevated triglyceride concentration [3]. Insulin resistance may be further assessed by completing an intact insulin, c-peptide, and a validated insulin resistance score [26]. Cardiovascular risk may be further assessed by completing testing of apolipoprotein B (Apo B), lipoprotein fractionation, lipoprotein (a), lipoprotein-associated phospholipase A2 (Lp-PLA2), and high-sensitivity C-reactive protein (hs-CRP) [26]. Endocrine function, such as blood glucose, thyroid levels, vitamin D, 25-hydroxy, and hepatic function, such as a comprehensive metabolic panel, may also be useful to assess risk for diseases impacting weight (e.g., hypo- or hyperthyroidism, Hashimoto's thyroiditis, vitamin D deficiency, insulin resistance, and T2D) and nonalcoholic fatty liver disease. Assess and screen for other common comorbidities of overweight or obesity, including osteoarthritis and sleep apnea using the Western Ontario McMaster (WOMAC) and STOP-BANG questionnaires, respectively [27–29]. For any positive results, further assessment and referral to appropriate specialist care is prudent. Assessing pregnancy status and current contraception method is recommended for females of childbearing age and potential at every visit due to its impact on assessing BMI and utility and safety of pharmacotherapy [30]. For example, glucagon-like peptide-1 (GLP-1) receptor agonists and GLP-1/glucose-dependent insulinotropic polypeptide (GIP) receptor agonists have the potential to improve fertility in males and females and reduce oral hormonal contraceptive absorption due to delayed gastric emptying, which can lead to contraception failure. Due to the increased risk of embryo-fetal toxicity with major congenital malformations, phentermine-topiramate (Qsymia) has an FDA-approved REMS program. In females of childbearing potential, a pregnancy test prior to phentermine-topiramate (Qsymia) initiation and monthly screening thereafter while on therapy is advised. Weight loss medications should be discontinued prior to conception [31].

In children and adolescents, assess associated comorbidities and secondary causes for overweight or obesity by checking blood pressure measurement(s), fasting lipid profile, fasting insulin, fasting glucose levels and oral glucose tolerance test, liver function, and endocrine function [1]. Interpret the results of any tests within the context of the level of the child's overweight or obesity, the child's age, history of comorbidities, possible genetic causes, and any family history of metabolic disease related to overweight or obesity [1].

Risk Stratification and Assessment

Obesity is associated with over 60 medical conditions and the leading causes of preventable death, the incidence and prevalence of which vary by BMI class, sex, age, and other patient factors [3]. Patients that are classified as very high risk and elicit the need for intense risk factor modification and management include those with established atherosclerotic diseases, T2D, sleep apnea, or metabolic syndrome [3]. Additionally, there is a direct relationship with increasing BMI categories and risk observed for diabetes mellitus, hypertension, and dyslipidemia [3].

Although BMI and WC are useful noninvasive quantitative markers to identify potential risk, both do not consistently accurately reflect the presence or severity of the health risk. The Edmonton Obesity Staging System (EOSS) is a risk-stratification tool that classifies individuals with obesity into five graded categories based on their morbidity and health-risk profile [3] (see Table 10.8). The EOSS has demonstrated ability to predict increased mortality; however, more studies need to determine whether it improves risk stratification over other tools, such as the Framingham Risk Score (FRS), Systematic Coronary Risk Evaluation (SCORE), ACC/AHA ASCVD Risk Estimator, or UK QRISK [3]. Given this, it remains beneficial to calculate a cardiovascular score using one or more of these tools as well.

Some conditions can improve after bariatric surgery, including CVD, hypertension, idiopathic intracranial hypertension, nonalcoholic fatty liver disease with or without steatohepatitis, obstructive sleep apnea, and T2D [1]. Consider a referral to a specialist weight management service if [1]:

- The person has complex disease states or needs that cannot be managed adequately in the current setting.
- Conventional treatment has been unsuccessful.
- Drug treatment is being considered for a person with a BMI of more than 50 kg/m^2.
- Specialist interventions (such as a very-low-calorie diet) may be needed.
- Bariatric surgery is being considered.

For those pursuing bariatric surgery intervention, the obesity surgery mortality risk score (OS-MRS) can be a useful clinical tool for the preoperative prediction of mortality risk in bariatric surgery [32]. This can help further assess the choice of the type of bariatric procedure, depending on the risk of postoperative complications.

Table 10.8 Assessment of obesity according to the EOSS tool stages and examples

	Stage 0 No clinical risk factors, physical symptoms, psychological symptoms, or functional limitations	Stage 1 Obesity-related subclinical clinical risk factors/mild symptoms	Stage 2 Established obesity-related comorbidities / moderate symptoms	Stage 3 Significant obesity-related end-organ damage	Stage 4 Severe/End-stage disease
Medical		Borderline HTN, impaired fasting glucose, elevated liver enzymes	HTN, type 2 diabetes, sleep apnea, PCOS, osteoarthritis	ASCVD, diabetes complications such as CKD or poor healing wounds	End-stage heart failure, dialysis, oxygen use, hepatic encephalopathy
Mental		Not requiring medical treatment for comorbidities. Occasional ache or fatigue	Depression, anxiety, eating disorder	Major and/or refractory depression, suicidal ideation	Severe and disabling psychological symptoms
Functional		Mild impairment of well-being but QOL not impacted	QOL beginning to be impacted with functional limitation on daily activities	Impairment of well-being and QOL significantly impacted; unable to work or complete routine activities	Severe functional limitations, such as wheelchair use due to disabling complication or immobility

Source: Ref. [3]

ASCVD Atherosclerotic cardiovascular disease, *CKD* chronic kidney disease, *HTN* hypertension, *PCOS* polycystic ovarian syndrome, *QOL* quality of life

Goals and Therapy Decision-Making

Weight loss goals are determined based on the severity of obesity-related complications and patient factors. Treatment selection and intensity of obesity intervention varies depending on the phase of prevention and treatment. The general goals of weight loss and management are at a minimum to prevent further weight gain, reduce body weight, and maintain a lower body weight long term. Further, the goals of therapy are to prevent, treat, and/or reverse the complications of overweight or obesity and improve the quality of life in patients by using appropriate non-pharmacological, pharmacological, and/or surgical therapy. Regarding weight loss, assessment using non-pharmacological and/or pharmacological approaches, the goal is to achieve 5–10% body weight loss or exceed 10% body weight loss, which are considered very good and excellent weight loss responses, respectively [30, 33, 34]. Bariatric surgery percent (%) body weight loss goals that require assessment post-surgery vary for each patient and type of surgery; therefore, the weight specialist team or surgeon should provide an estimated range for percent of excess body weight loss at various time points post-surgery. In general, pharmacotherapy should be discontinued if weight loss of at least 5% is not achieved after 12 weeks of maximum-dose therapy, and an alternative weight loss therapy should be considered [30]. Weight regain occurs with a high probability when pharmacotherapy and/or lifestyle modifications for obesity are discontinued. Weight regain following bariatric surgery is anticipated as soon as 12 months following surgery; however, there is no generally accepted criterion or definition for substantial weight gain. Therefore, appropriate chronic clinical assessment of care remains judicious to assess weight in relation to the patient's overall health, comorbidities, risk factors, lifestyle, and therapy decision-making.

Conclusion

Identifying, evaluating, and treating this prevalent and high-risk disease in all ages is vital for reducing morbidity and mortality. Clinical assessment of overweight and obesity comprises a multitude of factors, including a comprehensive history of subjective and objective parameters, physical examination, clinical and laboratory markers, risk stratification and classification, and goals of care and therapy decision-making. Due to the heterogeneity of disease, each individual's health should be uniquely assessed to provide evidence-based person-centered care. Despite current limitations to classifications and risk stratification regarding health outcomes, unique laboratory markers, tools to measure types of body mass, and therapeutic options continue to be developed and positively impact the assessment and management of overweight and obesity.

References

1. Obesity: identification, assessment and management. London: National Institute for Health and Care Excellence (NICE); 2023. (NICE Guideline, No. 189.) https://www.ncbi.nlm.nih.gov/books/NBK588750/. Accessed 18 Nov 2023.
2. Vallis M, Piccinini-Vallis H, Sharma AM, Freedhoff Y. Modified 5 as. Minimal intervention for obesity counseling in primary care. Can Fam Physician. 2013;59:27–31.
3. Kushner R. Clinical assessment and management of adult obesity. Circulation. 2012;126:2870–7.
4. Klein DA, Sylvester JE, Schvey NA. Eating disorders in primary care: diagnosis and management. Am Fam Physician. 2021;103(1):22–32.
5. NASDOH. Screening Tools and Tool Kits: Helpful screening tools and tool kits. National Alliance to impact the Social Determinants of Health (NASDOH).https://nasdoh.org/screening-tools-and-tool-kits/. Accessed 18 Nov 2023.
6. Deurenberg P, Deurenberg-Yap M, Guricci S. Asians are different from Caucasians and from each other in their body mass index/body fat percent relationship. Obes Rev. 2002;3:141–6.
7. Misra A, Khurana L. The metabolic syndrome in south Asians: epidemiology, determinants, and prevention. Metab Syndr Relat Disord. 2009;7:497–514.

8. Misra A, Vikram NK. Insulin resistance syndrome (metabolic syndrome) and obesity in Asian Indians: evidence and implications. Nutrition. 2004;20:482–91.
9. American Medical Association. Report 07 of the Council on Science and Public Health (A-23): Support Removal of BMI as a Standard Measure in Medicine and Recognizing Culturally-Diverse and Varied Presentations of Eating Disorders and Indications for Metabolic and Bariatric Surgery (Reference Committee D). American Medical Association. https://www.ama-assn.org/system/files/a23-handbook-refcom-d.pdf. Accessed 20 July 2024.
10. Ardeljan AD, Hurezeanu R. Sarcopenia. In: StatPearls. Treasure Island (FL): StatPearls Publishing; 2023. https://www.ncbi.nlm.nih.gov/books/NBK560813/. Accessed 30 Nov 2023.
11. World Health Organization. Waist circumference and waist-hip ratio: report of a WHO expert consultation, Geneva, 2008. https://iris.who.int/bitstream/handle/10665/44583/9789241501491_eng.pdf?sequence=1&isAllowed=y. Accessed 28 July 2024.
12. Ross R, Neeland IJ, Yamashita S, et al. Waist circumference as a vital sign in clinical practice: a consensus statement from the IAS and ICCR working group on visceral obesity. Nat Rev Endocrinol. 2020 Mar;16(3):177–89.
13. Alberti KG, Eckel RH, Grundy SM, et al. Harmonizing the metabolic syndrome: a joint interim statement of the international diabetes federation task force on epidemiology and prevention; National Heart, Lung, and Blood Institute; American Heart Association; world heart federation; international atherosclerosis society; and International Association for the study of obesity. Circulation. 2009;120:1640.
14. WHO. Body mass index-for-age (BMI-for-age): Charts & Tables. World Health Organization (WHO). https://www.who.int/toolkits/child-growth-standards/standards/body-mass-index-for-age-bmi-for-age. Accessed 20 Nov 2023.
15. Cronk C, Crocker AC, Pueschel SM, et al. Growth charts for children with down syndrome: 1 month to 18 years of age. Pediatrics. 1988;81(1):102–10.
16. Ranke MB, Pfluger H, Rosendahl W, et al. Turner syndrome: spontaneous growth in 150 cases and review of the literature. Eur J Pediatr. 1983;141(2):81–8.
17. Lyon AF, Preece MA, Grant DB. Growth curves for girls with turner syndrome. Arch Dis Child. 1985;60(10):932–5.
18. Pyeritz RE. In: Emery AH, Rimoirn DL, editors. Principles and practice of medical genetics. New York: Churchill Livingstone; 1983.
19. Pyeritz RE. In: Papadatas CJ, Bartsocas CS, editors. Endocrine genetics and genetics of growth. Alan R. Liss, Inc; 1985.
20. Kline AD, Barr M, Jackson LG. Growth manifestations in the Brachmann-deLange syndrome. Am J Med Genet. 1993;47(7):1042–9.

21. Morris CA, Demsey SA, Leonard CO, et al. Natural history of Williams syndrome: physical characteristics. J Pediatr. 1988;113(2):318–26.
22. Holm V. Overview of Prader-Willi syndrome. In: Greenswag LR, Alexander RC, editors. Management of Prader-Willi syndrome. 2nd ed. New York: Springer-Verlag; 1995.
23. Horton WA, Rotter JI, Rimoin DL, et al. Standard growth curves for achondroplasia. J Pediatr. 1978;93(3):435–8.
24. Hampl SE, Hassink SG, Skinner AC, et al. Clinical practice guideline for the evaluation and treatment of children and adolescents with obesity. Pediatrics. 2023;151(2):e2022060640.
25. Wharton S, Lau DCW, Vallis M, et al. Obesity in adults: a clinical practice guideline. CMAJ. 2020;192(31):E875–91.
26. Defining the intersection of chronic conditions: The evidence demonstrating the interrelationships between chronic cardiometabolic diseases continues to expand, supporting a personalized approach to reducing risk. Quest Diagnostics Incorporated: Quest Cardiometabolic Center of Excellence at ClevelandHeartLab. 2022.
27. McConnell S, Kolopack P, Davis AM. The Western Ontario and McMaster universities osteoarthritis index (WOMAC): a review of its utility and measurement properties. Arthritis Rheum. 2001;45:453–61.
28. Chung F, Abdullah HR, Liao P. STOP-Bang questionnaire: a practical approach to screen for obstructive sleep apnea. Chest. 2016;149(3):631–8.
29. Silva GE, Vana KD, Goodwin JL, et al. Identification of patients with sleep disordered breathing: comparing the four-variable screening tool, STOP, STOP-Bang, and Epworth sleepiness scales. J Clin Sleep Med. 2011;7(5):467–72.
30. Grunvald E, Shah R, Hernaez R, et al. AGA clinical practice guideline on pharmacological interventions for adults with obesity. Gastroenterology. 2022;163(5):1198–225.
31. American College of Obstetricians and Gynecologists. ACOG practice bulletin no. 230: obesity in pregnancy. Obstet Gynecol. 2021;137(6):e128–44.
32. Thomas H, Agrawal S. Systematic review of obesity surgery mortality risk score – preoperative risk stratification in bariatric surgery. Obes Surg. 2012 Jul;22(7):1135–40.
33. Garvey WT, Mechanick JI, Brett EM, et al. American Association of Clinical Endocrinologists and American College of endocrinology comprehensive clinical practice guidelines for medical care of patients with obesity. Endocr Pract. 2016;22(Suppl 3):1–203.
34. Apovian CM, Aronne LJ, Bessesen DH, et al. Pharmacological management of obesity: an endocrine society clinical practice guideline. J Clin Endocrinol Metab. 2015;100(2):342–62.

Non-pharmacologic Interventions for Overweight and Obesity

11

Rachel Basinger and Alaina Van Dyke

Introduction

Disease Burden

The World Health Organization (WHO) defines overweight and obesity as abnormal or excessive fact accumulation that presents a risk to health. Although often thought of as a human behavior problem, the WHO recognizes obesity as a medical condition due to malnutrition that affects most of the world. Excessive weight is no longer a burden seen only in high-income countries as the increased prevalence in adult and pediatric populations is growing rapidly in low- and middle-income countries. Worldwide obesity has almost tripled since 1975. In 2016, 39% of adults were overweight and 13% were living with obesity [1]. The prevalence of obesity in the United States exceeds global averages. In 2022, obesity in adults was 41.9% with 9.2% classified as severe obesity. Non-Hispanic Black adults account for 49.9% of the obesity rates, compared to 45.6%, 41.4%, and 16.1% among Hispanic

R. Basinger (✉) · A. Van Dyke
Jerry H. Hodge School of Pharmacy, Texas Tech University Health Sciences Center, Dallas, TX, USA
e-mail: Rachel.basinger@ttuhsc.edu; Alaina.VanDyke@ttuhsc.edu

© The Author(s), under exclusive license to Springer Nature Switzerland AG 2025

J. Clements (ed.), *The Pharmacist's Pocket Guide for Diabetes and Obesity*, https://doi.org/10.1007/978-3-031-88835-9_11

adults, non-Hispanic White adults, and non-Hispanic Asian adults, respectively. The financial burden of obesity is substantial. Medical cost associated with obesity was nearly 173 billion dollars in 2019 [2].

The health consequences of overweight and obesity are numerous. Excessive weight leads to metabolic disorders, cardiovascular disease, nonalcoholic fatty liver disease and nonalcoholic steatohepatitis, polycystic ovary syndrome, female infertility, male hypogonadism, obstructive sleep apnea, asthma, osteoarthrosis, urinary stress incontinence, depression, gastroesophageal reflux disease, and cancer [3]. Obesity has been associated with endometrial, breast, ovarian, prostate, liver, gallbladder, kidney, and colon cancers [1]. Obesity can also increase the risk of severe illness, complications, and death from infectious diseases, as seen in the recent COVID-19 pandemic [4].

The Pharmacist's Role in Non-pharmacological Interventions

The main treatment goal of weight management is to prevent or improve comorbid conditions. An initial 5–10% weight loss is necessary to achieve improvements in most weight-related conditions [3]. Along with physical health, improving emotional well-being and body composition for cosmetic benefits is important. Like any chronic condition, treatment is a lifelong challenge [1].

Pharmacists are well trusted by the public and are the most accessible health-care professionals. Education of pharmacists includes physical assessment skills required to assess and monitor weight and general knowledge of dietary and physical activity guidelines. As the medication experts, pharmacists can identify medications that cause weight gain or hinder weight loss. Common offenders include second-generation antipsychotics, hormonal contraceptives, systemic corticosteroids, anticonvulsants, sulfonylureas, thiazolidinedione, insulin, or beta blockers. Lastly, pharmacists are introduced to motivational interviewing, which can help improve adherence to lifestyle interventions and other components of a weight loss plan. When assistance is needed that falls outside the scope of practice or expertise of a pharmacist, a referral to the appropriate health-care provider can be placed [5].

Dietary Interventions

Dietary Guidelines

The purpose of the Dietary Guidelines for Americans is to provide guidance for the food and beverages that promote good health, reduce the risk of diet-related chronic disease, and meet nutrient needs. The document does comment on weight loss through a multimodal approach, including diet. One specific dietary recommendation made was to reduce food and beverages high in added sugars to reduce calories. The guidelines acknowledge the need for long-term solutions with adequate support from health-care providers, family, and social networks [6].

Caloric needs vary greatly between age, gender, body weight, and activity level. Creating a deficit of 500 kcal/day or more promotes about 1-pound weight loss per week. Diets that promote more than 2 pounds a week with severe caloric restrictions should be supervised by a provider to ensure adequate nutrition and safety. Supplements with multivitamins and multiminerals are often necessary to ensure adequate intake of key nutrients with very-low-calorie diets. Caloric restriction can be obtained through a variety of strategies.

Intermittent Fasting

Instead of focusing on what to eat, intermittent fasting focuses on when to eat. The goal is to force the body to utilize fat storage for energy during a prolonged period of fasting.

There are three main approaches. A daily fasting requires eating to occur only during a 6–8 h period while fasting the remaining 16–18 h. A weekly plan includes eating regularly for most days of the week but limiting to one meal a day for about

2 days a week. Lastly, complete fasts that last 24–72 h can be done. Longer durations of fasting, however, can lead to the body going into starvation mode and burning muscle instead of fat. At all times, hydration remains important. Intermittent fasting is considered safe for the general adult population, but those with certain conditions such as insulin-dependent diabetes or eating disorders should be referred to their providers for clearance [7].

A systematic review including 27 trials showed a range of weight loss benefit from 0.8% to 13% with no serious adverse events from intermittent fasting. Hunger was the highest reported symptom. The limitations with most of data for intermittent fasting are short study durations with most being only weeks to months and low numbers of participants. Short-term data is promising, but long-term sustainability and weight loss outcomes data is lacking [8].

Food Additives

The use of artificial sweeteners and fat substitutes does reduce caloric intake; however, the overall health benefits or potential harm is controversial. Artificial sweeteners include acesulfame potassium, advantame, aspartame, fructose, neotame, saccharin, sorbitol, stevia, sucralose, and xylitol. Most are considered zero caloric alternatives except fructose, sorbitol, and xylitol as they do have about 10 calories per serving. Aspartame can have a bitter taste when heated and is not ideal for cooking, but also contains phenylalanine, which is contraindicated in patients with phenylketonuria. Saccharin and acesulfame potassium have bitter tastes as well. Sorbitol causes osmotic diarrhea when used in excess.

Fat substitutes can cut calories in half. Microparticulated proteins may not be used in cooking due to instability when heated. Sucrose polyester can bind fat-soluble vitamins and cause gastrointestinal side effects since it is not absorbed. Soluble fiber is a common plant derived alternative to fat in a variety of foods, including meat alternatives.

Meal Replacements

Meal replacement strategies reduce caloric intake through portion control. With this plan, two meals are severely caloric restricted by means of a prepared shake, bar, or packaged meal. The third meal is determined by the patient but is encouraged to be healthy and of moderate calories. These programs are successful in initial weight loss, but often unobtainable for long-term adherence.

Altered Proportions of Food Groups

Daily calories can be reduced by swapping high-energy, low nutrition dense foods with low-energy, high nutrition dense foods. The main macronutrients of interest to decrease are fat and sugar.

Weight Loss Programs

The Atkins® diet promotes a low carbohydrate with high fiber diet. Developed by Dr. Robert C. Atkins, this diet gained popularity with his first publication in 1972. The Atkins® diet stresses eating better more than eating less and is generally thought to be safe for most patients. Pre-packaged meals and snacks are readily available for consumers [9]. A more severe low carbohydrate diet is the ketogenic diet. It was first described in 1921 as a dietary treatment for seizures, and the diet has been popular since the 1970s due to the weight loss benefits. When carbohydrate intake is restricted, insulin secretion decreases, which activates ketogenesis. Ketosis induced by nutritional deficits are typically safe as the production of ketone bodies is not significant enough to alter the pH of the blood. Short-term data show significant weight loss with acceptable adverse events. Patients may experience the "keto flu" temporarily. These flu-like symptoms usually last only a few days to weeks. Long-term compliance is challenging and though there is data up to 2 years, most study durations are weeks to months [10].

Commercial weight-loss programs provide structured guidance that may be appealing to some patients. Most programs include support groups or counseling, calorie-restricted pre-packaged meals and snacks, and tracking apps, but additional benefits such as health coaches, medical providers, body monitoring devices, or pharmacotherapy varies with each program. There are a variety of programs available. Patients choosing a commercial weight-loss program should pick a program that meets their desired support system, flexibility, meal choices, balance of diet and exercise, and costs. Well-known programs include Weight Watches®, Jenny Craig®, and Nutrisystem®. Programs show success while patients are enrolled and adherent to the plan, but little is known about long-term success after patients graduate from programs and continue their lifestyle changes on their own [11].

Comparison of Popular Diets

A 2020 systematic review of 14 various dietary patterns on weight loss included 121 trials. Weight reduction at 6 months was about 4–5 kg for low-carbohydrate or low-fat diets and 4 kg for moderate-carbohydrate or moderate-fat diets. For specific dietary plans, the Atkins® diet resulted in 5.5 kg weight loss, DASH diet in 3.6 kg weight loss, and Zone diet in 4.1 kg. If studies exceeded 6 months, weight-loss effects diminished over time [12]. Refer to Table 11.1 for the breakdown of macronutrients of popular dietary patterns.

Table 11.1 Macronutrients of popular diets

Type	Diet name	% kcal carb	% kcal protein	% kcal fat
Low carb	Atkins, South Beach, Zone	<40	30	30–55
Moderate macronutrients	Biggest Loser, DASH, Jenny Craig, Mediterranean, Portfolio, Slimming World, Volumetrics, Weight Watchers	55–60	15	21–30
Low fat	Ornish, Rosemary Conley	60	10–15	≤ 20

Source: Ref. [12]
kcal Kilocalorie

So, what is the best specific diet? The answer is it depends on your patient. In general, caloric intake should be restricted to promote energy deficit, but the exact method depends on the patient's ability to conduct and maintain new dietary patterns. Refer to Chap. 3, Table 3.1 for a more detailed overview of dietary patterns and their associated outcomes.

Physical Activity

Physical Activity Guidelines

The Physical Activity Guidelines for Americans mirrors the recommendations for weight loss seen in the dietary guidelines. These guidelines state that the combination of physical activity with reduced caloric intake must be considered for weight management as the combination is more beneficial than either alone. For weight loss of more than 5%, exceeding general recommendations to achieve more than 300 min of moderate-intensity activity a week is typically necessary. For the same benefit, 150 min of vigorous-intensity activity can be used to save time [13].

Resistance or muscle-strengthening activities at least 2 days of the week are essential to maintain muscle mass during weight loss. The acquired muscle is not only leaner in size than fat tissue but it also increases metabolic rate. It is beneficial to target all major muscle groups each week [3, 13].

Recommendations are for all adults, but those unable to meet recommendations are encouraged to incorporate what physical activity is achievable. If physical activity is limited, dietary changes have to be more severe to accommodate. The requirement of at least 10 min per session of physical activity has been removed with the current guidelines. Any activity is better than none, and it all adds up. Medical clearance is not required with the exception of those with cardiovascular, metabolic, or renal disease. These patients should be referred to the appropriate provider, but screening should not create a barrier. Starting with small goals and increasing in intensity, duration, or frequency is recommended to reduce the risk of injury or boredom when starting a new exercise routine. Over time, physical fitness will improve to allow for progression and introducing new activities that were not obtainable at baseline. For example, walking can be a good start for anyone, who is sedentary at baseline but desires to run. Where appropriate, referral to an exercise physiologist or a certified fitness professional can be included [13].

Behavioral Interventions

Intensive lifestyle interventions include more than just eating habits/choices and physical activity. Behavioral interventions play a key, but often overlooked, role in weight loss. A pharmacist may assist in general behavioral interventions, but patients will need to be referred for more specialty interventions. Patients should be given the autonomy for self-monitoring of weight, dietary intake, and physical activity through logs or apps and establishing their goals. Ethnic, cultural, socioeconomic factors, and educational background are important to consider when creating goals. The community where a patient lives may offer local resources [3].

Goals should be SMART goals, meaning specific, measurable, attainable, relevant, and time bound. Encouraging highly motivated patients to be more aggressive with goal setting has shown better outcomes. Setting higher goals such as at least 10% weight loss versus only 5–10% led to a greater weight loss in participants [14]. Goals should be intensified if at least 2.5% of weight loss is not achieved within a month to increase risk of long-term success [3].

Education during individual or shared medical appointments through in person or virtual visits should review the pathophysiology and health consequence of obesity, appropriate dietary choices, importance of physical activity, triggers of poor health decisions, problem-solving barriers, and stress reduction. Referral to another health-care provider is recommended when patients would benefit from cognitive behavioral therapy, behavior contracting, and psychosocial counseling, which is outside the scope of a pharmacy [3]. One study showed that mindfulness eating, the practice of paying attention to food without judgment, reduces food cravings and portion sizes [15]. Cognitive behavioral therapy for weight loss increases self-control over food intake and reduces emotional eating [16]. These are just two examples of behavioral interventions that have been shown to promote weight loss.

Bariatric Surgery

Patients with at least class 2 obesity and one severe weight-related complication can be referred for bariatric surgery, though this should generally be done only after lifestyle interventions have been unsuccessful. Patients with class 1 obesity with diabetes or metabolic syndrome can also be considered but data are more limited for this population.

Sleep

The link between sleep disturbances and obesity is well documented in the literature, specifically that of insufficient sleep duration and sleep fragmentation [17–19]. Sleep deprivation has been hypothesized to contribute to alterations in the appetite-regulating hormones, leptin and ghrelin. Leptin, known as a satiety hormone, and ghrelin, commonly referred to as a hunger hormone, have been studied in sleep restriction experiments. Although the results of these experiments varied, many studies found there to be a decrease in leptin levels and an increase in ghrelin levels when sleep was inadequate [19]. Furthermore, studies have failed to demonstrate an increase in energy expenditure during the extended period of wakefulness that one experiences with sleep restriction. Therefore, these changes in appetite regulation, which promote excessive caloric intake, and the lack of increased energy expenditure to counterbalance this, put individuals at a higher risk of obesity [19].

Sleep assessments should be conducted for all patients suspected of having sleep disturbances, especially those with overweight or obesity, and referrals to sleep medicine specialists and behavioral health professionals should be made as indicated. For additional information on sleep assessments, as well as strategies to promote sleep health, refer to Chap. 3: Non-Pharmacological Interventions for Type 2 Diabetes.

Multidisciplinary Teams

A 2019 systematic review of international guidelines concluded that most guidelines advocate for a multidisciplinary team for the treatment of overweight and obesity [20]. The composition of the team can vary to fit the needs of the practice, but teams often include physicians, dieticians, nurses, educators, physical trainers, psychologists, and pharmacists.

Summary and Key Takeaways

All patients should be prescribed therapeutic lifestyle interventions as part of a comprehensive plan to lose and maintain weight. An intensive therapeutic lifestyle plan includes dietary restriction, physical activity, and behavioral interventions. The macronutrient composition of the dietary plan has less impact than the restriction of calories for those with overweight and obesity. Patients adhere best to dietary and physical activity goals that are tailored to patient presences. Pharmacists have the knowledge and skills to participate in multidisciplinary teams to assist patients in obtaining and maintaining healthy body compositions to reduce the risk and burden of weight-related complications.

References

1. World Health Organization. Obesity. Available at https://www.who.int/health-topics/obesity#tab=tab_1. Accessed 9 Dec 2023
2. Centers for Disease Control and Prevention. Overweight and Obesity; 2023. Available at: https://www.cdc.gov/obesity/index.html. Accessed 19 Dec 2023

3. Garvey WT, Mechanick JI, Brett EM, et al. American Association of clinical endocrinologists and American College of endocrinology comprehensive clinical practice guidelines for medical care of patients with obesity. Endocr Pract. 2016;22(Suppl 3):1–203.
4. Pugliese G, Liccardi A, Graziadio C, et al. Obesity and infectious diseases: pathophysiology and epidemiology of a double pandemic condition. Int J Obes. 2022;46:449–65.
5. Jordan MA, Harmon J. Pharmacist interventions for obesity: improving treatment adherence and patient outcomes. Integr Pharm Res Pract. 2015;8(4):79–89.
6. U.S. Department of Agriculture and U.S. Department of Health and Human Services. Dietary Guidelines for Americans, 2020–2025. 9th Edition; 2020. Available at: DietaryGuidelines.gov
7. Cabo R, Mattson M. Effects of intermittent fasting on health, aging, and disease. N Engl J Med. 2019;381:2541–51.
8. Welton S, Minty R, O'Driscoll T, et al. Intermittent fasting and weight loss: systematic review. Can Fam Physician. 2020;66(2):117–25.
9. Atkins. Atkins diet. https://www.atkins.com/how-it-works. Accessed 19 Dec 2023
10. Masood W, Annamaraju P, Khan Suheb MZ, et al. Ketogenic. In: StatPearls. Treasure Island (FL): StatPearls Publishing; 2023. Available from: https://www.ncbi.nlm.nih.gov/books/NBK499830/
11. Obesity Action Coalition. Commercial weight-loss options; 2023. Available at: https://www.obesityaction.org/obesity-treatments/what-is-obesity-treatment/commercial-weight-loss-options/. Accessed 20 Dec 2023
12. Ge L, Sadeghirad B, Ball GDC, et al. Comparison of dietary macronutrient patterns of 14 popular named dietary programmes for weight and cardiovascular risk factor reduction in adults: systematic review and network meta-analysis of randomised trials. BMJ. 2020;369:m696.
13. USDHHS U.S. Department of Health and Human Services. Physical Activity Guidelines for Americans. 2nd ed. Washington: U.S. Department of Health and Human Services; 2018.
14. Wren GM, Koutoukidis DA, Scragg J, Whitman M, Jebb S. The association between goal setting and weight loss: prospective analysis of a community weight loss program. J Med Internet Res. 2023;25:e43869.
15. Dunn C, Haubenreiser M, Johnson M, et al. Mindfulness approaches and weight loss, weight maintenance, and weight regain. Curr Obes Rep. 2018;7(1):37–49.
16. Jacob A, Moullec G, Lavoie KL, et al. Impact of cognitive-behavioral interventions on weight loss and psychological outcomes: a meta-analysis. Health Psychol. 2018;37(5):417–32.
17. Gangwisch JE, Malaspina D, Boden-Albala B, Heymsfield SB. Inadequate sleep as a risk factor for obesity: analyses of the NHANES I. Sleep. 2005;28(10):1289–96.

18. Cappuccio FP, Taggart FM, Kandala NB, et al. Meta-analysis of short sleep duration and obesity in children and adults. Sleep. 2008;31(5):619–26.
19. Reutrakul S, Punjabi NM, Van Cauter E. Chapter 25: impact of sleep and circadian disturbances on glucose metabolism and type 2 diabetes. In: Cowie CC, Casagrande SS, Menke A, et al., editors. Diabetes in America. 3rd ed. Bethesda: National Institute of Diabetes and Digestive and Kidney Diseases; 2018.
20. Semlitsch T, Stigler FL, Jeitler K, Horvath K, Siebenhofer A. Management of overweight and obesity in primary care – a systematic overview of international evidence-based guidelines. Obes Rev. 2019;20(9):1218–30.

Pharmacotherapy 12

Nicole Slater

Managing obesity often warrants pharmacotherapy for many patients to achieve and maintain long-term weight loss [1]. Today, there are several medications available for managing obesity, many of which have become increasingly popular in recent years. Part of the selection process involves the overall assessment of obesity-related comorbidities and the selection of a therapy that will either assist with the comorbidity or not cause additional harm because of that comorbidity. The choice and intensity of obesity interventions vary according to the phase of prevention and treatment, becoming more aggressive and comprehensive as the severity of obesity and its complications increase. Medications for both short- and long-term management are available, but guideline recommendations prioritize long-term therapy because short-term treatment (6 months or less) has not been shown to produce health benefits or sustained weight loss. Pharmacotherapy should be offered to those with obesity for long-term treatment when the potential benefits outweigh the risks [1].

N. Slater (✉)
Department of Pharmacy Practice, Shenandoah University,
Bernard J Dunn School of Pharmacy, Winchester, VA, USA

© The Author(s), under exclusive license to Springer Nature Switzerland AG 2025

J. Clements (ed.), *The Pharmacist's Pocket Guide for Diabetes and Obesity*, https://doi.org/10.1007/978-3-031-88835-9_12

Pharmacotherapy Drug Classes

The available pharmacotherapy options for the management of overweight and obesity are indicated in addition to lifestyle modifications (defined as reduced caloric intake and increased physical activity) [1]. Current guidelines recommend that individuals who have attempted lifestyle modifications and continue to have a body mass index (BMI) ≥ 30 kg/m^2 or ≥ 27 kg/m^2 with an obesity-related comorbidity are eligible for pharmacotherapy [2, 3].

Additionally, the following individuals are also suitable for pharmacotherapy interventions [1]:

- Adults who are motivated to lose weight.
- Adults who have failed to achieve or sustain weight loss with lifestyle interventions alone.
- Adolescents 12 years of age and older with a BMI corresponding to 30 kg/m^2 or greater for adults, which equate to a child being greater than or equal to the 95th percentile for their age.

For overweight and obesity management, the approved medication by the Food and Drug Administration are outlined below [4]. Some of the medications are only approved for short-term use; however, several of the available medications are approved for long-term management (see Table 12.1).

Table 12.1 Pharmacotherapy for short- or long-term use

Short-term use	Long-term use
Phentermine (Adipex-P)	Bupropion with naltrexone extended release (Contrave)
Phendimetrazine (Bontril)	Phentermine with topiramate sustained release (Qsymia)
Diethylpropion (Tenuate)	Orlistat (Xenical, Alli)
	Liraglutide (Saxenda)
	Semaglutide (Wegovy)
	Tirzepatide (Zepbound)

Source: Ref. [4]

- Sympathomimetics are considered for short-term use only and include phentermine, phendimetrazine, and diethylpropion. One additional combination product, marketed for long-term use, includes extended release topiramate plus low-dose phentermine (Qsymia). Topiramate is a carbonic anhydrase inhibitor that decreases appetite and binge-eating behaviors when combined with low-dose phentermine [4].
- Bupropion-naltrexone sustained release combination (Contrave) utilizes two separate medications that have other indications beyond weight loss when used individually. This combination product includes a dopamine/norepinephrine reuptake inhibitor and a mu-opioid receptor antagonist, which when used together helps to decrease appetite and reduce cravings for food [4].
- High-dose glucagon-like peptide-1 (GLP-1) receptor agonists, liraglutide (Saxenda) and semaglutide (Wegovy), are also used in diabetes management at lower doses. This class of medications work to reduce appetite, slow gastric emptying, and improve insulin sensitivity. Additionally, tirzepatide (Zepbound) is a dual GLP-1/GIP (glucose-dependent insulinotropic polypeptide) medication that has recently been approved for long-term management of overweight and obesity as well and acts in a fashion similar to GLP-1 receptor agonist [4].
- Orlistat (Xenical, Alli) is a pancreatic lipase inhibitor that decreases the absorption of dietary fat. Orlistat is approved for long-term use as well but is often limited by its side-effect profile of fecal incontinence, bloating, and anal leakage and is not tolerated by most [4].
- Setmelanotide (Imcivree) is a melanocortin 4 (MC4) receptor agonist approved for long-term use in patients 6 years and older with a genetically confirmed test of proopiomelanocortin (POMC), proprotein convertase subtilisin/kexin type 1 (PCSK1), or leptin receptor (LEPR) deficiency, or for patients with Bardet-Biedl syndrome [4, 5].

Medications approved for short-term use are generally not recommended and have limited clinical utility in practice given that obesity is a long-standing disease that often requires long-term management; however, phentermine (Adipex-P) is often used off-label as a long-term solution in patients without contraindications or those who are able to tolerate it. This has been endorsed by the American Gastroenterology Association (AGA) and mentioned in the American Association of Clinical Endocrinology guidelines as well [1, 2].

Phentermine is a stimulant that increases the release of several neurotransmitters (dopamine, serotonin, norepinephrine) in the brain to reduce appetite, allowing patients to lose weight due to a reduction in overall caloric intake, which is why many patients often regain the weight they lose once phentermine therapy is discontinued. This medication is a federally controlled substance (C-IV) because it does have the ability for misuse and/or cause drug dependence; so, most states have a limitation on how much can be given in a specified time frame. Phentermine is available as both an extended release capsule and as a tablet. The 15- or 30-mg capsule or 37.5-mg tablet is usually taken once a day in the morning, 1–2 hours before breakfast. The immediate release of 8 mg can be taken up to 3 times daily, 30 min before a meal. Both have been shown to have comparable effectiveness [6]. Despite recommendations against phentermine for long-term management, it continues to be one of the most widely prescribed weight-loss medication in select patients due to low cost and lack of serious long-term adverse medication reactions reported over the past 20 years [6, 7]. Pharmacotherapy management guidelines recommend against the use of sympathomimetic agents in patients with uncontrolled hypertension or a history of cardiovascular disease (CVD) [8].

The selection of medications for long-term use should be individualized based on clinical weight loss goals, weight-related comorbidities, as well as medication cautions and contraindications (Table 12.2). Discontinuation should be considered in patients, who fail to lose sufficient amounts of body weight after 3 months and in patients, who experience significant adverse medication reactions. Consider potential alternative weight-loss agents in those who are unable to lose weight or tolerate the initial treatment regimen [8].

Table 12.2 Pharmacotherapy for long-term use

Medication	Dosing	Contraindication(s)	Key adverse reactions	Additional comments
Orlistat (Alli)*	60 mg 3 times daily with each main meal containing fat	Organ transplant or are taking medicine to reduce organ rejection, patients who are taking cyclosporine, and in patients with known problems absorbing food	Stomach cramping Bloating Diarrhea/loose stool Anal leakage/fecal incontinence	*available without a prescription Take during or up to 1 hour after the meal. Omit dose if meal is occasionally missed or contains no fat. Absorption of oral contraceptives may be reduced and may directly interfere with the absorption of other narrow therapeutic range medications, such as cyclosporine, levothyroxine, and antiretrovirals
Orlistat (Xenical)	120 mg 3 times daily with each main meal containing fat	See above	See above	See above

(continued)

Table 12.2 (continued)

Medication	Dosing	Contraindication(s)	Key adverse reactions	Additional comments
Phentermine with topiramate extended release (Qsymia)	3.75 mg phentermine / 23 mg topiramate once daily for 14 days 7.5 mg phentermine / 46 mg topiramate once daily Maximum dose of phentermine 15 mg with topiramate 92 mg once daily	Pregnancy, glaucoma, hyperthyroidism, patients receiving treatment or within 14 days following treatment with monoamine oxidase inhibitors (MAOIs)	Paresthesia Dizziness Dysgeusia Insomnia Constipation Dry mouth	Take in the morning to avoid insomnia Consider limitations in prescribing as it is a controlled substance (C-IV). Taper 15/92 mg dose when discontinuing

Bupropion with naltrexone sustained release (Contrave)	Week 1: 8 mg naltrexone / 90 mg bupropion (1 tablet) once daily in the morning Week 2: 8 mg naltrexone / 90 mg bupropion twice daily (morning and evening) Week 3: 16 mg naltrexone / 180 mg bupropion in the morning and 8 mg naltrexone / 90 mg bupropion in the evening Week 4: 16 mg naltrexone / 180 mg bupropion twice daily (morning and evening)	Uncontrolled high blood pressure, seizures, eating disorder, opioid addiction, pregnancy, concomitant opioids, abrupt discontinuation of alcohol, seizure medication, or a sedative	Nausea Constipation Headache Vomiting Dizziness Insomnia Dry mouth Diarrhea	Bupropion lowers seizure threshold. Naltrexone has a rare report of hepatotoxicity. Consider limitations due to drug interactions with opioids and CYP2D6 substrates / inducers

(continued)

Table 12.2 (continued)

Medication	Dosing	Contraindication(s)	Key adverse reactions	Additional comments
Liraglutide (Saxenda)	Weekly titration schedule: 0.6 mg once daily 1.2 mg once daily 1.8 mg once daily 2.4 mg once daily 3.0 mg once daily	Personal or family history of medullary thyroid carcinoma or in patients with multiple endocrine neoplasia syndrome type 2	Nausea Diarrhea Constipation Vomiting Injection site reaction Headache Hypoglycemia in combination with sulfonylureas or insulin	Utilize proper technique for administration into abdomen, back of the arm, or thigh. Encourage to reduce portion sizes, avoid fatty/greasy/spicy foods, and be mindful of carbonated beverage intake

Semaglutide (Wegovy)	Monthly titration schedule: 0.25 mg once weekly 0.5 mg once weekly 1 mg once weekly 2 mg once weekly 2.4 mg once weekly	Personal or family history of medullary thyroid carcinoma or in patients with multiple endocrine neoplasia syndrome type 2	Nausea Diarrhea Constipation Vomiting Injection site reaction Headache Hypoglycemia when used concomitantly sulfonylureas or insulin	See liraglutide. Reduce dose from 2.4 to 1.7 mg if maximum dose cannot be tolerated

(continued)

Table 12.2 (continued)

Medication	Dosing	Contraindication(s)	Key adverse reactions	Additional comments
Tirzepatide (Zepbound)	Monthly titration schedule: 2.5 mg once weekly 5 mg once weekly 7.5 mg once weekly 10 mg once weekly 12.5 mg once weekly 15 mg once weekly	Personal or family history of medullary thyroid carcinoma or in patients with multiple endocrine neoplasia syndrome type 2	Nausea Diarrhea Vomiting Constipation Abdominal pain Dyspepsia Injection site reactions Hypoglycemia when used concomitantly sulfonylureas or insulin	See liraglutide. Maintenance doses include 5, 10, and 15 mg doses

Sources: Refs. [9, 12, 14, 16, 21, 22]

*Alli

Orlistat (Alli, Xenical) promotes weight loss by inhibiting gastrointestinal lipases, thereby decreasing the absorption of fat from the gastrointestinal tract. On average, 120 mg of orlistat taken 3 times per day will decrease fat absorption by 30%. It is important to note that this medication must be taken within 1 hour of consuming foods that contain fat to exert its effect and patients should be counseled that if they plan to skip a meal or consume a meal that does not contain fat, the dose of orlistat can be skipped [9]. In addition to weight loss, orlistat has also been shown to improve insulin sensitivity and lower serum glucose levels, and can also reduce serum cholesterol, low density lipoprotein (LDL) cholesterol, triglycerides, and apolipoprotein B levels [10, 11]. While orlistat can be quite effective, it also promotes several unwanted side-effects that make this medication quite difficult to tolerate. The main adverse effects include fatty/oily stool, fecal urgency, oily spotting, increased defecation, fecal incontinence, flatulence with discharge, and oily evacuation [11]. Orlistat may also decrease the absorption of other medications as well as fat-soluble vitamins A, D, E, and K, and supplementation with a multivitamin may be required during treatment with orlistat. Orlistat is approved for the chronic treatment of obesity in adults and adolescents between ages 12 and 16 years and can also be purchased over the counter (Alli) by patients 18 years of age and older [9–11].

Phentermine plus topiramate (Qsymia) is a combined, controlled-release tablet that works by increasing norepinephrine (NE) and dopamine neurotransmission, resulting in appetite-suppressing effects, leading to a decrease in food intake. This medication also acts as an adrenergic agonist that activates the sympathetic nervous system to increase energy expenditure, which in turn ultimately burns more calories [12, 13]. The recommended dosing strategy for the phentermine plus topiramate extended-release tablets involves a gradual titration and is available in four doses: 3.75/23 mg (starting dose), 7.5/46 mg (recommended treatment dose), 11.25/69 mg, or 15/92 mg (maximum treatment dose). Likewise, when discontinuing therapy, the dose should be gradually decreased by taking a dose every other day for at least 1 week to prevent the possible development of seizures [13]. This medication can cause insomnia; so, it is recommended that individuals take it in the morning to prevent sleep deprivation and it is also considered to be a federally controlled substance (because of the phentermine component).

Bupropion with naltrexone (Contrave) is a combination tablet with two distinct mechanisms that work together to reduce cravings and appetite [14]. Bupropion is a reuptake inhibitor of dopamine and NE, which enhances activation of the central melanocortin pathways. Naltrexone, an opioid receptor antagonist, and disrupts the mu-opioid receptor's auto-inhibitory feedback on anorexigenic neurons in the hypothalamus that are stimulated by bupropion. This disruption helps sustain the weight-loss effects induced by bupropion and further promote those effects with continued use. Bupropion/naltrexone comes in tablets containing 90 mg of bupropion hydrochloride sustained-release and 8 mg of naltrexone [15]. The recommended starting dose is 1 tablet daily and increasing by 1 tablet each week until a total dose of 2 tablets twice daily is reached (total daily dose: bupropion 360 mg/naltrexone 32 mg) [14].

Semaglutide 2.4 mg (Wegovy) was FDA-approved for the treatment of adult obesity in June 2021 and is a long-acting GLP-1 (glucagon-like peptide-1) receptor agonist that is administered as weekly subcutaneous injections at doses of 0.25, 0.5, 1.0, 1.7, and 2.4 mg [16]. It promotes weight loss through multiple mechanisms including slowed gastric emptying, thereby reducing hunger and energy intake, in addition to direct anorexigenic effects on the brain leading to increased satiety [17]. Semaglutide is also approved for adolescents 12 years of age and older with obesity. The most common side effects noted are nausea, diarrhea, vomiting, and constipation [16]. The efficacy of semaglutide has been studied in those with and without diabetes mellitus and has been associated with the greatest amount of weight loss when compared to all other approved weight-loss medications to date [18]. Additional studies suggest that semaglutide offers superior weight loss compared to other agents like phentermine-topiramate (Qsymia) and naltrexone-bupropion (Contrave), which have reported average weight losses of 7–10% in their respective trials [19, 20].

Liraglutide 3.0 mg (Saxenda) is another GLP-1 agonist that was approved by the FDA in December 2014 for adults as well as adolescents ages 12 and older [21]. Both liraglutide and semaglutide are contraindicated in a personal or family history of medullary thyroid carcinoma or multiple endocrine neoplasia syndrome type 2. Additionally, women of childbearing age should complete a pregnancy test prior to starting semaglutide and be using contraception when in use. Furthermore, semaglutide 2.4 mg should be discontinued at least 2 months prior to conception per manufacturer's recommendation in the package insert [16].

Lastly, tirzepatide, a dual glucose-dependent insulinotrophic peptide (GIP) and GLP-1 receptor agonist, has shown the greatest efficacy for weight loss compared to all other obesity medications listed above [22]. In the SURMOUNT-1 trial, participants treated with tirzepatide achieved significant weight reductions, with the average weight loss ranging from 15% to 22.5% (dose dependent) of their body weight over 72 weeks [23–25]. This degree of weight loss is greater than what has been observed with other agents, even semaglutide, which in the STEP trials resulted in an average weight loss of about 15% of body weight at the 2.4 mg dose [18, 26]. The efficacy of tirzepatide in achieving such substantial weight loss marks it as a potential game-changer in obesity management, offering new hope for patients, who struggle with achieving meaningful weight reductions with existing therapies.

Overall, pharmacotherapy has demonstrated significant efficacy in the management of obesity, as evidenced by numerous clinical trials. Long-term outcomes from these studies suggest that sustained weight loss can be achieved, particularly when pharmacotherapy is combined with ongoing lifestyle interventions. However, the durability of weight loss varies among medications, with some patients experiencing weight regain upon discontinuation, which is why it is imperative to also utilize lifestyle changes alongside of pharmacotherapy that can help someone achieve and sustain long-term weight loss [1].

Patient Selection and Individualization of Therapy

Selecting the appropriate candidates for pharmacotherapy in obesity management is crucial for achieving optimal outcomes. As stated above, pharmacotherapy is recommended for adult patients with a BMI $\geq$30 kg/m^2 or $\geq$ 27 kg/m^2 in the presence of obesity-related comorbidities. Individualized therapy should be prioritized based on the clinical characteristics and obesity-related disease states that a patient may have at the time of therapy initiation. Pharmacotherapy is also recommended when lifestyle interventions alone have not been sufficient to achieve weight loss over time. Individualizing treatment involves considering the patient's unique health profile, preferences, and potential risks. Any medication selected for individuals trying to lose weight should be selected based on their overall efficacy, side-effect profile, and the presence of any contraindications. Special populations require additional consideration: pediatric patients may benefit from lifestyle modifications as first-line treatment, with pharmacotherapy reserved for severe cases; geriatric patients may need therapies that avoid exacerbating age-related conditions like osteoporosis or cardiovascular disease; and individuals with comorbidities such as diabetes might benefit from medications like GLP-1 receptor agonists, which offer both weight loss and glycemic control. Careful monitoring and regular reassessment ensure that the chosen therapy continues to align with the patient's evolving needs and health status and ensures consistent and sustained weight loss over time.

Conclusion

Overall, pharmacotherapy for overweight and obesity is a valuable tool for individuals struggling with weight loss, particularly when tailored to individual needs and used as part of a comprehensive treatment plan. It is important to weigh the risks and benefits before choosing a medication therapy and ensuring that the chosen therapy will aid in long-term overall health and wellness.

References

1. Garvey WT, Mechanick JI, Brett EM, et al. American Association of Clinical Endocrinologists and American College of endocrinology comprehensive clinical practice guidelines for medical care of patients with obesity. Endocr Pract. 2016;22(Suppl 3):1–203.
2. Grunvald E, Shah R, Hernaez R, et al. AGA clinical practice guideline on pharmacological interventions for adults with obesity. Gastroenterology. 2022;163(5):1198–225.
3. Jensen MD, Ryan DH, Apovian CM, American College of Cardiology/American Heart Association Task Force on Practice Guidelines; Obesity Society, et al. 2013 AHA/ACC/TOS guideline for the management of overweight and obesity in adults: a report of the American College of Cardiology/American Heart Association Task Force on Practice Guidelines and The Obesity Society. J Am Coll Cardiol. 2014;63(25 Part B):2985–3023.
4. Tchang BG, Aras M, Kumar RB, et al. Pharmacologic treatment of overweight and obesity in adults. [Updated 2021 Aug 2]. In: Feingold KR, Anawalt B, Blackman MR, et al. . Endotext [Internet]. South Dartmouth (MA): MDText.com, Inc; 2000. Available from: https://www.ncbi.nlm.nih.gov/books/NBK279038/#
5. Imcivree (Setmelanotide) [package insert]. Boston, MA: Rhythm Pharmaceuticals, Inc; 2021.
6. Saunders KH, Umashanker D, Igel L, et al. Obesity pharmacotherapy. Med Clin N Am. 2018;102:135–48.
7. Velazquez A, Apovian CM. Update on obesity pharmacotherapy. Ann N Y Acad Sci. 2018;1411:106–19.
8. Apovian CM, Aronne LJ, Bessesen DH, et al. Pharmacological management of obesity: an endocrine society clinical practice guideline. J Clin Endocrinol Metab. 2015;100(2):342–62.
9. Xenical (Orlistat) [package insert]. South San Francisco, CA: Genentech USA, Inc.; 2019.
10. Yanovski SZ, Yanovski JA. Long-term drug treatment for obesity: a systematic and clinical review. JAMA. 2014;311(1):74–86.
11. Sahebkar A, Simental-Mendia LE, Reiner Z, et al. Effect of orlistat on plasma lipids and body weight: a systematic review and meta-analysis of 33 randomized controlled trials. Pharmacol Res. 2017;122:53–65.
12. Qsymia (phentermine and Topiramate extended-release). [package insert]. Mountain View, CA: VIVUS, Inc.; 2020.
13. Hirsch J, Mackintosh RM, Aronne LJ. The effects of drugs used to treat obesity on the autonomic nervous system. Obes Res. 2000;8(3):227–33.
14. Contrave (naltrexone and bupropion) [package insert]. La Jolla, CA: Currax Pharmaceuticals LLC; 2020.

15. Yanovski SZ, Yanovski JA. Naltrexone extended-release plus bupropion extended-release for treatment of obesity. JAMA. 2015;313(12):1213–4. https://doi.org/10.1001/jama.2015.1617.
16. Novo Nordisk. Wegovy (semaglutide 2.4mg) [package insert]. Plainsboro, NJ; 2021.
17. Knudsen LB, Lau J. The discovery and development of Liraglutide and Semaglutide. Front Endocrinol (Lausanne). 2019;10:155.
18. Wilding JPH, Batterham RL, Calanna S, et al. Once-weekly semaglutide in adults with overweight or obesity. N Engl J Med. 2021;384:989–1002. https://doi.org/10.1056/NEJMoa2032183.
19. Rubino DM, Greenway FL, Khalid U, et al. Effect of semaglutide 2.4 mg once-weekly on body weight in adults with overweight or obesity: STEP 8. Diabetes Obes Metab. 2023;25(3):663–74.
20. Kushner RF, Bray GA, Ryan DH, et al. Clinical experience with lorcaserin: comparative weight loss in patients treated with phentermine/topiramate, lorcaserin, and liraglutide. Obesity (Silver Spring). 2018;26(6):1075–81.
21. Saxenda (Liraglutide) [package insert]. Plainsboro, NJ: Novo Nordisk Inc.; 2020.
22. Zepbound (tirzepatide) [package insert]. East Hanover, NJ: Novartis Pharmaceuticals Corporation; 2023.
23. Jastreboff AM, Aronne LJ, Ahmad NN, et al. Tirzepatide once weekly for the treatment of obesity. N Engl J Med. 2022;387(3):205–16.
24. Frias JP, Davies MJ, Rosenstock J, et al. Tirzepatide versus semaglutide once weekly in patients with type 2 diabetes. N Engl J Med. 2021;385(6):503–15.
25. Rubino DM, Greenway FL, Khalid U, et al. Effect of tirzepatide once-weekly on body weight in adults with overweight or obesity: SURMOUNT-1. Diabetes Obes Metab. 2022;24(11):2101–12.
26. Pi-Sunyer X, Astrup A, Fujioka K, et al. A randomized, controlled trial of 3.0 mg of liraglutide in weight management. N Engl J Med. 2015;373(1):11–22.

Management of Comorbid Conditions

13

Cynthia M. Phillips

Introduction

The chronic condition of obesity is a multifaceted disease state associated with various comorbidities. According to 2024 data, a body mass index (BMI) of ≥25 kg/m^2 contributes to death related to cardiovascular disease (CVD), stroke, diabetes, and cancer in around 4 million adults yearly [1]. Historically, clinical practice guidelines have identified the need for weight loss in individual with a BMI of 25–29.9 kg/m^2 and at risk for CVD or those with a BMI ≥ 30 kg/m^2 [2–4]. Various assessment methods can be conducted at baseline and subsequent visits to assess weight loss; as a marker of body fat, waist circumference is important to identify mortality risk [5].

The 2013 American Heart Association/American College of Cardiology/the Obesity Society Guideline for Overweight and Obesity emphasized that individuals classified as overweight or are living with obesity, hypertension, dyslipidemia, prediabetes, diabetes or other weight-related comorbidities should be

C. M. Phillips (✉)
Department of Clinical Pharmacy and Outcomes Sciences,
University of South Carolina College of Pharmacy, Columbia, SC, USA
e-mail: phillips@cop.sc.edu

© The Author(s), under exclusive license to Springer Nature Switzerland AG 2025

J. Clements (ed.), *The Pharmacist's Pocket Guide for Diabetes and Obesity*, https://doi.org/10.1007/978-3-031-88835-9_13

intensively managed with comprehensive lifestyle intervention as well as pharmacotherapy [3]. The American Association of Clinical Endocrinology/American College of Endocrinologists Comprehensive Clinical Practice Guidelines for Medical Care of Patients with Obesity identified that a weight loss of 10%–15% is needed for improvement in clinical goals of therapy for comorbidities in persons with existing overweight or obesity [4]. While a myriad of comorbidities affects body systems in the person who is overweight or obese, clinical trials typically underrepresent this demographic [2]. Therefore, clinical practice guidelines for the management of common disease states typically focus on individuals represented within clinical trials. Guidelines for the management of obesity address medical decision-making for comorbid conditions and scientific statements may focus on specific comorbid conditions in people living with obesity [3–5]. The risks and benefits of pharmacological treatment in overweight, obesity, and associated comorbidities are increasingly important [6]. Pharmacists involved in chronic disease management should be aware of treatment options for obesity with associated comorbidities as well as how those medications may contribute to weight gain and other adverse effects in this patient population [7].

Cardiovascular Disease

Obesity is a well-known risk factor in CVD. The Dallas Heart Study highlighted that increased visceral fat tissue is independently related to an increase in CVD [8]. Researchers note that CVD contributes to at least 41% of deaths in people living with obesity [9]. Nonpharmacological recommendations for cardiovascular comorbidities identify weight loss through healthy eating choices and physical activity [10]. Standards of care for CVD prioritize outcomes with pharmacological treatment; clinical trials investigating the benefits of weight loss medications incorporate disease state markers corresponding to cardiovascular benefits [11, 12].

Hypertension

Visceral adiposity modifies mechanisms involved in the maintenance of normal blood pressure. Alterations in insulin sensitivity, renal sodium absorption, the sympathetic nervous system, and the renin-angiotensin-aldosterone system can increase blood pressure [13, 14]. Physical compression of the kidneys by intrarenal fat and structural changes in the vasculature also contribute to elevations in blood pressure [5–16]. There is a strong relationship between a decrease in waist-to-hip ratio and the development of hypertension [16].

Weight loss medications (also known as antiobesity medications) can vary in their effects on blood pressure markers. Heart rate should be monitored when using phentermine with topiramate extended release (ER) and naltrexone with bupropion ER [4]. Short-term use of antiobesity medications, such as orlistat and phentermine with topiramate, is associated with a 1–3 mm Hg mean change in systolic blood pressure [17]. While the use of naltrexone with bupropion is associated with weight loss of 4%, it can result in a mean increase in 2 mm Hg in systolic blood pressure [17]. The use of glucagon-like peptide-1 (GLP-1) receptor agonists is associated with greater reductions of weight as well as mean change in blood pressure; for every 1 kg of weight lost, there is an associated drop of 1 mmHg in blood pressure measurement [16, 17].

The treatment of obesity-related hypertension in individuals who are overweight or have obesity should not only incorporate medications that address expected pathophysiological targets but also consider the contributions of weight-related adverse effects [16, 18]. Nevertheless, large clinical trials that investigate the benefits of a targeted approach to hypertension in the overweight or obese are lacking [16]. Angiotensin converting enzyme inhibitors (ACEi), angiotensin II receptor blockers (ARBs), and calcium channel blockers (CCBs) target the physiological contributions without the metabolic consequences associated with thiazides, thiazide-like diuretics, or beta blockers [15].

Dyslipidemia

In regards to obesity, the dyslipidemia profile of an individual with a higher body weight or living with obesity is characterized by normal to moderately elevated low-density lipoprotein (LDL); other changes in the lipid panel include increased small dense LDL, decreased high-density lipoprotein (HDL), and increased triglycerides [19]. Atherogenic alterations reflect insulin resistance and inflammation associated with adipokines [10, 20, 21]. Central adiposity is also associated with increased cardiometabolic risk [18]. In addition, risk enhancers of atherosclerotic cardiovascular disease (ASCVD) include metabolic syndrome, which is associated with at least three of the following risk factors: increased waist circumference, elevated triglycerides, low HDL, elevated blood pressure, and/or increased serum glucose [18].

Established guidelines do address alterations in LDL as well as increased triglycerides in the non-HDL measurement [22, 23]. Therapy for dyslipidemia in individuals with obesity should follow evidence-based guidelines to lower the risk for ASCVD [20, 24]. Lifestyle modifications that focus on weight loss are prioritized in the recommendations. Those individuals who are between 20 and 39 years of age are encouraged to maintain a lifestyle that involves heart-healthy eating as well as regular physical activity [18]. Healthy lifestyle habits continue to be essential for those aged 40–75 for primary prevention as well as those with established ASCVD. For individuals with hypertriglyceridemia, lifestyle modifications are encouraged for individuals living with obesity [18]. A weight reduction of 5% or more can reduce triglyceride levels; in a meta-analysis, lifestyle interventions resulting in a 1 kg weight loss are associated with a 4 mg/dL decrease in triglycerides [21, 24]. The greater the weight loss, the greater reductions in triglycerides [21].

The effects of antiobesity medications on lipid profiles demonstrate greater reductions in the lipid profile than lifestyle modifications alone. Phentermine with topiramate and naltrexone with bupropion do demonstrate reductions in triglycerides, decreases in LDL-C, and increases in HDL. Liraglutide, semaglutide, and tirzepatide result in more pronounced decreases in lipid levels due to more substantial weight loss [21].

Coronary Artery Disease

Adipose tissue is involved in endocrine functions, such as lipid and glucose metabolism and immune functions involving cytokines. Atherosclerosis, endothelial dysfunction, and insulin resistance can develop with dysregulation of adipose tissue [21]. Structural and hemodynamic changes occur because of fat accumulation around body organs and within the cardiovascular system compounding the risk of coronary artery disease [25]. The resulting alterations with dyslipidemia, hypertension, and altered glucose metabolism create an environment for the development of atherosclerosis [21].

With the development of incretin mimetics, significant changes in cardiovascular outcomes were observed in people with type 2 diabetes mellitus (T2D) [26]. Cardiovascular outcomes trials for GLP-1 receptor agonists in people with T2D demonstrate clinically significant improvements in the three-point major adverse cardiovascular events (MACE) of a composite endpoint (cardiovascular death, nonfatal myocardial infarction, nonfatal stroke) [26]. Certain GLP-1 receptor agonists (e.g., liraglutide, semaglutide, dulaglutide) are now considered first-line therapies for individuals with T2D with high risk for or have existing ASCVD [27].

Liraglutide was approved in 2010 as an adjunct to diet and exercise for the treatment of T2D [28]. As a GLP-1 receptor agonist, researchers saw significant weight reduction associated with liraglutide in people with T2D in the Liraglutide Effect and Action in Diabetes Studies (LEAD) [29]. Liraglutide was the first GLP-1 receptor agonist to receive approval specifically for weight loss in 2014 [28]. The SCALE (Satiety and Clinical Adiposity-Liraglutide Evidence) trials investigated liraglutide's effects on change in body weight in those individuals who were overweight or obesity with and without T2D [12, 30]. Glycemic and cardiometabolic variables (e.g., change in A1C, fasting glucose, blood pressure, lipid panel) demonstrated greater improvement within the liraglutide group compared to the placebo groups over the 56-week trial for those individuals without T2D [12, 30]. The Liraglutide Effect and Action in Diabetes: Evaluation of Cardiovascular Outcome Results (LEADER) trial demonstrated cardiovascular benefits for people with T2D [31]. A post hoc analysis of the SCALE trials demonstrated that a liraglutide 3.0 mg dose was not associated with excess cardiovascular risk for the primary composite outcome of the first occurrence of cardiovascular death, nonfatal myocardial infarction, or nonfatal stroke [32].

Injectable semaglutide was approved for the treatment of T2D in 2017 and weight loss in 2021 [28]. Injectable semaglutide at doses of 0.5 or 1 mg demonstrated cardiovascular benefit for those individuals with T2D for the primary outcome of the first occurrence of cardiovascular death, nonfatal myocardial infarction, or nonfatal stroke in the SUSTAIN-6 trial (Trial to Evaluate Cardiovascular and Other Long-term Outcomes with Semaglutide in Subjects with Type 2 Diabetes) [33]. Statistically significant changes for decrease in body weight occurred in the treatment arm [33]. The STEP (Semaglutide Treatment Effect in People) trials investigated subcutaneous semaglutide and its benefits on weight loss [34]. For example, the STEP 1 trial included people living with obesity or those who were overweight with a weight-related condition (no diabetes). Participants receiving semaglutide experienced statistically significant benefits for the co-primary outcomes of mean change in body weight and weight reduction of 5% in the treatment group in STEP 1. Individuals randomized to the treatment group also exhibited benefits in cardiometabolic risk factors such as decreases in blood pressure, lipid levels, and A1C [34].

Additional studies were designed to investigate the cardiovascular benefits of injectable semaglutide 2.4 mg in adult individuals who were overweight without diabetes but with preexisting heart disease. The primary endpoint of composite death from cardiovascular causes, nonfatal myocardial infarction, and nonfatal stroke was reduced by 20% in those individuals receiving the injectable semaglutide 2.4 mg weekly over a mean duration of 33 months [35]. Researchers noted that the benefits of those in the trial with prediabetes (approximately two-thirds of participants) were noteworthy and should spur a greater therapeutic focus in this patient population [35].

Tirzepatide, a glucose-dependent insulinotropic polypeptide (GIP) and GLP-1 receptor agonist was approved for the treatment of T2D in conjunction with diet and exercise in May 2022 [36]. The SURPASS trials investigated tirzepatide in a variety of patients who were newly diagnosed with T2D as monotherapy, persons with T2D inadequately controlled on other anti-diabetic agents, or with insulin [37]. Dose-dependent reductions in the primary endpoint of A1C occurred with each of the tirzepatide treatment arms. Clinically significant weight loss occurred with each of the treatment arms across the trials in persons with T2D [37]. As with other incretin mimetics, tirzepatide demonstrated benefits for weight loss in the SURPASS trials.

The SURPASS-CVOT trial is an ongoing trial investigating the cardiovascular benefits of tirzepatide titrated to 15 mg once weekly versus dulaglutide 1.5 mg once weekly in persons with T2D with a BMI of ≥ 25 kg/m^2, age 40 or older with established ASCVD. The trial's primary outcome is the first event of a major adverse cardiovascular event (MACE) [38].

Injectable tirzepatide, dosed at 5, 10, or 15 mg once weekly over 72 weeks versus placebo, was investigated in persons without diabetes and with BMI $\geq$ 30 kg/m^2 or $\geq$ 27 kg/m^2 and one weight-related symptom (sleep apnea, hypertension, hyperlipidemia, or cardiovascular) in the SURMOUNT trials. The co-primary endpoints were changes in body weight from baseline and 5% or more weight loss at week 72 [39]. Individuals receiving tirzepatide 5–15 mg doses experienced a mean percentage change in weight from −15.0% to −20.9% as compared to −3.1% with placebo. A statistically significant difference was observed between the tirzepatide arm (5% or more) and placebo (35%) for those experiencing 5% or more weight loss at week 72. Prespecified cardiometabolic measures including waist circumference, systolic blood pressure, fasting insulin, and lipid levels were assessed. Waist circumference decreased by −14.0 cm in the 5 mg tirzepatide group, −17.7 cm in the 10 mg tirzepatide group, and − 18.5 cm in the tirzepatide 15 mg group compared to

−4.0 cm in the placebo group. Pooled tirzepatide groups (5, 10, and 15 mg doses) showed decreases in the following measures from baseline: −7.2 mmHg decrease in systolic blood pressure, −4.8 mmHg decrease in diastolic blood pressure, −24.8 mg/dL percent change in triglycerides, and an increase of 8.0 mg/dL percent change in HDL cholesterol [39].

A post hoc analysis of the SURMOUNT-1 trial was conducted to assess tirzepatide's effect on the risk for atherosclerotic heart disease. Researchers calculated the baseline, week 24, and week 72 10-year ASCVD risk scores using the American College of Cardiology/American Heart Association scoring system for the various treatment arms of tirzepatide 5, 10, 15 mg, and placebo. Those with existing CVD were excluded. Risk scores for all groups were categorized into low (<5.0%), borderline (5.0 to <7.5%), intermediate (≥7.5% to <20.0%), and high (≥20.0%). While most individuals were in the low-risk category (80.4%), the borderline (8.6%) and intermediate (10.0%) groups were similar in distribution. The relative change in risk score with tirzepatide treatment for the intermediate to high-risk groups at week 24 was −22.2% to −16.05% compared to the placebo at −0.7%. The indirect measure of cardiometabolic risk reduction identifies the benefit of tirzepatide over the length of the study [40].

Congestive Heart Failure

Risk factors for congestive heart failure include hypertension, CVD, and left ventricular hypertrophy, for which obesity is a risk factor [5]. Persons with overweight and obesity develop heart failure with preserved ejection fraction (HFpEF) to a greater degree [5]. A distinct phenotype of heart failure with preserved ejection fraction is identified with obesity [41]. Individuals with obesity-related HFpEF possess larger left and right ventricles, higher right atrium (RA) pressures, higher pulmonary capillary wedge pressures (PCWPs), and higher epicardial fat thickness [41]. Yet, an obesity paradox exists, as those with heart failure with reduced ejection fraction (HFrEF) have better outcomes than those with normal weight [5].

The STEP HFpEF trial investigated obesity-related heart failure in patients without diabetes using subcutaneously administered semaglutide 2.4 mg or a matching placebo with standard of care. Individuals included those with left ventricular ejection fraction (LVEF) ≥45%, BMI ≥ 30 kg/m^2, New York Heart Association (NYHA) functional class II–IV, and no diabetes. Medication effect on symptoms, physical limitations, and body weight compared to placebo demonstrated improved symptoms and physical limitations as assessed by the Kansas City Cardiomyopathy Questionnaire Clinical Summary Score (KCCQ-CSS) and decreased body weight and inflammation. Researchers identified that the combination of the standard of care with sodium glucose cotransporter 2 (SGLT2) inhibitors and GLP-1 receptor agonists would benefit those with the obesity-related phenotype of HFpEF [42].

At the time of writing this chapter, ongoing trials are investigating tirzepatide in persons with a BMI ≥ 30 kg/m^2 and HFpEF in the Study of Tirzepatide in Participants with Heat Failure with Preserved Ejection Fraction and Obesity (SUMMIT) and in those with overweight and obesity with or at high risk for cardiovascular conditions in the Study of Tirzepatide on the Reduction on Morbidity and Mortality in Adults with Obesity (SURMOUNT-NMO) [43].

Conclusion

The management of obesity and its associated comorbidities requires a comprehensive and collaborative approach. Pharmacists are integral, providing medication management, patient education, and support for lifestyle modifications. By optimizing pharmacotherapy and ensuring adherence to treatment plans, pharmacists can significantly improve patient outcomes. Pharmacists can help address the unique needs of each patient living with obesity, including comorbid conditions, to enhance their quality of life and overall health.

References

1. World Obesity Federation. World obesity atlas 2024. World Obesity Federation. 2024. [Internet]. 2024 [cited 2024 July 2024]. Available from https://data.worldobesity.org/publications/?cat=22. p 8.
2. Pagarkar D, Harrop E, Erlanger L. How should we approach body size diversity in clinical trials? AMA J Ethics. 2023;25(7):E517–27. https://doi.org/10.1001/amajethics.2023.517.
3. Donato KA, Hu FB, Hubbard VS, Jakicic JM, Kushner RF, Loria CM, Millen BE, Nonas CA, Pi-Sunyer FX, Stevens J, Stevens VJ, Wadden TA, Wolfe BM, Yanovski SZ. 2013 AHA/ACC/TOS guideline for the management of overweight and obesity in adults: a report of the American College of Cardiology/American Heart Association task force on practice guidelines and the Obesity Society. Circulation. 2014;129(Suppl 2):S102–38.
4. Garvey WT, Mechanick JI, Brett EM, Garber AJ, Hurley DL, Jastreboff AM, Nadolsky K, Pessah-Pollack R, Plodkowski R. Reviewers of the AACE/ ACE obesity clinical practice guidelines. American association of clinical endocrinologists and American college of endocrinology comprehensive clinical practice guidelines for medical care of patients with obesity. Endocr Pract. 2016;22(Suppl 3):1–203. https://doi.org/10.4158/EP161365.GL.
5. Powell-Wiley TM, Poirier P, Burke LE, Després JP, Gordon-Larsen P, Lavie CJ, Lear SA, Ndumele CE, Neeland IJ, Sanders P, St-Onge MP. Obesity and cardiovascular disease: a scientific statement from the American Heart Association. Circulation. 2021;143(21):e984–e1010. https://doi.org/10.1161/CIR.0000000000000973.
6. Guglielmi V, Bettini S, Sbraccia P, Busetto L, Pellegrini M, Yumuk V, Colao AM, El Ghoch M, Muscogiuri G. Beyond weight loss, added benefits could guide the choice of anti-obesity medications. Curr Obes Rep. 2023;12:127–46. https://doi.org/10.1007/s13679-023-00502-7.
7. Clements JN, Albanese NP, D'Souza JJ, Mishner A, Reece S, Trujillo J, Whitely HP. Clinical review and role of clinical pharmacists in obesity management: An opinion of the endocrine and metabolism practice and research network of the American College of Clinical Pharmacy. J Am Col Clin Pharm. 2021;4:1469–84. https://doi.org/10.1002/jac5.1512.
8. Victor RG, Haley RW, Willett DL, Peshock RM, Vaeth PC, Leonard D, Basit M, Cooper RS, Iannacchione VG, Visscher WA, Staab JM, Hobbs HH. The Dallas heart study: a population-based probablilty sample for the multidisciplinary study of ethnic differences in cardiovascular health. Am J Cardiol. 2004;93:1473. 10.1016/j.amjcard.2004.02.058
9. Afshin A, Forouzanfar MH, Reitsma MB, Sur P, Estep K, Lee A, Marczak L, Mokdad AH, Moradi-Lakeh M, Naghavi M, et al. Health effects of overweight and obesity in 195 countries over 25years. N Engl J Med. 2017;377:13–27. https://doi.org/10.1056/NEJMoa1614362.

10. Grundy SM, Stone NJ, Bailey AL, Beam C, Birtcher KK, Blumenthal RS, Braun LT, de Ferranti S, Faiella-Tommasino J, Forman DE, Goldberg R, Heidenreich PA, Hlatky MA, Jones DW, Lloyd-Jones D, Lopez-Pajares N, Ndumele CE, Orringer CE, Peralta CA, Saseen JJ, Smith SC Jr, Sperling L, Virani SS, Yeboah J. 2018 AHA/ACC/AACVPR/AAPA/ABC/ACPM/ADA/AGS/APhA/ASPC/NLA/PCNA guideline on the management of blood cholesterol: a report of the American College of Cardiology/American Heart Association task force on clinical practice guidelines. Circulation. 2019;139:e1082–143. https://doi.org/10.1161/CIR.0000000000000625.
11. Heidenreich PA, Bozkurt B, Aguilar D, Allen LA, Byun J, Colvin MM, Deswai A, Drazner MH, Dunlay SM, Evers LR, Fang JC, Fedson SE, Fonarow GC, Hayek SS, Hernandez AF, Khaznie P, Kittleson MM, Lee CS, Link MS, Milano CA, Nnacheta LC, Sandhu AT, Stevenson LW, Vardeny O, Vest AR, Yancy CW. 2022 AHA/ AA/ HFSA guideline for the management of heart failure: a report of the American College of Carediology/ American heart Asociation joint committee on clinical practice guidelines. Circulation. 2022;145:e895–e1032. https://doi.org/10.1161/CIR.0000000000001063.
12. Michos ED, Lopez-Jimenez F, Gulati M, MD, MS. Role of glucagon-like peptide-1 receptor agonists in achieving weight loss and improving cardiovascular outcomes in people with overweight and obesity. J Am Heart Assoc. 2023;12:e029282. https://doi.org/10.1161/JAHA.122.029282.
13. Landsberg L, Aronne LJ, Beilin LJ, Burke V, Igel LI, Lloyd-Jones D, Sowers J. Obesity-related hypertension: pathogenesis, cardiovascular risk, and treatment. J Clin Hypertens. 2013;15:14–33. https://doi.org/10.1111/jch.12049.
14. Parvanova A, Reseghetti E, Abbate M, Ruggenenti P. Mechanisms and treatment of obesity related hypertension-part 1: mechanisms. Clin Kidney J. 2024;17:1–18. https://doi.org/10.1093/ckj/sfad282.
15. Shams E, Kamalumpundi V, Peterson J, Gismondi RA, Oigman W, de Gusmao Correia ML. Highlights of mechanisms and treatment of obesity related hypertesnon. J Hum Hypertens. 2022;36:785–93. https://doi.org/10.1038/s41371-021-00644-y.
16. Whelton PK, Carey RM, Aronow WS, Casey DE Jr, Collins KJ, Dennison Himmelfarb C, DePalma SM, Gidding S, Jamerson KA, Jones DW, MacLaughlin EJ, Muntner P, Ovbiagele B, Smith SC Jr, Spencer CC, Stafford RS, Taler SJ, Thomas RJ, Williams KA Sr, Williamson JD, Wright JT Jr. 2017 ACC/AHA/AAPA/ABC/ACPM/AGS/APhA/ASH/ASPC/NMA/PCNA guideline for the prevention, detection, evaluation, and management of high blood pressure in adults: a report of the American College of Cardiology/American Heart Association task force on clinical practice guidelines. J Am Coll Cardiol. 2018;71:e127–248.

17. Hall ME, Cohen JB, Ard JD, Egan BM, Hall JE, Laive CJ, Ma J, Ndumele CE, Schuaer PR, Shimbo D. Weight-loss strategies for prevention and treatment of hypertension. Hypertension. 2021;78:e38–50. https://doi.org/10.1161/HYP.0000000000000202l.
18. Nussbaumerova B, Rosolova H. Obesity and dyslipidemia. Curr Atheroscler Rep. 2023;25:947–55. https://doi.org/10.1007/s11883-023-01167-2.
19. Vekic J, Zeljkovic A, Stefanovic A, Jelic-Ivanovic A, Spasojevic-Kalimanovska V. Obesity and dydlipidemia. Metabolism Clinical and Experimental. 2019;92:71–81. https://doi.org/10.1016/j.metabol.2018.11.00.
20. Franssen R, Monajemi H, Stroes ESG, JJP K. Obesity and dyslipidemia. Med Clin North Am. 2011;95:893–902. https://doi.org/10.1016/j.mcna.2011.06.003.
21. Bays HE, Toth PP, Kris-Etherton PM, Abate N, Aronne LJ, Brown WV, Gonzalez-Campoy JM, Jones SR, Kumar R, La Forge R, Samuel VT. Obesity, adiposity and dyslipidemia: a consensus statement from the National Lipid Association. J Clin Lipidol. 2013;7:304–83. https://doi.org/10.1016/j.jacl.2013.04.001.
22. Arnett DK, Blumenthal RS, Albert MA, Buroker AB, Goldberger ZD, Hahn EJ, Himmelfarb CD, Khera A, Lloyd-Jones D, McEvoy JW, Michos ED, Miedema MD, Muñoz D, Smith SC Jr, Virani SS, Williams KA Sr, Yeboah J, Ziaeian B. 2019 ACC/AHA guideline on the primary prevention of cardiovascular disease: executive summary: a report of the American College of Cardiology/American Heart Association task force on clinical practice guidelines. Circulation. 2019;140:e563–95. https://doi.org/10.1161/CIR.0000000000000677.
23. Lloyd-Jones DM, Morris PB, Ballantyne CM, Birtcher KK, Covington AM, DePalma SM, Minissian MB, Orringer CE, Smith SC Jr, Waring AA, Wilkins JT. 2022 ACC expert consensus decision pathway on the role of nonstatin therapies for LDL-cholesterol lowering in the management of atherosclerotic cardiovascular disease risk: a report of the American College of Cardiology Solution set Oversight Committee. J Am Coll Cardiol. 2022;80:1366–418. https://doi.org/10.1016/j.jacc.2022.07.006.
24. Hasan B, Nayfeh T, Alzuabi M, Wang Z, Kuchkuntla AR, Prokop LJ, Newman CB, Murad MH, Rajjo TI. Journal of Clinical Endocrinology & Metabolism. 2020;105(12):3695–703. https://doi.org/10.1210/clinem/dgaa673.
25. Chandrasekaran P, Wieskirchen R. The signaling pathways in obesity-related complications. J Cell Commun. Signal. 2024;18:E12039. https://doi.org/10.1002/ccs3.12039.
26. Marx N, Husain M, Lehrke M, Verma S, Sattar N. GLP-1 receptor agonists for the reduction of atherosclerotic cardiovascular risk in patients with type 2 diabetes. Circulation. 2022;146:1882–94. https://doi.org/10.1161/CIRCULATIONAHA.122.059595.

27. American Diabetes Association Professional Practice Commitee. Pharmacologic approaches to glycemic treatment-standards of care in diabetes-2024. Diabetes Care. 2024;47(1):S158–78. https://doi.org/10.2337/dc24-S009.
28. Elmaleh-Sachs A, Schwartz JL, Gramante CT, Nicklas JM, Gudzune KA, Jay M. Obesity Management in Adults. JAMA. 2023;330(20):2000–25. https://doi.org/10.1001/jama.2023.19897.
29. Blonde L, Rusell-Jones D. The safety and efficacy of liraglutide with or without antidiabetic drug therapy in type 2 diabetes: an overview of the LEAD 1-5 studies. Diabetes Obes Metab. 2009;11:26–34. https://doi.org/10.1111/j.1463-1326.2009.01075.x.
30. Pi-Sunyer A, Astrup A, Fujioka K, Greenway F, Halpern A, Krempf M, Lau DCW, le Roux CW, Ortiz RV, Jensen BB, Wilding JPH. A randomized controlled trial of 3.0 mg of liraglutide in weight management. N Engl J Med. 2015;373:11–22. https://doi.org/10.1056/NEJMoa1411892.
31. Marso SP, Daniels GH, Brown-Frandsen K, Kristensen P, Mann JFE, Nauck MA, Nissen SE, Pocock S, Poulter NR, Ravn LS, Steinberg WM, Stockner M, Zinman B, Bergenstal RM, Buse JB. Liraglutide and cardiovascular outcomes in type 2 diabetes. N Engl J Med. 2016;375:311–22. https://doi.org/10.1056/NEJMoa1603827.
32. Davies MJ, Aronne LJ, Caterson ID, Thomsen AB, Jacobsen PB, Marso SP. Liraglutide and cardiovascular outcomes in adults with overweight or obesity: a post hoc analysis from SCALE randomized controlled trials. Diabetes Obes Metab. 2018;20:734–9. https://doi.org/10.1111/dom.13125.
33. Marso SP, Bain SC, Consoli A, Eliaschewitz FG, Jódar E, Lawrence AL, Lingvay I. Semaglutide and cardiovascular outcomes in type 2 diabetes 2016. N Engl J Med. 2016;375:1834–44. https://doi.org/10.1056/NEJMoa1607141.
34. Wilding JPH, Batterham RL, Calanna S, Davies M, Van Gaal LF, Lingvay I, McGowan BM, Rosenstock J, Tran MTD, Wadden TA, Wharton S, Yokote K, Zeuthen N, Kushner RF. Once weekly semaglutide in adults with overweight or obesity. N Engl J Med. 2021;384:989–1002. https://doi.org/10.1056/NEJMoa2032183.
35. Lincoff AM, Brown-Frandsen K, Colhoun HM, Deanfield J, Emerson SS, Esbjerg S, Hardt-Lindberg S, Hovingh GK, Kahn SE, Kushner RF, Lingvay I, Oral TK, Michelsen MM, Plutzky J, Tornøe CW, Ryan DH. Semaglutde and cardiovascular outcome in obesity without diabetes. N Engl J Med. 2023;389:2221–32. https://doi.org/10.1056/NEJMoa2307563.
36. Syed Y. Tirzepatide: first approval. Drugs. 2022;82:1213–20.
37. De Block C, Bailey C, Wysham C, Hemmingway A, Allen SE, Peleshok J. Tirzepatide for the treatment of adults with type 2 diabetes: an endocrine perspective. Diabetes Obes Metab. 2023;25:3–17. https://doi.org/10.1111/dom.14831.

38. Nicholls SJ, Bhatt DL, Buse JB, Del Prato S, Kahn SE, Lincoff AM, McGuire DK, Nauck MA, Nissen SE, Sattar N, Zinman B, Zoungas S, Basile J, Bartee A, Miller S, Nishiyama H, Pavo I, Weerakkody G, Wiese RJ, D'Alessio D. Comparison of tirzepatide and dulaglutide on major adverse cardiovascular events in participants with type 2 diabetes and atherosclerotic cardiovascular disease: SURPASS-CVOT design and baseline characteristics. Am Heart J. 2024;267:1–11.
39. Jastreboff AM, Aronne LJ, Ahmad NN, Wharton S, Connery L, Alves B, Kiyosue A, Zhang S, Liu B, Munch MC, Stefanski A. Tirzepatide once weekly for the treatment of obesity. N Engl J Med. 2022;387:205–16.
40. Hankosky ER, Wang H, Neff L, Kan H, Wang F, Ahmad NN, Griffin R, Stetanski GWT. Tirzepatide reduces the predicted risk of atherosclerotic cardiovascular disease and improves cardiometabolic risk factors in adults with obesity or overweight: SURMOUNT-1 post hoc analysis. Diabetes Obes Metab. 2024;26:310–28. https://doi.org/10.1111/dom.15318.
41. Okokata M, Reddy YNV, Pislaru SV, Melenovsky V, Borlaug BA. Evidence supporting the existence of a distinct obese phenotype of heart failure with preserved ejection fraction. Circulation. 2017;136:6–19. https://doi.org/10.1161/CIRCULATIONAHA.116.026807.
42. Butler J, Abildstrøm SZ, Borlaug BA, Davies MJ, Kitzman DW, Petrie MC, Shah SJ, Verma S, Abhayaratna WP, Chopra V, Ezekowitz JA, Fu M, Ito H, Lelonek M, Núñez J, Perna E, Schou M, Shenni M, van der Meer P, von Lewinski D, Wolf D, Altschul RL, Rasmussen S, Kosiborod MN. Semaglutide in patients with obesity and heart failure across mildy reducted or preserved ejection fraction. J Am Coll Cardiol. 2023;82:2087–96. https://doi.org/10.1016/j.jacc.2023.09.811.
43. Harrington J, Sattar N, Felker GM, Januzzi JL, Lam CSP, Pagidipati NJ, Pandey A, Van Spall HGC, McGuire DK. Putting more weight on obesity trials in heart failure. Curr Heart Fail Rep. 2024;21:194–202. https://doi.org/10.1007/s11897-024-00655z.

Bariatric Surgery

14

Martin Gordon and Katy Wolfe

Introduction

During the mid-to-late twentieth century, bariatric surgical procedures began to be developed by physicians for various disease states. However, it was not until the 1990s declaration of an obesity epidemic that the rise and prominence of bariatric surgeries gained national attention [1]. The earliest bariatric procedures had significant complications, though refinement of technique and the development of laparoscopic surgery have helped lower these associated risks [1]. Currently, it is estimated that the risk of death and major complications is 0.1 and 4%, respectively [2]. Due to the growing patient population with obesity, the annual number of bariatric surgeries has increased over the past decade, with the only decline seen in 2020, amid the COVID-19 epidemic [3].

M. Gordon (✉)
Department of Pharmacy, Spartanburg Regional Healthcare System, Spartanburg, SC, USA
e-mail: pgordon@srhs.com

K. Wolfe
Department of Pharmacy, Duke University Hospital, Durham, NC, USA
e-mail: katherine.wolfe@duke.edu

© The Author(s), under exclusive license to Springer Nature Switzerland AG 2025

J. Clements (ed.), *The Pharmacist's Pocket Guide for Diabetes and Obesity*, https://doi.org/10.1007/978-3-031-88835-9_14

Although pharmacotherapy for obesity has evolved with the development of new medications in recent years, bariatric surgery remains one of the most effective weight loss strategies for severe obesity. Additionally, bariatric surgery has been shown to reduce cardiovascular risk, microvascular disease, and cancer, while improving glycemic control and quality of life, and suggesting a lower all-cause mortality [4–6]. Bariatric surgery is associated with higher initial costs, but data suggest the long-term cost-effectiveness of the procedure with possible cost savings for individuals [6]. Individuals who undergo bariatric procedures may also see remission in multiple comorbid conditions, including type 2 diabetes (T2D), hypertension, dyslipidemia, and obstructive sleep apnea [7].

Patient Selection

One of the first clinical guidance documents on bariatric surgery for people with obesity was published by the National Institutes of Health (NIH) in 1991. This NIH Consensus Statement established the criteria for bariatric surgery among those with a body mass index (BMI) $\geq$40 kg/m^2 without any comorbid conditions and BMI $\geq$35 kg/m^2 with comorbid conditions [8]. Although various clinical guidelines and further NIH Consensus Statements have been released since this time, the NIH BMI criteria have remained the basis of candidacy for bariatric surgical procedures over the past three decades [6, 9]. However, new guidelines have challenged this BMI framework and have included additional factors to determine individualized appropriateness of a procedure. The American Diabetes Association (ADA) Standards of Care contain such personalized recommendations, such as specific BMI criteria for Asian Americans that are lower than the general population criteria [6]. Historically, the ADA recommendations contained separate selection criteria based on BMI and the inability of individuals to achieve durable weight loss and/or improvement in comorbid conditions with nonsurgical therapies [6]. However, the newest ADA recommendations were updated to reflect the American Society for Metabolic and Bariatric Surgery (ASMBS) recommendations for people with T2D. The ADA recommends that clinicians consider metabolic surgery in people with diabetes with a BMI of 30.0 kg/m^2 or greater (or BMI of 27.5 kg/m^2 in Asian American individuals) [6]. The ASMBS and the International Federation for the Surgery of Obesity and Metabolic Disorders (IFSO) released a joint statement in 2022 that contained major updates to the NIH guidance [10]. The joint statement recommends bariatric surgery for individuals with a BMI $\geq$35 kg/m^2 regardless of comorbid conditions and consideration for those with a BMI of 30.0–34.9 kg/m^2 in the presence of metabolic disease [10]. The lowering of BMI criteria is reflective of recent data demonstrating significant long-term weight reduction and remission of comorbid conditions including hypertension, diabetes, and dyslipidemia. The new BMI criteria from ASMBS/IFSO have the potential to expand the number of eligible candidates for bariatric surgery. Table 14.1 contains a summary of the individual selection criteria between different clinical guidance documents available for bariatric surgery.

Table 14.1 Selection criteria for bariatric surgery

Guideline	Individual without comorbid condition (kg/m^2)	Individual with comorbid condition (kg/m^2)	Asian American without comorbid condition	Asian American with comorbid condition	No improvement with nonsurgical therapies
1991 NIH consensus statement [8]	BMI ≥40	BMI ≥35	Not addressed	Not addressed	Not addressed
2019 AACE joint statement [9]	BMI ≥40	BMI ≥35	Not addressed	Not addressed	BMI 30.0–34.9 kg/m^2
2022 ASMBS/IFSO joint statement [10]	BMI ≥35	BMI 30.0–34.9	BMI ≥27.5 kg/m^2	Not addressed	Not addressed
2024 ADA Standards of Care [6]	Not addressed	BMI ≥30.0	Not addressed	BMI ≥27.5 kg/m^2	Not addressed

Adapted from sources: Refs. [6, 8–10]

AACE American association of clinical endocrinology, *ADA* American diabetes association, *ASMBS* American society for metabolic and bariatric surgery, *BMI* body mass index, *IFSO* international federation for the surgery of obesity and metabolic disorders, *NIH* national institutes of health

Types of Bariatric Surgeries

In the field of bariatric surgery, a range of procedures has been developed to address the challenges faced by individuals dealing with obesity. Commonly performed surgeries include Roux-en-Y gastric bypass, sleeve gastrectomy, biliopancreatic diversion with duodenal switch (BPD/DS), and single-anastomosis duodeno-ileal bypass with sleeve gastrectomy (SADI-S). Each surgery operates on distinct principles, promoting weight loss through diverse mechanisms.

Roux-en-Y Gastric Bypass

Roux-en-Y gastric bypass is a widely used method known for its irreversibility and has a targeted weight loss of 30–35% [9]. This procedure involves dividing the stomach into two segments—a small upper pouch and a larger lower section—limiting food intake and reducing fat and calorie absorption. The subsequent connection of the pouch directly to the small intestine redirects the digestive process, decreasing food intake and modifying nutrient absorption, ultimately facilitating weight loss [11]. Diabetes remission has been noted in up to 63% of patients within 1–5 years after undergoing the Roux-en-Y gastric bypass surgery. However, up to 50% of these individuals experience recurrence of diabetes, as the median duration for this diabetes-free life period is approximately 8 years [6]. The Roux-en-Y gastric bypass surgery has also been shown to prevent reflux esophagitis, gastritis, and gastric cancer in the residual. Some disadvantages include stomal ulcers, internal hernias, and long-term micronutrient deficiencies [9].

Sleeve Gastrectomy

Sleeve gastrectomy involves removing approximately 80% of the stomach, creating a tubular structure that restricts food capacity. A significant aspect is the decrease in ghrelin, the hormone regulating appetite. This procedure offers benefits such as substantial weight loss and a shorter hospital stay without the need to reroute the intestines [12]. Targeted weight loss for a sleeve gastrectomy is 25–30% and approximately 23% of individuals achieve an A1C of 6.0% or lower after surgery [6]. This procedure is generally considered to be easy to perform and has fewer long-term complications as compared to other procedures. It does, however, carry a higher risk of gastroesophageal reflux disease (GERD) [9].

Biliopancreatic Diversion with Duodenal Switch

BPD/DS follows a two-phase surgical approach, starting with a sleeve gastrectomy. The subsequent duodenal switch involves closing off a section of the small intestine and reconnecting it to the duodenum. While effective for weight loss, this procedure carries an increased risk of malnutrition and vitamin deficiencies due to reduced nutrient absorption [13]. Targeted weight loss after BPD/DS is 35–45% and is a procedure that is effective for individuals with a BMI above 40 kg/m^2. Disadvantages include GERD, internal hernias, and micronutrient deficiencies that are even more pronounced than those seen in individuals undergoing the Roux-en-Y gastric bypass [9].

Single-Anastomosis Duodeno-Ileal Bypass with Sleeve Gastrectomy

Similar to BPD/DS, the SADI-S procedure follows a two-step process, beginning with a sleeve gastrectomy and progressing to a duodeno-ileal bypass. This rerouting diverts food through a shorter segment of the small intestine, reducing the time and distance available for calorie and fat absorption [14]. It has been described as an easier procedure to perform compared to BPD/DS, with targeted weight loss also in the 35–45% range. There is little long-term data currently available, but similar to BPD/DS, nutritional deficiencies can be seen [9].

In summary, the varied landscape of bariatric surgeries mirrors the evolving nature of weight loss interventions. Each procedure presents unique advantages and considerations, underscoring the importance of a comprehensive evaluation of individual patient profiles to determine the most suitable option. As with any medical intervention, the decision to undergo bariatric surgery should be made in consultation with health-care professionals, considering the potential risks and benefits associated with each procedure.

Clinical Perspective Pre-surgery

Management Months Prior to Surgery

After an individual is identified as a potential bariatric surgery candidate based on BMI and the potential presence of comorbid conditions, the individual must undergo an extensive pre-procedure evaluation. The evaluation must include a comprehensive medical history, psychosocial history, physical exam, and other appropriate laboratory testing to assess the surgical risk [9]. A thorough risk and benefit discussion is a key component of the pre-procedure evaluation to provide the individual with details on procedural options, choice of surgeon/medical institution, and requirement to maintain appropriate long-term follow-up and nutrient supplementation post-surgery [9]. Individuals may be considered for a referral to a specialist in obesity medicine, as pre-procedure weight loss can reduce liver volume and help improve the technical parts of the surgery as well as other comorbid conditions, such as glycemic control and blood pressure management [9].

In the months prior to surgery, comorbid disease state control is important for optimizing the overall health of the patient for surgery. Clinicians can assist patients with implementing lifestyle modifications, including healthy low-calorie dietary patterns and physical activity, in addition to their pharmacotherapy [9]. For people with diabetes, a comprehensive care plan must be implemented to achieve optimal pre-procedure glycemic control [9, 15].

Clinicians should account for individual-specific factors in determining the pre-procedure A1C goal. In general, targeting an A1C of 6.5 7% (or less) is reasonable and may be associated with shorter hospital stays and improved bariatric procedure outcomes [9]. In those with advanced diabetes complications and/or difficulty to reach the general target, a goal A1C of 7–8% is reasonable [9]. Individuals with a pre-procedure A1C of 8% or greater will require special consideration with determining the timing of surgery [9]. Individuals should be treated with appropriate glucose-lowering medications according to the ADA clinical guidelines, with consideration of glucagon-like peptide-1 (GLP-1) receptor agonists, due to their associated weight-loss outcomes [15]. As part of the pre-procedure evaluation, a fasting lipid panel will need to be obtained, and dyslipidemia treated appropriately with cholesterol-lowering therapies [9]. Additionally, blood pressure should be managed appropriately to achieve optimal management in the months prior to surgery. Tobacco cessation is another important consideration for optimizing health for surgery ideally stopping smoking 1 year but at least 6 weeks prior to the bariatric procedure [9]. Individuals who are candidates for bariatric procedures are recommended to avoid pregnancy pre-procedure and women of reproductive age should be counseled on contraception options before surgery [9].

Management Immediately Prior to Surgery

In the weeks and days leading up to bariatric surgery, individuals should be counseled by the clinician on the perioperative management of medications. Most glucose-lowering medications may be continued until surgery with consideration for holding medications such as sodium-glucose cotransporter-2 inhibitors (SGLT-2i) and metformin immediately prior to surgery [15]. For SGLT-2i specifically, it is recommended to hold canagliflozin, dapagliflozin, and empagliflozin 3 days before a scheduled surgery and ertugliflozin for at least 4 days prior to surgery [16]. The American Society of Anesthesiologists provides guidance for consideration to hold GLP-1 receptor agonist on the day of the procedure for daily dosing and a week prior for weekly dosing [17]. Individuals can continue their blood pressure and heart failure medications until surgery, though they may be counseled on holding an angiotensin-converting enzyme inhibitor or angiotensin-receptor blocker immediately prior, due to the potential risk for intraoperative hypotension [18]. Antithrombotic management in the immediate preoperative period should take into consideration the thrombotic risk of the patient and the associated high bleeding risk of bariatric procedures. It is required to hold warfarin 5 days prior to the scheduled surgery or direct oral anticoagulants for at least 2 days prior to bariatric surgery [19]. Individuals receiving estrogen therapy should hold at least one cycle of oral contraceptives and 3 weeks of hormone replacement therapy to reduce the risk of post-procedure thromboembolic complications [9].

Clinical Perspective Post-surgery

Bariatric surgeries cause significant changes in the gastrointestinal tract and other parts of the body, which can impact how medications are processed. The absorption of medication is affected, but distribution in tissues, metabolism, and elimination may also change. It is challenging to separate the effects of surgery and weight loss on medication effectiveness. Notably, various procedures have different impacts, and there is variability among individuals in how medications are absorbed after surgery. Unfortunately, there is limited data to fully understand this complex issue [20]. The potential impacts of any bariatric procedure on medication absorption and effectiveness should be carefully considered post-surgery, especially for critical drugs like anticoagulants and antiepileptics. Regular monitoring of plasma drug levels, especially for medications requiring periodic checks, is essential after surgery. Individuals should receive clear instructions on modifying their medication regimen, including prescription drugs, over-the-counter drugs, nutrient supplements, and homeopathic drugs upon hospital discharge [20]. Whenever possible, oral liquid forms should be preferred over solid forms for at least 2 months post-surgery; however, liquid forms with absorbable sugars should be avoided to prevent dumping syndrome [21]. If only solid forms are available, opening capsules and dispersing the powder in liquid can be considered. Caution is advised with extended-release formulations, as they may be unsuitable for crushing [22]. If product availability allows for it, immediate-release formulations are preferential to extended-release formulations due to absorption changes that are expected with bariatric surgery [21]. Individuals with diabetes may experience reduced medication needs initially after surgery, but long-term monitoring is crucial. Insulin requirements may decrease for up to 12 months or until weight loss stabilizes [23]. Adjustments should be made based on the basal insulin dose, with considerations for discontinuation or significant reduction. If basal insulin doses are <30 units/day before surgery, then it is reasonable to discontinue therapy after surgery. If the basal insulin dose is ≥30 units/day before surgery, then it is reasonable to decrease the dose by 50–80% after surgery [21, 23]. Short-acting insulin can be used for managing elevated glucose levels. Oral glucose-lowering agents may be discontinued or adjusted based on A1C levels, with a preference for metformin. If an individual is taking more than 1 oral medication and A1C is <9%, then metformin is the preferred single-agent therapy whereas, in those with an A1C ≥9%, a second agent can be coupled with metformin [21]. It is recommended to avoid oral medications that increase the risk of hypoglycemia such as sulfonylureas [20]. Continuous glucose monitors are recommended if hypoglycemia is a risk for the individual [9].

For individuals requiring anticoagulation, warfarin is preferred over DOACs, with dose adjustments based on INR results [24]. Limited evidence suggests rivaroxaban and apixaban may not require dose adjustment post-bariatric surgery, while information on dabigatran and edoxaban is lacking [25]. Drug-specific laboratory monitoring is recommended to ensure therapeutic levels.

Within 5 days of surgery, individuals should attempt moderate aerobic exercise between 150 and 300 min per week, unless an individual has a contraindication. In addition to exercise, individuals are encouraged to join support groups [9].

Individuals are recommended to avoid pregnancy post-procedure for 12–18 months and should be counseled on contraception options after bariatric procedures [9]. Individuals undergoing a malabsorptive procedure, including RYGB, should be counseled about non-oral contraceptive options [9]. Individuals who become pregnant following a bariatric procedure should undergo nutritional lab monitoring every trimester in addition to monitoring for appropriate weight gain and fetal health [9]. For individuals who become pregnant post-adjustable gastric band procedure, band adjustments may be required for appropriate weight gain for fetal development [9].

Conclusion

In summary, this exploration of bariatric surgery provides an understanding of its historical development, evolving surgical landscape, patient selection criteria, and clinical perspectives before and after the procedure. The mid-to-late twentieth century witnessed the inception of bariatric surgeries, gaining prominence in the 1990s amid the declared obesity epidemic. Advances in surgical techniques have significantly improved outcomes for weight-related comorbid conditions.

Despite the emergence of pharmacotherapy for obesity, bariatric surgery remains a highly effective strategy for severe obesity, demonstrating not only substantial weight loss but also significant improvements in cardiovascular risk, microvascular disease, cancer risk, glycemic control, and overall quality of life. The remission of comorbid conditions, including T2D, hypertension, dyslipidemia, and obstructive sleep apnea, underscores its multifaceted benefits.

Patient selection criteria, initially established by the NIH in 1991, has evolved with additional factors considered by newer guidelines, reflecting the dynamic nature of this field. The recent joint statement from the ASMBS and the IFSO further broadens eligibility criteria, potentially expanding the pool of candidates. The diverse landscape of bariatric surgeries, including Roux-en-Y gastric bypass, sleeve gastrectomy, BPD/DS, and SADI-S, presents health-care professionals with a range of options to encompass the needs of this growing patient population. The choice of procedure should be tailored to individual patient profiles, emphasizing the need for a comprehensive evaluation.

The clinical perspectives outlined in this chapter shed light on the management of individuals both before and after surgery, addressing pre-surgery evaluations, lifestyle modifications, and the potential impact of bariatric procedures on medication absorption and effectiveness. The post-surgery period requires vigilant monitoring and adjustments to medication regimens, emphasizing the importance of providing clear patient instructions upon hospital discharge.

As bariatric surgery continues to evolve, ongoing research and collaboration between medical societies are crucial for refining guidelines, improving patient outcomes, and advancing our understanding of the complex interplay between surgery, weight loss, and medication effectiveness.

References

1. Faria GR. A brief history of bariatric surgery. Porto Biomed J. 2017 May;2(3):90–2.
2. Flum DR, Belle SH, King WC, et al. Perioperative safety in the longitudinal assessment of bariatric surgery. N Engl J Med. 2009;361(5):445–54.
3. Clapp B, Ponce J, DeMaria E, et al. American Society for Metabolic and Bariatric Surgery 2020 estimate of metabolic and bariatric procedures performed in the United States. Surg Obes Relat Dis. 2022;18(9):1134–40.
4. Rubino F, Nathan DM, Eckel RH, et al. Metabolic surgery in the treatment algorithm for type 2 diabetes: a joint statement by international diabetes organizations. Diabetes Care. 2016;39(6):861–77.
5. O'Brien R, Johnson E, Haneuse S, et al. Microvascular outcomes in patients with diabetes after bariatric surgery versus usual care: a matched cohort study. Ann Intern Med. 2018;169(5):300–10.
6. Professional Practice Committee. 8. Obesity and weight management for the prevention and treatment of type 2 diabetes: standards of Care in Diabetes—2024. Diabetes Care. 2024;47(Suppl. 1):S145–57.
7. Chang SH, Stoll CR, Song J, et al. The effectiveness and risks of bariatric surgery: an updated systematic review and meta-analysis, 2003-2012. JAMA Surg. 2014;149(3):275–87.
8. Consensus Development Conference Panel. Gastrointestinal surgery for severe obesity. Ann Intern Med. 1991;115(12):956–61.

9. Mechanick JI, Apovian C, Brethauer S, et al. Clinical practice guidelines for the perioperative nutrition, metabolic, and nonsurgical support of patients undergoing bariatric procedures—2019 update: cosponsored by American Association of Clinical Endocrinologists/American College of Endocrinology, the Obesity Society, American Society for Metabolic and Bariatric Surgery, obesity medicine association, and American Society of Anesthesiologists - executive summary. Endocr Pract. 2019;25(12):1346–59.
10. Eisenberg D, Shikora SA, Aarts E, et al. 2022 American Society for Metabolic and Bariatric Surgery (ASMBS) and International Federation for the Surgery of obesity and metabolic disorders (IFSO): indications for metabolic and bariatric surgery. Surg Obes Relat Dis. 2022;18(12):1345–56.
11. Wittgrove AC, Clark GW. Laparoscopic gastric bypass, Roux en-Y—500 patients: technique and results, with 3-60 month follow-up. Obes Surg. 2000;10(3):233–9.
12. Cottam D, Qureshi FG, Mattar SG, et al. Laparoscopic sleeve gastrectomy as an initial weight-loss procedure for high-risk patients with morbid obesity. Surg Endosc. 2006;20(6):859–63.
13. Marceau P, Hould FS, Simard S, et al. Biliopancreatic diversion with duodenal switch. World J Surg. 1998;22(9):947–54.
14. Sánchez-Pernaute A, Herrera MAR, Pérez-Aguirre ME. Single anastomosis duodeno-ileal bypass with sleeve gastrectomy (SADI-S). One to three-year follow-up. Obes Surg. 2010;20(12):1720–6.
15. Alabduljabbar K, le Roux CW. Pharmacotherapy before and after bariatric surgery. Metabolism. 2023;148:155692.
16. FDA Drug Safety Communication. FDA revises label of SGLT2 inhibitors for diabetes to include warnings about too much acid in the blood and serious urinary tract infections. 2022. https://www.fda.gov/drugs/drug-safety-and-availability/fda-revises-labels-sglt2-inhibitors-diabetes-include-warnings-about-too-much-acid-blood-and-serious. Accessed 26 Feb 2024.
17. Ushakumari DS, Sladen RN. ASA consensus-based guidance on preoperative management of patients on glucagon-like peptide-1 receptor agonists. Anesthesiology. 2024;140(2):346–8.
18. Salim F, Khan F, Nasir M, Ali R, Iqbal A, Raza A. Frequency of intraoperative hypotension after the induction of anesthesia in hypertensive patients with preoperative angiotensin-converting enzyme inhibitors. Cureus. 2020;12(1):e6614.
19. Douketis JD, Spyropoulos AC, Murad MH, et al. Perioperative management of antithrombotic therapy: an American College of Chest Physicians Clinical Practice Guideline. Chest. 2022;162(5):e207–43.
20. Busetto L, Dicker D, Azran C, et al. Obesity management task force of the European Association for the study of obesity released "Practical

recommendations for the post-bariatric surgery medical management". Obes Surg. 2018;28(7):2117–21.
21. Lorico S, Colton B. Medication management and pharmacokinetic changes after bariatric surgery. Can Fam Physician. 2020;66(6):409–16.
22. Brocks DR, Ben-Eltriki M, Gabr RQ, Padwal RS. The effects of gastric bypass surgery on drug absorption and pharmacokinetics. Expert Opin Drug Metab Toxicol. 2012;8(12):1505–19.
23. Kheniser KG, Kashyap SR. Diabetes management before, during, and after bariatric and metabolic surgery. J Diabetes Complicat. 2018;32(9):870–5.
24. Martin KA, Lee CR, Farrell TM, Moll S. Oral anticoagulant use after bariatric surgery: a literature review and clinical guidance. Am J Med. 2017;130(5):517–24.
25. Kushnir M, Gali R, Alexander M, Billett HH. Direct oral Xa inhibitors for the treatment of venous thromboembolism after bariatric surgery. Blood Adv. 2023;7(2):224–6.

Special Populations 15

Ha Phan

Pediatrics and Adolescents

Epidemiology and Pathophysiology

Obesity affects 14.7 million children in the United States (19.7%). Prevalence is greatest among children ages 6–19 [1]. Obesity affects 26.2% of Hispanic children, 24.8% of non-Hispanic Black children, 16.6% of non-Hispanic white children, and 9% of non-Hispanic Asian children [1].

Commodities include hypertension, hyperlipidemia, type 2 diabetes (T2D), metabolic dysfunction-associated fatty liver disease (MAFLD), and sleep apnea [1, 2].

Health equities should be considered when discussing prevalence and outcomes in the pediatric population as well as weight biases and stigma associated with obesity. This may also include access to food, communication about weight using non-stigmatizing language, access to safe physical activity, and school environments [2].

H. Phan (✉)
Department of Pharmacy Practice, University of Mississippi School of Pharmacy, Jackson, MS, USA
e-mail: hkphan@umc.edu

© The Author(s), under exclusive license to Springer Nature Switzerland AG 2025

J. Clements (ed.), *The Pharmacist's Pocket Guide for Diabetes and Obesity*, https://doi.org/10.1007/978-3-031-88835-9_15

Assessment

The body mass index (BMI) is used in children and teens based on age and sex and is determined using percentiles for BMI instead of category cutoffs used in adults. Children and adolescents with overweight are at or above the 85th percentile and below the 95th percentile for age and sex [2]. Obesity is defined as a BMI at or above the 95th percentile for age and sex. Severe obesity is defined as a BMI at or above 120% above the 95th percentile. Class 2 obesity is defined as <140% of the 95th percentile to ≥120% or BMI ≥35 kg/m^2 to <40 kg/m,[2] whichever is lower based on the patient's age and sex. Class 3 obesity is ≥140% of the 95th percentile or BMI ≥40 kg/m^2. A z score is used to describe the relationship to the population mean, derived from Centers for Disease Control (CDC) Growth Charts. The z score may not be able to detect changes in adipose over time; however, an extended method was created to account for the limitations of the CDC Growth Charts [2].

In the assessment of obesity, medications that contribute to weight gain should be evaluated. Some common medications are listed in Table 15.1.

Table 15.1 Common medications contributing to weight gain

Therapeutic classifications	Medications
Antihistamines	Cetirizine and hydroxyzine
Antidepressants	Amitriptyline, nortriptyline, paroxetine, sertraline
Antiepileptics	Carbamazepine, gabapentin, pregabalin, valproate, vigabatrin
Antipsychotics	Aripiprazole, olanzapine, quetiapine, risperidone, ziprasidone, clozapine, haloperidol, mirtazapine
Glucocorticoids	Systemic hydrocortisone, prednisone, dexamethasone, and prednisolone

Source: Refs. [2, 3]

Guidelines

As stated previously, children and adolescents with obesity have an increased incidence of developing dyslipidemia, hypertension, and insulin resistance. There are different guidelines that recommend the diagnosis, assessment, and treatment of these comorbidities (Tables 15.2 and 15.3).

Table 15.2 Summary of diagnosis, assessment and treatment of comorbidities

Comorbidity	Diagnosis	Assessment	
Dyslipidemia (DLD)	FLP in children 10 years and older with BMI ≥85th percentile to <95th percentile FLP in children with BMI ≥95th percentile in ages 2–9 with obesity	Children ≥10 years of age with an LDL-C persistently >190 mg/dL or >160 mg/dL with familial hypercholesterolemia who does not respond to lifestyle treatment should be initiated on medication	
Hypertension (HTN)	≥90th percentile for age and height, needs to be repeatedly elevated ×3 on separate visits for elevated BP and stage 1 HTN and ×2 for stage 2 HTN should also work up additional secondary causes of HTN	Children 1–13 years of age Normal: <90th percentile Elevated: ≥90th to <95th percentile Stage 1: ≥95th percentile to <95th percentile +12 mmHg Stage 2: ≥95th percentile +12 mmHg	Children ≥13 years of age Normal: <120/80 mmHg Elevated: 120–129/<80 mmHg Stage 1: 130–139/80–89 mmHg Stage 2: ≥140/90 mmHg

(continued)

Table 15.2 (continued)

Comorbidity	Diagnosis	Assessment
Prediabetes and T2D	Considered after the onset of puberty or ≥10 years of age Oral glucose tolerance test (OGTT) Hemoglobin A1C Symptom(s) present of polydipsia, polyuria, bed wetting, polyphagia, unexplained fatigue	2-h OGTT 140 to 199 mg/dL (prediabetes or impaired glucose tolerance) ≥200 mg/dL = diabetes 5.7–6.4% = prediabetes or impaired glucose tolerance ≥6.5% = diabetes
MAFLD	ALT starting at ≥10 years of age	ALT 2× the ULN Hepatomegaly
PCOS	Total testosterone, free testosterone should be an early morning blood draw	First year post-menarche is >90 days in between cycles After second year post-menarche <21 days or >45 days in between cycles Lack of menses by 15 years of age or 2–3 years after breast budding Elevated free testosterone, total testosterone, and DHEA-sulfate
Mood disorders (depression)	PHQ-9	Scores of 10–20 on PHQ-9 indicate moderate—Severe depression

Source: Refs. [2–10]

ALT alanine transaminase, *FLP* fasting lipid panel, *LDL-C* low-density lipoprotein—cholesterol, *MAFLD* metabolic dysfunction-associated fatty liver disease, *OGTT* oral glucose tolerance test, *PCOS* polycystic ovary syndrome, *PHQ-9* patient health questionnaire, *T2D* type 2 diabetes, *ULN* upper limit of normal

Table 15.3 Summary of treatment of comorbidities

Comorbidity	Non-pharmacological treatment	Pharmacological treatment	Clinical pearls
Dyslipidemia (DLD)	Dietary modifications, daily physical activity, change in body weight if applicable	≥6 years of age rosuvastatin ≥8 years of age pravastatin and pitavastatin ≥10 years of age simvastatin, atorvastatin and fluvastatin	Note teratogenicity of statin therapy and should be discontinued at conception or 4 weeks prior to conception
Hypertension (HTN)	Dietary approaches to stop HTN (DASH) = high in fruits, vegetables, low-fat milk products, whole rains, fish, poultry, nuts, and lean red meats Weight loss and stress reduction. Strategies above should be implemented 3 to 6 months prior to initiation of medication but should be ongoing even if medication is initiated	Appropriate initiated agents: ACEis, ARBs, thiazide diuretics, CCBs	Medications should be increased every 2–4 weeks once adherence is verified until BP is controlled, patients should be seen every 4–6 weeks until BP has normalized Note teratogenicity of ACEi/ARB therapy and should be switched to CCB or other therapy by conception or by the 13th week of pregnancy

(continued)

Table 15.3 (continued)

Comorbidity	Non-pharmacological treatment	Pharmacological treatment	Clinical pearls
Prediabetes and T2D	Self-management education and support as appropriate, which, may include 60 min of moderate-to-vigorous physical activity	Metformin is preferred as initial treatment followed by GLP-1 receptor agonist or empagliflozin (if 10 year of age or older) then insulin If patient presents in ketosis/ ketoacidosis, insulin will be initiated immediately	Follow-up every 3 months, monitor with A1C
MAFLD	Weight loss of ≥10% of total body weight	None currently available	Annual AST and ALT measurement
PCOS	Patient-centered and address patient's priorities in partnership with patient and families Lifestyle counseling	OCPs with low androgenic activity Metformin Spironolactone	Follow up in 3–6 months on symptoms and adverse effects of medications Routine monitoring of serum androgens is not recommended
Mood disorders (depression)		Fluoxetine 5 mg or 10 mg ≥8 years of age Escitalopram 10 mg ≥12 years of age	Follow-up on medication efficacy in 4 weeks

Source: Refs. [4–9, 11–13]

ACEi angiotensin-converting enzyme inhibitors, *ALT* alanine transaminase, *AST* aspartate transaminase, *ARB* angiotensin receptor blockers, *CCB* calcium channel blocker, *GLP*-1 glucagon-like peptide-1, *MAFLD* metabolic dysfunction-associated fatty liver disease, *OCPs* oral contraceptives, *PCOS* polycystic ovary syndrome, *T2D* type 2 diabetes

Nutrition

First-line treatment usually includes motivational interviewing as well as intensive health behavior and lifestyle treatment (IHBLT). This usually includes multiple components and time which may all be limitations of successful treatment. IHBLT includes a longitudinal approach, which involves family-based interaction. IHBLT involves aligned expectations, self-management, non-stigmatizing care, and mutual engagement and participation. Management of more than or equal to 26 h of this described care may lead to a loss of 1.6–8.1 kg over 1 year [2].

Behavioral strategies are listed in Table 15.4.

Medications may be offered to children ages 8–11 years of age as a discussion of the indications, risks, benefits and as an adjunct to health behavior and lifestyle. For children younger than 12 years of age, there is no sufficient evidence to recommend pharmacotherapy solely for the indication of obesity [2]. Table 15.5 includes the medications that have been discussed in the management of pediatrics living with obesity.

Bariatrics

There is not a set age for qualification for bariatric surgery in pediatric patients and adolescent patients. Criteria for bariatric surgery in pediatric patients may include BMI ≥35 kg/m^2 or 120% of the 95th percentile for age and sex or a BMI ≥40 kg/m^2 or 140% of the 95th percentile for age and sex. The discussion of bariatric surgery may lead to shared decision-making that discusses through a multidisciplinary assessment of risks, benefits, psychosocial assessment, potential contraindications, pregnancy, and ongoing substance use disorder in pediatric patients. A laparoscopic Roux-en-Y gastric bypass is considered the gold standard [30]. Vertical sleeve gastrectomy is another procedure for the pediatric population. Following surgery, a reduction in BMI and improvement in comorbidities, such as hypertension, diabetes, and dyslipidemia, has been reported in the pediatric population

Table 15.4 Behavior strategies

Reduce sugary beverages to no more than 25 g each day of added sugar and no more than 1 8-oz serving of a sugary beverage per week
Utilize MyPlate as a tool created by the US Department of Agriculture used for encouraging low added sugar, low in concentrated fat, nutrient dense, with no calorie restriction.
Engage in moderate to vigorous physical activity for at least 60 min per day
Avoid skipping breakfast
Follow the 5–2–1-0 strategy: At least 5 fruits or veggies per day, less than 2 h of screen time, 1 h or more of moderate-to-vigorous physical activity and 0 sugary beverages
Strive for the appropriate amount of sleep according to age[a]

Source: Ref. [14]

[a]Infants (4–12 months) 12–16 h per 24 h, Toddler (1–2 years) 11–14, Preschool (3–5 years) 10–13 h, School Age (6–12 years) 9–12 h, Teen (13–18 years) 8–10 h

[31]. Complications postoperatively may include nausea, and dehydration [32]. Following surgery, adolescents were followed for 5 years following a Roux-en-Y and found to have similar weight loss as adults who had undergone a Roux-en-Y. Adolescents were found to have remission of T2D (86% vs 53%) and hypertension (68% vs 41%) more often than adults [33].

Monogenic Syndromes

Monogenic syndromes may include gene deficiencies with the melanocortin 4 receptor heterozygous mutation occurring in 2–5% of children living with severe obesity. Below in Table 15.6 is a summary of selective common mutations and their symptoms [2]. There are some medications approved such as setmelanotide that are targeting some of the deficiencies stated below, but this is still a developing area of practice. This can be identified utilizing a genetic test that is administered if the patient presents with symptoms during initial intake into a weight management clinic.

Table 15.5 Summary of medications used to manage weight

Medication	Indication(s)	Mechanism of action	Dose	Change in weight	Common adverse effects and warnings
Metformin	T2D, PCOS, prediabetes	Decreasing intestinal absorption, decreasing blood glucose production in the liver, and increasing insulin sensitivity	1000 mg one tablet twice daily	1 kg/m^2	Nausea, bloating, flatulence, diarrhea Lactic acidosis (rare)
Orlistat	Long-term treatment of obesity in children ages 12 and older	Inhibiting gastric and pancreatic lipases—inhibiting dietary fats by 30%	≥12 years of age 120 mg 3 times daily with each meal or up to 1 hour after eating	0.5–4.2 kg/m^2	Oily spotting, flatus with discharge, fecal urgency, fatty/oily stool

(continued)

Table 15.5 (continued)

Medication	Indication(s)	Mechanism of action	Dose	Change in weight	Common adverse effects and warnings
Phentermine	Weight management—Short-term those who have a BMI ≥30 kg/m² or ≥27 kg/m² with ≥1 weight-associated comorbidity ages 16 and older	Stimulating of hypothalamus to release norepinephrine	≥16 years of age 37.5 mg daily before breakfast	1.6–4.1% change in BMI	Caution in patients with structural cardiac abnormalities, and seizure disorders May cause insomnia, anxiety, increased BP, tachycardia
Liraglutide (subcutaneous injectable)	T2D, long-term treatment of children with obesity in ages 12 years and older	Slowing gastric emptying and promoting satiety	Diabetes: ≥10 years of age Obesity: ≥12 years of age 0.6 mg daily × 7 days then increase to, 1.2 mg daily × 7 days, 1.8 mg daily × 7 days, 2.4 mg daily × 7 days, 3.0 mg daily	5% BMI reduction	Caution in patients with a personal or family history of MTC, or in patients with MEN2

Dulaglutide (subcutaneous injectable)	T2D	Slowing gastric emptying and promoting satiety	Diabetes: ≥10 years of age 0.75 mg once weekly × 4 weeks, then increase to 1.5 mg once weekly	0.6% decrease in A1C, 0.9% decrease in A1C at 26 weeks at 1.5 mg dose	Diarrhea, vomiting, nausea, abdominal pain, hypoglycemia Caution in patients with a personal or family history of MTC, or in patients with MEN2
Semaglutide (subcutaneous injectable)	T2D, adjunct to reduced calorie diet and increased physical activity for chronic weight management ≥12 years of age with an initial BMI at the 95th percentile or greater for age and sex	Slowing gastric emptying and promoting satiety	≥12 years of age 0.25 mg once weekly × 4 weeks, then increase to 0.5 mg once weekly × 4 weeks, then increase to 1.0 mg weekly × 4 weeks, then increase to 1.7 mg once weekly × 4 weeks then increase to 2.4 mg once weekly	At 68 weeks was a change in 16.1% in BMI	Diarrhea, nausea, vomiting, constipation, abdominal pain, dyspepsia Caution in patients with a personal or family history of MTC, or in patients with MEN2

(continued)

Table 15.5 (continued)

Medication	Indication(s)	Mechanism of action	Dose	Change in weight	Common adverse effects and warnings
Phentermine with topiramate	In addition to lifestyle changes in patients ≥12 years of age with an initial BMI 95th percentile or higher	Stimulating of hypothalamus to release norepinephrine and suppressing appetite through satiety enhancement	3.75 /23 mg daily for 14 days then increase to 7.5 /46 mg daily for 12 weeks, then may increase to 11.25 /69 mg daily for 14 days then increase to 15 /92 mg daily for 12 weeks	10.44% change in BMI at the high dose of 15/92 mg	Cautions similar to phentermine above with the added caution of causing metabolic acidosis in patients who are predisposed to acidosis and ocular effects within 1 month of initiation, increase in HR, dry mouth, and headache
Lisdexamfetamine	Binge eating disorder in patients ≥18 years	Not known	30 mg daily, max 70 mg/day	Decrease in scores relating to binge eating disorder	Abdominal pain, dry mouth, insomnia

Empagliflozin	T2D	Inhibiting sodium-glucose cotransporter 2 in the proximal renal tubules, reduces reabsorption of glucose	10 or 25 mg daily	0.83% decrease in A1C at 26 weeks	Headache, hypoglycemia, urinary tract infection
Dapagliflozin	T2D	Inhibiting sodium-glucose cotransporter 2 in the proximal renal tubules, reduces reabsorption of glucose	5 or 10 mg daily	1.03% decrease in A1C at 26 weeks	Headache, hypoglycemia, urinary tract infections

Source: Refs. [15–29]

BMI body mass index, *BP* blood pressure, *MEN2* multiple endocrine neoplasia type 2, *MTC* medullary thyroid carcinoma, *PCOS* polycystic ovary syndrome, *T2D* type 2 diabetes

Table 15.6 Summary of common monogenic deficiencies

Monogenic deficiency	Symptoms
MC4R	Increased lean body mass, sometimes presents with low blood pressure and hyperinsulinemia
Leptin deficiency	Normal linear growth with reduced adult height. Quick onset obesity with hypothalamic dysfunction such as hypothyroidism, and hypogonadism. Responds to leptin treatment
Leptin receptor deficiency	Like above, however not responsive to leptin treatment
POMC deficiency	Adrenocorticotropic hormone deficiency, light skin in non-Hispanic white individuals

Source: Ref. [2]
MC4R melanocortin 4 receptor, *POMC* proopiomelanocortin

Geriatrics

There are no current practice guidelines that specifically address older adults (>60 years of age) who are living with obesity. There are systematic reviews that have looked at pharmacotherapy use and bariatric surgery among this population, concluding that there is not as much data surrounding pharmacotherapy. It is found that older age as one factor should not be a contraindication to intensive lifestyle recommendations or surgical intervention for obesity [33]. Intentional weight loss that combines caloric restriction, aerobic activity, and resistance exercises can assist with improving physical function and health in older adults. The potential for the negative impacts of weight loss on muscle and bone physiology can be mitigated by resistance exercise to minimize the potential harms of intentional weight loss in older adults [34]. The use of glucagon-like peptide-1 (GLP-1) receptor agonists for diabetes has been extrapolated and reviewed and was found to be consistent in safety compared to adults taking GLP-1 receptor agonists. Weight loss is still seen in older adults, but it does not seem to be different from adults taking GLP-1 receptor agonists for diabetes [35, 36]. There are no long-term studies that look at weight loss and GLP-1 receptor agonists use in older adults without diabetes regarding bone health or bone density.

Pregnancy and Lactation

With any sensitive population there is little data given the ethical considerations when providing medications to a population of patients that may be harmed during the process. Typically, weight loss is not advised during pregnancy but could be recommended during the preconception period. Many medications are not recommended for use during pregnancy due to the lack of data. In a systemic review of human trials and animal trials, it was found that GLP-1 receptor agonists that were used during pregnancy in animals led to reduced fetal weight and/or growth, delayed ossification and skeletal variants, and reduced maternal weight. In human studies, there was no significant maternal-to-fetal transfer, but GLP-1 receptor agonists were excreted in the breast milk. Therefore, this class of medications should be discontinued during pregnancy and potentially used with caution during lactation [37–40].

Lactation data on the use of topiramate at doses up to 200 mg showed low levels in the infant serum. Sedation and diarrhea was reported in breastfed infants, but otherwise there seemed to be no long-term adverse effects on long-term development in the infants that were exposed to topiramate during lactation; however, the use of phentermine in combination with topiramate is not recommended during breastfeeding [41, 42].

Conclusion

There have been developments in pharmacotherapy over the last few years that have expanded the role of pharmacists in the management of obesity. Specifically, several medications previously approved for obesity management in adults has now been approved for use in pediatric patients. A need in this area is more long-term data on how these medications affect adolescents, older adults, and patients who are pregnant and lactating. Additionally, as more adolescents are seeking bariatric surgery, the role for pharmacists in post-surgery management may also expand in clinical practice. Pharmacists should have a baseline understanding of the initiation, monitoring, and follow-up needed in the management of obesity in special populations.

References

1. Stierman BD, Afful J, Carroll MD. Prevalence of overweight, obesity, and severe obesity among children and adolescents aged 2–19: United States, 1963–1965 through 2017–2020. NCHS E-Health Stats. 2021. Available from: https://www.cdc.gov/obesity/data/childhood.html
2. Hampl SE, Hassink SG, Skinner AC, et al. Clinical practice guideline for the evaluation and treatment of children and adolescents with obesity. Pediatrics. 2023;151(2):e2022060640.
3. Ratliff JC, Barber JA, Palmese LB, Reutenauer EL, Tek C. Association of prescription H1 antihistamine use with obesity: results from the National Health and nutrition examination survey. Obesity. 2010;18(12):2398–400.
4. Grundy SM, Stone NJ, Bailey AL, et al. 2018 AHA/ACC/AACVPR/AAPA/ABC/ACPM/ADA/AGS/APhA/ASPC/NLA/PCNA guideline on the management of blood cholesterol: executive summary: a report of the American College of Cardiology/American Heart Association task force on clinical practice guidelines. J Am Coll Cardiol. 2019;73(24):3168–209.
5. Flynn JT, Kaelber DC, Baker-Smith CM, et al. Clinical practice guideline for screening and management of high blood pressure in children and adolescents. Pediatrics. 2017;140(3):e20171904.
6. Professional Practice Committee. 14. Children and adolescents: standards of care in diabetes – 2024. Diabetes Care. 2024;47(Suppl. 1):S258–81.
7. Sweeny KF, Lee CK. Nonalcoholic fatty liver disease in children. Gastroenterol Hepatol (N Y). 2021;17(12):579–87.
8. Cree-Green M, Torchen, L, Bernier A, Burgert T. PCOS Toolkit. Pediatric Endocrine Society; 2021. Available from: https://pedsendo.org/wp-content/uploads/2021/04/PCOS_Provider_Toolkit-4.2021.pdf
9. Kamboj MK, Bonny AE. Polycystic ovary syndrome in adolescence: diagnostic and therapeutic strategies. Transl Pediatr. 2017;6(4):248–55.
10. Cheung AH, Zuckerbrot RA, Jensen PS, et al. Guidelines for adolescent depression in primary care (GLAD-PC): part II. Treatment and ongoing management. Pediatrics. 2018;131(3):e20174082.
11. Lundberg GP, Mehta LS. Familial hypercholesterolemia and pregnancy. American College of Cardiology; 2018. Available from: https://www.acc.org/Latest-in-Cardiology/Articles/2018/05/10/13/51/Familial-Hypercholesterolemia-and-Pregnancy
12. Bullo M, Tschumi S, Bucher BS, Bianchetti MG, Simonetti GD. Pregnancy outcome following exposure to angiotensin-converting

enzyme inhibitors or angiotensin receptor antagonists. Hypertension. 2012;60(2):444–50.
13. Screening and Management of the Hyperandrogenic Adolescent. ACOG Committee opinion no. 789. American college of obstetricians and gynecologists. Obstet Gynecol. 2019;134:e106–14.
14. Paruthi S, Brooks LJ, D'Ambrosio C, et al. Recommended amount of sleep for pediatric populations: a consensus statement of the American Academy of sleep medicine. J Clin Sleep Med. 2016;12(6):785–6.
15. Pu R, Shi D, Gan T, et al. Effects of metformin in obesity treatment in different populations: a meta-analysis. Ther Adv Endocrinol Metab. 2020;21(11):2042018820926000.
16. Rogovik AL, Goldman RD. Pharmacologic treatment of pediatric obesity. Can Fam Physician. 2011;57(2):195–7.
17. Xenical. Food and Drug Administration; 2012. Available from: https://www.accessdata.fda.gov/drugsatfda_docs/label/2012/020766s029lbl.pdf. Accessed 27 Nov 2023.
18. Ryder JR, Kaizer A, Rudser KD, et al. Effect of phentermine on weight reduction in a pediatric weight management clinic. Int J Obes. 2017;41(1):90–3.
19. Kelly AS, Auerbach P, Barrientos-Perez M, et al. A randomized, controlled trial of liraglutide for adolescents with obesity. N Engl J Med. 2020;382(22):2117–28.
20. Saxenda. Food and Drug Administration; 2014. Available from: https://www.accessdata.fda.gov/drugsatfda_docs/label/2014/206321orig1s000lbl.pdf. Accessed 27 Nov 2023.
21. Arslanian SA, Hannon T, et al. Once-weekly dulaglutide for the treatment of youths with type 2 diabetes. N Engl J Med. 2022;387:433–43.
22. Weghuber D, Barrett T, Barrientos-Pérez M, et al. Once-weekly semaglutide in adolescents with obesity. N Engl J Med. 2022;387(24):2245–57.
23. Wegovy. Food and Drug Administration; 2023. Available from: https://www.accessdata.fda.gov/drugsatfda_docs/label/2023/215256s007lbl.pdf. Accessed 27 Nov 2023.
24. Kelly AS, Bensignor MO, Hsia DS, et al. Phentermine/topiramate for the treatment of adolescent obesity. NEJM Evid. 2022;1(6):10.
25. Qsymia. Food and Drug Administration; 2012. Available from: https://www.accessdata.fda.gov/drugsatfda_docs/label/2012/022580s000lbl.pdf. Accessed 27 Nov 2023.
26. Fornaro M, Solmi M, Perna G, et al. Lisdexamfetamine in the treatment of moderate-to-severe binge eating disorder in adults: systematic review and exploratory meta-analysis of publicly available placebo-controlled, randomized clinical trials. Neuropsychiatr Dis Treat. 2016;12:1827–36.
27. Vyvanse. Food and Drug Administration; 2017. Available from: https://www.accessdata.fda.gov/drugsatfda_docs/label/2017/208510lbl.pdf. Accessed 27 Nov 2023.

28. Laffel LM, Danne T, Klingensmith GJ, et al. Efficacy and safety of the SGLT2 inhibitor empagliflozin versus placebo and the DPP-4 inhibitor linagliptin versus placebo in youth with type 2 diabetes: a multicentere, randomised, double-blind parallel group, phase 3 trial. Lancet Diabetes Endocrinol. 2023;11(3):161–81.
29. Shehadeh N, Barrett T, Galassetti P, et al. T2NOW study group. Dapagliflozin or saxagliptin in pediatric type 2 diabetes. NEJM Evid. 2023;2(12)
30. Alqahtani AR, Elahmedi M, Abdurabu HY, Alqahtani S. Ten-year outcomes of children and adolescents who underwent sleeve gastrectomy: weight loss, comorbidity resolution, adverse events, and growth velocity. J Am Coll Surg. 2021;233(6):657–64.
31. Armstrong SC, Bolling CF, Michalsky MP, Reichard KW. Pediatric metabolic and bariatric surgery: evidence, barriers, and best practices. Pediatrics. 2019;144(6):e20193223.
32. Inge TH, Courcoulas AP, Jenkins TM, et al. Five-year outcomes of gastric bypass in adolescents as compared with adults. N Engl J Med. 2019;380(22):2136–45.
33. Haywood C, Sumithran P. Treatment of obesity in older persons – a systemic review. Obes Rev. 2019;20:588–98.
34. DiMilia PR, Mittman A, Batsis JA. Benefit-to-risk balance of weight loss intervention in older adults with obesity. Curr Diab Rep. 2019;19(100):114.
35. Karagiannis T, Tsapas A, Athanasiadou E, et al. GLP-1 receptor agonists and SGLT2 inhibitors for older people with type 2 diabetes: a systematic review and meta-analysis. Diabetes Res Clin Pract. 2021;174:108737.
36. Huynh G, Runeberg H, Weideman R. Evaluating weight loss with semaglutide in elderly patients with type 2 diabetes. J Pharm Technol. 2023;39(1):10–5.
37. Liraglutide. Drugs and Lactation Database (LactMed®); 2020. Available from: https://www.ncbi.nlm.nih.gov/books/NBK500977/. Accessed 27 Nov 2023.
38. Semaglutide. Drugs and Lactation Database (LactMed®; 2023.Available from: https://www.ncbi.nlm.nih.gov/books/NBK500980/. Accessed 27 Nov 2023.
39. Wajtryt O, Dedecjus M. Pregnancy after exposure to GLP-1 receptor angoists. A case report and literature review. Endocr Abstr. 2023;90(EP532) Available from: https://www.endocrine-abstracts.org/ea/0090/ea0090ep532
40. Muller DR, Stenvers DJ, Malekzadeh A, et al. Effects of GLP-1 agonists and SGLT2 inhibitors during pregnancy and lactation on offspring outcomes: a systematic review of the evidence. Front Endocrinol. 2023;14:1215356.

41. Topiramate. Drugs and Lactation Database (LactMed®); 2022.Available from: https://www.ncbi.nlm.nih.gov/books/NBK501259/. Accessed 27 Nov 2023.
42. Phentermine. Drugs and Lactation Database (LactMed®); 2022. Available from: https://www.ncbi.nlm.nih.gov/books/NBK582102/. Accessed 27 Nov 2023.

Part IV

The Role of the Pharmacist in Clinical Scenarios

16

Allison Presnell

Pharmacists play a vital role in the health-care team, regardless of the practice setting. For the management of diabetes and obesity, pharmacists can pursue a variety of certificate training and/or board certifications to stay up to date with best practices in the care of persons living with diabetes and obesity [1]:

- American Pharmacists Association: https://www.pharmacist.com/Education/Certificate-Training-Programs
  - Pharmacy-Based Immunization Delivery Medication Therapy Management
  - Patient-Centered Diabetes Care
  - Pharmacists Getting Paid Through Collaborative Clinical Services
- American Society of Health System Pharmacists
  - Diabetes Management Certificate: https://elearning.ashp.org/products/10824/diabetes-management-certificate
  - Weight Management Certificate: https://elearning.ashp.org/products/9695/weight-management-certificate

A. Presnell (✉)
Department of Pharmacy Practice, Campbell University College of Pharmacy & Health Sciences, Buies Creek, NC, USA
e-mail: apresnell@campbell.edu

© The Author(s), under exclusive license to Springer Nature Switzerland AG 2025

J. Clements (ed.), *The Pharmacist's Pocket Guide for Diabetes and Obesity*, https://doi.org/10.1007/978-3-031-88835-9_16

- Association of Diabetes Care and Education Specialists: https://www.adces.org/dces-career
    - Certified Diabetes Care and Education Specialist
    - Board-Certified in Advanced Diabetes Management
- Board of Pharmacy Specialties.
    - Board-Certified Ambulatory Care Pharmacist: https://bpsweb.org/ambulatory-care-pharmacy/
    - Board-Certified Pharmacotherapy Specialist: https://bpsweb.org/pharmacotherapy/
    - Board-Certified Pediatric Pharmacy Specialist: https://bpsweb.org/pediatric-pharmacy/
    - Board-Certified Geriatric Pharmacist: https://bpsweb.org/geriatric-pharmacy/
- Centers for Disease Control National Diabetes Prevention Program https://www.cdc.gov/diabetes/prevention/program-providers.htm
    - Lifestyle Change Program Provider
- RxCE.com, LLC: https://rxce.com/CertificatePrograms/Diabetes-ACPE-Pharmacy-Certificate-Program
    - ACPE-Approved Diabetes Management Certificate for Pharmacists
- University of North Carolina Eshelman School of Pharmacy
    - Diabetes Certificate Course: www.pharmacy.unc.edu/ce

Pharmacists provide care for people living with diabetes and obesity in a variety of practice settings:

- Academia
    - Creating/delivering content and providing direct training to student pharmacists
- Association Management
    - Delivering relevant content to pharmacists for continuing education and workplace toolkits, lobbying for pharmacists' role in health-care, advocating for pharmacist profession to other health-care associations, and developing certifications and certificate programs for advancing pharmacy practice

- Community Outreach (diabetes screening initiative)
  - Screening in a community outreach event or health fair for diabetes and obesity, educating on diabetes prevention, and lifestyle education
- Community Pharmacy
  - Appropriately dispensing medications, providing drug and medication device education, counseling on glucometer/continuous glucose monitor use, and educating on over-the-counter (OTC) weight loss medication
- Compounding Pharmacy
  - Following quality standards and industry guidelines to appropriately compound medications in diabetes that promote weight loss and/or weight loss medications in people with weight classified as overweight or are living with obesity, especially during FDA shortages
- Consultant Pharmacy
  - Educating health-care providers on genomics testing and personalized medicine, along with conducting chart reviews in long-term care facilities for appropriate medication use
- Inpatient Pharmacy
  - Reviewing trends with blood glucose monitoring, providing medication management during hospitalization to ensure appropriate weight-based medication dosing and dispensing, and providing medication and device education
- Managed Care Pharmacy
  - Conducting medication formulary management, medication authorization criteria/determinations, and disease state-related quality measures
- Pharmaceutical Industry
  - Authoring medical articles or answering drug information questions, providing support to health-care providers as educators, pharmaceutical representatives, or medical science liaisons
- Pharmacy Administration
  - Leading medication management in population health initiatives, identifying viable practice models for pharmacists' presence in direct and non-direct patient care opportunities

for disease state management, and overseeing clinical outcomes data

- Primary Care or Specialty Clinic (outpatient).
  - Completing direct patient care visits for medication management through protocol or collaborative practice agreement (prescribing medications, ordering/interpreting labs, medication device education, glucose interpretation through glucometer or continuous glucose monitoring device, follow-up)

Pharmacists are well positioned to provide recommendations for medications in diabetes that promote weight loss and/or weight loss medication strategies in people with weight classified as overweight or living with obesity. Medication management is crucial during the weight loss period to minimize the risk of:

- Discontinuation of medication due to side effects (nausea, vomiting, diarrhea, constipation, etc.)
- Ineffectiveness/unrealistic patient expectations for blood glucose lowering or weight loss
- Pill burden
- Hypoglycemia
- Medication cost burden
- Hypotension

Consideration for medications that promote weight loss but also have cardioprotective or renal protective properties should be a priority for patients with diabetes and chronic kidney disease, heart failure, atherosclerotic cardiovascular disease (ASCVD) or high-risk ASCVD [2]. Selection of medication based on efficacy for glucose-lowering and potential for weight loss should be prioritized in people with diabetes and those who are overweight or have obesity [3–5].

The pharmacist plays a key role in each step of comprehensive, clinical care of persons living with diabetes and obesity to ensure the best clinical outcomes.

1. Patient Interaction

Pharmacists can conduct and complete direct patient care scenarios (referral, shared clinical appointment, patient counseling) through in-person or virtual appointments. Pharmacists can also conduct and complete non-direct patient care scenarios, such as consults or phone calls from other health-care providers.

2. Evaluation of Patient

When making clinical recommendations, pharmacists will often review an electronic medical record or patient intake form to determine the appropriateness of medication management for diabetes and obesity. With respect to diabetes and obesity, the pharmacist conducts at comprehensive review of the following information, among other relevant data:

- Past medical history
- Inactive and active medications
- Medical problem list
- Insurance status
- Current body mass index (BMI)
- Weight changes
- Blood pressure
- Electrocardiogram
- Recent health-care provider progress notes
- Labs
- Presence of diabetes or history of diabetes/prediabetes

3. Patient Interview and Medication Recommendations

Medication recommendations are made by the pharmacist through evaluation of the efficacy and safety of the medication for the individual patient with their specific drug-drug or drug-disease interactions in mind. During the interview, the pharmacist evaluates for appropriate medication adherence and addresses and concerns about the current treatment plan. If multiple options are viable for the individual, the pharmacist reviews the pros and cons of each medication with the individual to determine the best option through shared decision-making. Because of the potential high cost of some brand name medications for diabetes and obesity, affordability can be a barrier to utilization of guideline-directed medication therapy. Pharmacists can discuss which medications are covered and what the copayment will be, what table to expect with the deductible, etc. The pharmacist can also assess for barriers to medication adherence related to cost.

4. Medication Education

   When a medication is started for diabetes and obesity, the pharmacist can review all aspects of medication in patient-friendly language. This includes brand and generic name, mechanism of action, route of medication administration (oral, daily injectable, weekly injectable), storage, missed dose instructions, side effects, anticipated weight loss results, contraindications/exclusions from medication use, and counseling points to help reduce risk of side effects. The pharmacist can answer questions and employ the teach-back method to ensure communication about the medication was comprehended by the individual.

5. Development of Patient Education Materials

   Pharmacists can utilize available resources created by pharmaceutical companies and national/state pharmacy organizations as well as organizations for diabetes and obesity to create a comprehensive list of educational materials for the patient. These resources can be provided in print, video, and electronic resources. Suggestions for development of effective education materials are as follows:

- Reading level:
  - Aim for a sixth grade reading level as approximately 75% of adult Americans can comfortably read materials at this level.
- Language and vocabulary:
  - Choose simple, common words over medical jargon. For instance, use "pill" instead of "medication," "eat" instead of "consume," and "weigh" instead of "measure."
  - Keep sentences short (around 10 words) and use the active voice.

- Paragraphs and organization:
  - Keep paragraphs short, focusing on one important issue per paragraph.
  - Present information in a logical sequence.
  - Use headings to break up content and make it easier to navigate.

- Visual aids:
  - Include photos, illustrations, and graphics to enhance understanding.
  - Share videos from a reputable source, such as the manufacturer or a national organization.
  - Ensure visual elements align with the content and reinforce key points.
- Typography and layout:
  - Use a font size between 10 and 14 points. Larger fonts benefit elderly individuals and those with impaired vision.

6. Development of Electronic Medical Records

Pharmacists can develop shortcuts for clinical documentation, templates, order sets, and other resources to streamline patient care and medication ordering for management of diabetes and obesity.

7. Follow-Up

When medications are started for diabetes and obesity that promote weight loss, close follow-up is necessary between appointments to assess for safety and efficacy of medication use. For people with diabetes, blood glucose evaluation is necessary within 1–2 weeks of starting a new medication [3–5]. When insulin is initiated or started as an add-on therapy, close follow-up is necessary to prevent hyperglycemia or hypoglycemia. For people experiencing or desiring weight loss, medications for comorbidities, such as hypertension, may need to be adjusted or de-escalated.

Pharmacists can communicate with individuals through electronic medical record, phone calls, in-person visits or telemedicine to assess for medication benefits (weight loss, glucose-lowering effect), side effects, adherence, dietary, and lifestyle changes. Based on patient communication between office visits, pharmacists under collaborative practice agreement or protocols may advise increasing, decreasing, or maintaining current doses of medications for diabetes and obesity until the next office follow-up.

8. Medication Access
   Medications for the treatment of diabetes and obesity often require a prior authorization from the insurance. Pharmacists can review medication formulary, perform insurance benefits investigation, assist with medication prior authorization (along with pharmacy technicians, medical assistants, or nursing support). If an individual is uninsured or underinsured, the pharmacist can work with clinical support staff to complete manufacturer-based medication patient assistance program applications when appropriate.

9. Patient Cost Savings
   Beyond prescribing, pharmacists are aware of the cost burden that many medications for diabetes and obesity can impose on patients. Pharmacists can recommend manufacturer coupons, discount plans through a pharmacy, online discount pharmacy platforms, or other means necessary to facilitate access to the lowest available cost for medications.

10. Comprehensive Care
    Pharmacists provide comprehensive care for people living with diabetes and obesity. Pharmacists ensure appropriate follow-up with referrals to nutrition, ophthalmology, endocrinology, social work, primary care, podiatry, cardiology, nephrology, as well as recommend consultation for nonsurgical and surgical interventions for weight loss. Pharmacists help to achieve quality measures by ensuring patients are up to date with routine labs,

vaccinations, and preventative screenings, facilitating care in people living with diabetes and obesity.

Patient Case Example

A 74-year-old female (she/her) comes to the pharmacist-run outpatient clinic for diabetes management. She has type 2 diabetes mellitus and has recently started using a continuous glucose monitor. She is also interested in medications to help with weight loss.

Vitals	Problem list	Medications	Labs
Height: 5′ 8″ Weight: 240 lb BMI 36.5 kg/m^2 BP: 110/70 mm hg P: 82 bpm	Hypertension History of myocardial infarction (2015) Type 2 diabetes Dyslipidemia Osteoarthritis	Insulin glargine 50 units SubQ in the evening Insulin aspart 15 units SubQ TID before meals Valsartan 160 mg PO QAM Metoprolol succinate ER 25 mg PO QAM Atorvastatin 40 mg PO QAM Aspirin 81 mg PO QAM Acetaminophen 650 mg PO PRN	A1C: 7.4% Glucose: 165 mg/dL LDL-C: 52 mg/dL eGFR: 58 mL/min/1.73 m^2 Microalbumin/creatinine: 12 mg/g

BMI body mass index, *BP* blood pressure, *eGFR* estimated glomerular filtration rate, *ER* extended release, *LDL-C* low-density lipoprotein cholesterol, *P* pulse, *PO* by mouth, *PRN* as needed, *QAM* in the morning, *SubQ* subcutanously, *TID* three times daily

Because the individual has a goal for improved blood glucose with potential for weight loss, the best medication to add at this time is a glucagon-like peptide-1 (GLP-1) or GLP-1/glucose-dependent insulinotropic peptide (GIP) receptor agonist once weekly subcutaneous injection. Since the patient has established atherosclerotic cardiovascular disease, guidelines recommend a GLP-1 receptor agonist or sodium-glucose co-transporter-2 inhibitor with demonstrated cardiovascular disease risk reduction as a part of the glucose-lowering plan. Therefore, semaglutide (oral or subcutaneous (SubQ) injection) or dulaglutide SubQ injection would be preferred in this scenario. Semaglutide SubQ injection proved superiority over dulaglutide SubQ injection in improving glycemic control and reducing body weight and would be the preferred choice in the case scenario [6]. The individual would be recommended to start semaglutide 0.25 mg SubQ once weekly.

Another consideration is the risk of hypoglycemia when adding semaglutide to the individual's regimen with a current A1C of 7.4%. The total daily dose of insulin regimen may be decreased 10–20% before initiation of semaglutide, or blood glucose levels can be monitored closely if the insulin dose is not proactively reduced at the initiation of a GLP or GLP/GIP. A continuous glucose monitor can be utilized to provide frequent blood glucose monitoring or trends with multiple daily injections of insulin [7]. Blood glucose levels and trends can be reevaluated in 4 weeks before it is recommended to titrate semaglutide to 0.5 mg weekly. At that time, an additional 10–20% reduction in insulin may be recommended to prevent hypoglycemia.

Conclusion

Pharmacists are knowledgeable health-care professionals and can provide valuable care to people living with diabetes and obesity in a variety of practice settings.

References

1. Council on Credentialing in Pharmacy. Credentialing and privileging of pharmacists: a resource paper from the council on credentialing in pharmacy. Am J Health Syst Pharm. 2014;71:1891–900.
2. Professional Practice Committee. 10. Cardiovascular disease and risk management: standards of care in diabetes – 2024. Diabetes Care. 2024;47(Suppl. 1):S179–218.
3. Professional Practice Committee. 9. Pharmacologic approaches to glycemic treatment: standards of care in diabetes – 2024. Diabetes Care. 2024;47(Suppl. 1):S158–78.
4. Professional Practice Committee. 8. Obesity and weight management for the prevention and treatment of type 2 diabetes: standards of care in diabetes – 2024. Diabetes Care. 2024;47(Suppl. 1):S145–57.

5. Davies MJ, Aroda VR, Collins BS, et al. Management of hyperglycemia in type 2 diabetes, 2022. A consensus report by the American Diabetes Association (ADA) and the European association for the study of diabetes (EASD). Diabetes Care. 2022;45(11):2753–86.
6. Pratley RE, Aroda VR, Lingvay I, et al. Semaglutide versus dulaglutide once weekly in patients with type 2 diabetes (SUSTAIN 7): a randomised, open-label, phase 3b trial. Lancet Diabetes Endocrinol. 2018;6(4):275–86.
7. Professional Practice Committee. 7. Diabetes technology: standards of care in diabetes – 2024. Diabetes Care. 2024;47(Suppl. 1):S126–44.

Future Research and Practice Changes

17

Meagen Rosenthal

Background

Patient-centered care is defined as "the care that accounts for the values, preferences, and expressed needs of patients when considering how to proceed with specific care and management of individuals' health" [1]. Pharmacists have an essential role in patient-centered outcomes research, along with comparative effectiveness research and implementation science for both diabetes and obesity. For example, pharmacists can develop and support diabetes care and education as training that teaches patients personalized strategies for managing diabetes. Topic areas would include healthy eating, physical activity, monitoring blood sugar, medication adherence, problem-solving skills, health-coping skills, and risk-reduction behavior [2, 3]. Pharmacists can also address social determinants of health, which are conditions where people are born, live, work, play, worship, and age that affect health functioning and quality of life [4].

M. Rosenthal (✉)
Pharmacy Administration, University of Mississippi,
University, MS, USA
e-mail: mmrosent@olemiss.edu

© The Author(s), under exclusive license to Springer Nature Switzerland AG 2025

J. Clements (ed.), *The Pharmacist's Pocket Guide for Diabetes and Obesity*, https://doi.org/10.1007/978-3-031-88835-9_17

The prevalence of both type 2 diabetes (T2D) and obesity has continued to rise in the United States since 2000 [5, 6]. The impact of these conditions has not been equal across all populations in the United States. For example, most recent data show that American Indian or Alaskan Native, non-Hispanic peoples over 18 years of age have a prevalence of diabetes that is roughly 16%, compared to Black, non-Hispanic (12.5%), Asian, non-Hispanic (9.2%), Hispanic (10.3%), or White, non-Hispanic (8.5%) peoples [5]. Furthermore, even with these broad racial categories, there are important subgroup differences (e.g., Asian Indian, non-Hispanic peoples = 10.8% prevalence) [5]. Similar data can also be seen in the prevalence of obesity. Most recent findings suggest that non-Hispanic Black adults have a prevalence of obesity that is 50%, compared to Hispanic adults (45.6%), non-Hispanic White adults (41.4%), and non-Hispanic Asian adults (16.1%) [6].

There are numerous proven behavioral health interventions and medications that slow, and sometimes reverse these conditions. For example, consider diabetes self-management education and support (DSMES). Several recent systematic reviews and meta-analyses have shown that DSMES training has positive impacts on glycemic control, weight loss, diabetes knowledge, self-efficacy, quality of life, dietary behavior, physical activity, smoking cessation, and medication adherence [7, 8]. The strength of this evidence has led to widespread endorsement of DSMES training by a variety of health-care professionals including family physicians, physician assistants, nurse practitioners, and pharmacists [9].

However, access to, and use of, DSMES is not universal. One estimate from 2019 suggested that there were roughly 6000 accredited DSMES sites in the United States to provide services to the more than 30 million people currently diagnosed with diabetes [10]. Furthermore, rates of referral to these existing programs continues to be low, with estimates ranging from fewer than 5–54% of eligible patients being approached [10, 11]. Yet, even among those patients who do manage to receive a referral, it is not uncommon for them to underutilize these programs. For example, in one study, 66% of those referred did not receive any

DSMES training at all, and just 13% received 8 or more hours of the needed training [11].

There are several explanations that have been put forward as to why patients fail to follow through when referred to DSMES programming. A systematic review by Horigan et al., examining why patients declined available placements in diabetes education programs, found two broad categories of reasons [12]. The first set centered around logistical, medical, or financial constraints [12]. For example, some patient education sessions were being held during times or in locations they simply could not access. The second set of reasons for nonattendance to diabetes education programs was related to lack of perceived benefit and emotional or cultural acceptance. Studies found that some patients did not feel that diabetes was a significant problem to worry about in their lives [12]. A similar set of barriers was replicated in a 2021 study and included timing and location of programming, as well as psychological stigma within patients themselves [13].

Efforts to address these barriers have led to calls for DSMES programming to be tailored to the specific needs of various populations, including, but not limited to, disproportionally impacted racial and ethnic groups, people with low health literacy, people who have developmental disabilities, and those people for whom English is a second language [14]. One such program developed to address these concerns is the DEEP™ Program [15]. This program was designed to be used in low-income, racial, and ethnic minority populations, and employs a train-the-trainer model designed to engage community members as resources for others within their own communities [15].

Despite these efforts, patient access and attrition from DSMES programs continues to be problematic. Taking into consideration current reimbursement models tend to focus on the provision of group sessions (REF), it is worth considering whether the access problem could potentially be solved by addressing patient attrition. The remainder of this chapter outlines how understanding patients' perspectives on DSMES programming and diabetes self-management, as well as creation of an approach to integrating new services into pharmacy practice, can help minimize attrition issues and potentially spread DSMES programing more broadly.

Person-Centered Care

Practicing pharmacists are very familiar with the term *person- (or patient-) centered care* [16]. In the most basic sense, person-centered care emphasizes that providers account for the values, preferences, and expressed needs of patients when considering how to proceed with the specific care and management of an individual's health [1]. Pharmacy practice within the United States has encapsulated this process in the pharmacists patient care process, wherein pharmacists are implored to provide holistic care to the people with whom they engage, including considering and making efforts to account for the impact of the social determinants of health [4, 16].

While clinical evidence is mixed on the impact of this model of care regarding patient outcomes, the spirit of person-centered care has permeated all aspects of patient care delivery [17]. Importantly, patients have expressed perceived value in personalized care. For instance, a recent study found that perceptions of patient centeredness by hospitalized patients increased the sense of patient safety [18]. Such findings have prompted many recent works attempting to better measure and understand the perception of patient centeredness from the perspective of patients [19].

Pharmacy-based studies have found that patient-centered medication reviews have been well received by physician collaborators and resulted in improved medication outcomes for patients [20, 21]. Moreover, data show that pharmacists are interested in and willing to integrate these approaches to care within their practices. A recent qualitative study concluded that pharmacists are already actively providing patient-centered care services and are interested in providing more services in the future [22]. This same principle of person centeredness has further made its way into approaches to research design.

Person-Centered Research

This process of melding person-centered care with person-centered research began in 2010, with the passing of the Affordable Care Act [23]. An important part of this legislation was the establishment of the Patient Centered Outcomes Research Institute (PCORI) [24]. PCORI is an independent nonprofit research organization with the mission to generate knowledge to help patients and their families make better informed health decisions [24]. The knowledge generated by PCORI-funded projects primarily comes from comparative effectiveness research (CER) [24]. CER compares two or more evidence-based medical treatments, services, or health-care practices to provide patients, families, and other stakeholders more comprehensive data when making decisions about which treatment or practice might be best for them [24].

As of the writing of this chapter, PCORI has funded nearly 2400 research and related projects. One recent example of a PCORI-funded CER project compared two treatments for myasthenia gravis (an autoimmune disorder) and found that no difference in patient-perceived quality of life (QoL) or clinical outcomes was established [25]. While one treatment found more serious adverse events associated with its use, authors were able to determine that a dose reduction could prevent these outcomes, while maintaining efficacy [25]. When presented in this fashion, data could be helpful to patients when making decisions on a course of treatment. For example, knowledge that QoL and clinical outcomes were similar for each course may provide clinicians confidence in choosing the lower cost option, which would then allow them to maintain the treatment protocol for a longer period.

Another recent study compared the effectiveness of tailored interventions to increase screening for colorectal cancer (CRC) [26]. This study found that patients, who received a mailed DVD containing a tailored message, plus a phone call from a patient navigator, were 4 times more likely to complete CRC screening than those in usual care, and two-and-a-half times more likely to screen compared to those who received only the DVD. In this example, a clinic or health system might be apt to hire a patient navigator, seeing that the time and effort would be offset by increased revenue for the higher quantity of CRC screenings, in addition to improved patient satisfaction given earlier detection in the disease process and improved outcomes [26].

Turning to pharmacy practice, a recent systematic review compared implementation strategies for pharmacist-delivered professional services in the community setting [27]. This systematic review identified six studies: two focused on improved use of medications, three focused on primary care and public health, and one focused on the implementation of services in both categories [27]. The review found that some form of staff training was effective; however, the risk of bias was moderate to critical. Tools used to report outcomes of implementation studies (StaRI tool [28]) were unclear and harms, published protocols, and economic evaluations were not reported [27]. This suggests that there are great opportunities to expand the use of CER research within the pharmacy practice research domain.

Another form of award offered by PCORI focuses on stakeholder engagement research [24]. From the institute's perspective, the engagement of patients and caregivers ensures that the research being funded is more likely to address their specific concerns, and by extension, is more likely to be enacted by stakeholders [29]. Approaches to address engagement can vary along a wide spectrum. Thus, a ten-step framework for continuous patient engagement has been adopted by PCORI and includes the following opportunities for patients to provide feedback [30]:

1. Soliciting topics
2. Prioritizing research
3. Framing the question
4. Selecting comparators and outcomes
5. Creating a conceptual framework
6. Analyzing the plan
7. Collecting the data
8. Reviewing and interpreting results
9. Translating results
10. Disseminating findings

However, the authors recognize that patient-engaged research is relatively new and go on to provide additional details on the kinds of patient-engagement methods that are most appropriate for achieving each of these steps [30]. Authors advocate for the use of focus group meetings for identifying research questions that are important to participants, while interdisciplinary meetings, which include patients, researchers, and other stakeholders, are more appropriate for developing a research plan [30].

A recent scoping review assessed the impact of patient partnerships on research outcomes identified in 14 distinct articles and covered topic areas like chronic conditions, cancer, primary care, and youth [31]. The authors identified six roles for patients in research including steering committee membership, advisory board membership, consultation, codesign, knowledge translation, and research tasks [31]. Looking across each of those forms of patient engagement codesign represents the approach with the greatest amount of patient involvement in the research process. Many included studies had patients sitting on advisory boards or as members of governance structures (nine studies), followed by dissemination efforts (nine studies), and enacting consultant-type roles (eight studies) [31]. A total of six studies had patients involved in research-related processes that include generating research questions or reviewing interview guides [31].

This final observation is not that surprising. Patient codesign runs counter to the historical approach used to conduct research at academic institutions. The traditional model has highly trained individuals making observations in clinical practice and/or via literature scan to identify gaps in practice and proposing and conducting research to address those deficiencies. Patient codesign has the potential to reorient the power structure of research teams by placing the patients in a position of authority by virtue of their lived experience with the condition under investigation. This approach, however, demands more time and greater investment from researchers. With their knowledge of the larger literature, researchers may need to educate patients about existing literature and negotiate with patients about priorities for research questions. In the next section, an example of a project wherein patients were invited to participate in research question writing will be outlined to shed light onto how this process looks like in practice.

The PaRTIClpate Project

The Patient Centered Research to Improve Community Involvement (PaRTICIpate) in diabetes self-management project combined community-based participatory research (CBPR) principles with the indigenous consensus method to emphasize the voice and perspective of patients living with diabetes. This was accomplished through a series of meetings that culminated in the creation of 15 patient-driven research questions. The creation of the research questions took place over 2 years, with six patient team-member meetings across three communities, two additional meetings with researchers and clinicians, and a final day-long large group meeting [32]. The first round of patient team-member meetings was structured to allow patient participants to explore diabetes management broadly and learn about the research process (one meeting was held in each of the participating communities) [32]. These meetings allowed the patient members to get to know the research team. Aside from demographic information collected from participants, no other data was gathered in these meetings [32]. The second patient-team member meetings allowed them to more specifically explore areas wherein they wanted to increase their knowledge around diabetes management, as well as to share how this information would need to be delivered to maximize its benefit to patients [32]. Researchers, clinicians, and other stakeholders were asked to meet just once, given their previous exposure to the content area. During this meeting, these stakeholder participants were asked to share their perspectives on patient needs [32]. The findings from the patient team member and stakeholder meetings were then analyzed and aggregated across the participating communities using qualitative content analysis [33].

Once this data was aggregated and summarized, it was shared with the participants of a day-long event designed to write patient-driven research questions [32]. Patient team members and other stakeholders, who had participated in the previous meetings, were invited to take part in this event, which took place on a university campus [32]. In this meeting, groups of patients were partnered with clinicians, researchers, and stakeholders to write patient-driven research questions using the summaries of second round meeting discussions as a guide [34]. At the conclusion of this meeting, 15 research questions were identified.

The 15 research questions were split into thematic groups, which allowed for further investigation of what information was already available to answer these questions. The thematic groups included: "communication"; "patient knowledge and perceptions"; "diabetes prevention"; and "diabetes management." There were five research questions that fell into the communication theme, two questions in the patient knowledge and perceptions theme, two questions in the diabetes prevention theme, and six questions in the diabetes management theme. An example of a communication research question was, "Can we develop a training program that would better prepare patients for meetings with health-care providers?" [35]. An example of a patient knowledge and perception question was, "How does family history of diabetes affect a patient's diabetes knowledge and motivation for self-care?" [35]. An example of a diabetes prevention question was, "How do we manage weight and diet in younger people with diabetes to prevent long-term complications?" [35]. An example of a diabetes management question was, "How do we tackle the stigma associated with starting insulin?" [36]. Given the broadness of the research questions, the research team decided to apply the scoping review methodology, which enabled the inclusion of a variety of research study designs, from experimental interventions to observational studies, for consideration [37].

After consideration, the research team decided to conduct two scoping reviews. The first scoping review lumped the questions from the communication, patient knowledge and perceptions, and diabetes prevention themes together [35]. The second scoping review focused specifically on diabetes management [36]. This decision was made after completing the first systematic search of the literature and learning that more than 1400 articles were already published about the questions focused on diabetes management specifically [36].

Taken together, these scoping reviews identified three research opportunities. Data showed that for roughly one-third of the research questions, there was already substantial evidence that could be implemented by patients and providers. However, it was clear that patients had either not received this guidance, or had not received it in a way that made it usable to them on daily basis.

The second grouping of cocreated questions offered new insights into previously held notions about a particular topic area. For example, one of the questions, "What is the effect of health-care provider (e.g., general medicine physician vs. specialist), and educational method (patient counseling vs. pamphlets) on patient outcomes?" identified three related studies. The addition of the type of health-care provider (i.e., generalist versus specialist) offered the potential for new insights that were more meaningful to patients and their families [36].

For the final groups of questions, the scoping reviews found that no previous research had been conducted (e.g., How does the provider understanding of the American Diabetes Association treatment guidelines affect patient stress and confusion?) [36]. When considering the magnitude of research conducted for diabetes self-management, this was a truly surprising finding. While it is not clear what the impact of this potential data would be, these questions certainly offer a new perspective on how to assist patients and families in managing this condition.

It is to this first group of questions that the final section of this chapter will draw particular attention toward. Specifically, this section will offer one approach for streamlining and scaling the uptake and use of existing evidence by both patients and providers in the future.

Implementation Science and Pharmacy

Implementation science is a relatively new field of study. Its focus is on, "the scientific study of methods to promote the systematic uptake of research findings and other [evidence based practices

(EBP)] into routine practice" to improve the provision of medicine and by extension, health outcomes [38]. It has been estimated that it takes on average 17 years for an EBP to become part of routine care in health service delivery [39]. This implies that during the intervening years, patients are not benefiting from these practices. Yet, new evidence continues to be developed further extending the timeline for improved health outcomes for all.

Implementation science, like patient-centered research, works to fill a gap in the traditional research paradigm. In the traditional research paradigm, the focus has been exclusively on whether an intervention works in rarified, usually academic medical center-based populations [38]. While this approach does provide a degree of certainty about the efficacy of a treatment or other clinical intervention, it does not provide any information about how that treatment or intervention is best applied to other environments or clinical settings. In fact, a fundamental assumption made by these traditional research approaches is, if the evidence is sound, it will simply be adopted. As a result, treatments and interventions that were meant to have large population health impacts have shown to be disappointing [38]. This has led to increasing criticisms of EBPs and evidence-based medicine, which overlook the fact that these trials, subsequent reviews, and meta-analyses were never intended to account for implementation [40].

At a population health level, implementation science has been seen as a mechanism for health systems to maximize value in the distribution of health-care resources [41]. One of the best-known examples of implementation science integration into a health system is the US Department of Veterans Affairs (USVA) Quality Enhancement Research Initiative (QUERI) [41]. QUERI, which has partnered system administrators with academic researchers, was created to more rapidly implement effective interventions to improve the health of military veterans [41]. Through this partnership, system administrators are exposed to best practices in a clinical area, while academic researchers learn about and account for environmental factors in the design and implementation of their studies. These environmental factors can include limitations with budget, clinical culture, staffing, and variations in the populations of patients being served.

Between 2015 and 2019, QUERI has supported 49 EBPs' implementation across 465 facilities, in collaboration with 71 operations partners, to develop 71 toolkits to support the training of 5147 VA staff members, who serve more than 250,000 Veterans [42]. While data collection on health outcomes for many of these programs was ongoing at the time this evaluation was published, authors could already point to increases in disease screening, appropriate diagnoses, referrals, increased workflow efficiencies, provider satisfaction, improved Veteran satisfaction, and cost savings from avoided hospitalizations [42]. Moreover, two of the EBPs (inpatient walking and a data-driven approach to enhance quality of care for Veterans with transient ischemic attack) have already been selected to for scale-up and spread across the region [42].

Within pharmacy practice, there have been an increasing number of studies and articles that employ aspects of implementation science into their design. For example, there have been studies examining pharmacist-led deprescribing initiatives [43], practice-based research networks [44], the implementation of medication therapy management services [45], medication reviews [46], and the addition of professional services more generally [27]. Two recent reviews of professional service implementation and medication review implementation shed light on additional opportunities for advancing pharmacy practice using implementation science principles [27, 46].

A systematic review designed to assess the comparative effectiveness of implementation strategies for community pharmacist delivered professional services identified six eligible papers [27]. Most of these papers were focused on primary care or public health services and used some form of staff training as the implementation strategy [27]. To evaluate the quality of these studies' descriptions of the implementation strategy, they applied the Standards for Reporting Implementation Studies (StaRI) tool [28]. This tool is broken down into two main sections, the "implementation strategy" and the other being the "intervention" to be implemented and contains a total of 27 items across these categories [28]. The authors of the systematic review found on the implementation strategy level that none of the articles reported any economic evaluation, harms, or a published protocol [27]. They also found no report regarding level of economic evaluation [27].

In a recent scoping review on the implementation of medication reviews within community pharmacy, authors identified 40 original research articles [46]. Only nine of the studies utilized a theoretical framework, model, or tool to guide the implementation strategy and 35 of the studies used an active implementation strategy, characterized by direct involvement from the research team [46]. Of the included articles, 19 used a single implementation strategy, while the remainder were multifaceted, and most measured adoption as the primary outcome. The authors of the scoping review concluded that more experimental research designs are needed to meaningfully evaluate implementation strategies [46].

As such, there appear to be many opportunities for pharmacy practice research, the advancement of integration, and application of implementation science principles in understanding how to scale and spread well-founded EBPs. Whether through the integration of one of the many theoretical models or frameworks [47], partnering with a health economist to evaluate the cost of implementations strategies, or including an implementation scientist on the study team will ensure the best possible design approaches are taken and implementation strategy chosen.

Conclusion

Both person-centered research and implementation science offer unique and innovative approaches for the advancement of pharmacy practice, the benefit of patients, and population health. In this chapter is presented the background and definitions of both person-centered research and implementation science while providing several examples of research projects and literature reviews for each of these approaches from both the general health literature and pharmacy practice perspectives. Finally, opportunities to advance research using each of these methodological perspectives were also outlined. The future of pharmacy practice and related research continue to be bright opportunities to think about our work differently from other disciplines. It is only through this interdisciplinary approach can we hope to truly realize improved health for all.

References

1. Davis K, Schoenbaum SC, Audet AM. A 2020 vision of patient-centered primary care. J Gen Intern Med. 2005;20(10):953.
2. CDC. Diabetes Self-Management Education and Support (DSMES) Toolkit | Diabetes | CDC; 2023. https://www.cdc.gov/diabetes/dsmes-toolkit/index.html. Accessed 20 Nov 2023.
3. Shrivastava SR, Shrivastava PS, Ramasamy J. Role of self-care in management of diabetes mellitus. J Diabetes Metab Disord. 2013;12(1):14.
4. Social Determinants of Health – Healthy People; 2030 | health.gov. https://health.gov/healthypeople/priority-areas/social-determinants-health. Accessed 20 Mar 2024.
5. CDC. Prevalence of Diagnosed Diabetes | Diabetes | CDC; 2022. https://www.cdc.gov/diabetes/data/statistics-report/diagnosed-diabetes.html. Accessed 8 Sep 2023.
6. CDC. New Adult Obesity Maps. Centers for Disease Control and Prevention; 2023. https://www.cdc.gov/obesity/data/prevalence-maps.html. Accessed 14 Sep 2023.
7. Tanaka R, Shibayama T, Sugimoto K, Hidaka K. Diabetes self-management education and support for adults with newly diagnosed type 2 diabetes mellitus: a systematic review and meta-analysis of randomized controlled trials. Diabetes Res Clin Pract. 2020;169:108480.
8. Enricho Nkhoma D, Jenya Soko C, et al. Impact of DSMES app interventions on medication adherence in type 2 diabetes mellitus: systematic review and meta-analysis. BMJ Health Care Inform. 2021;28(1):e100291.
9. Powers MA, Bardsley JK, Cypress M, et al. Diabetes self-management education and support in adults with type 2 diabetes: a consensus report of the American Diabetes Association, the Association of Diabetes Care & Education Specialists, the Academy of Nutrition and Dietetics, the American Academy of Family Physicians, the American Academy of PAs, the American Association of Nurse Practitioners, and the American Pharmacists Association. J Am Pharm Assoc. 2020;60(6):e1–e18.
10. Youssef GA. It's all about access! Diabetes Spectr. 2020;33(1):82–8.
11. Alsayed Hassan D, Curtis A, Kerver J, Vangsnes E. Diabetes self-management education and support: referral and attendance at a patient-centered medical home. J Prim Care Community Health. 2020;11:2150132720967232.
12. Horigan G, Davies M, Findlay-White F, Chaney D, Coates V. Reasons why patients referred to diabetes education programmes choose not to

attend: A systematic review. Diabet Med J Br Diabet Assoc. 2017;34(1):14–26.
13. Hadjiconstantinou M, Quinn LM, Tippins F, et al. A perspective piece on Diabetes Self-Management Education and Support (DSMES) programmes for under-represented groups with T2DM in the UK. Br J Diabetes. 2021;21(1):3–10.
14. Blanchette JE, Aaron SP, Allen NA, Litchman ML. Equity in the provision of diabetes self-management education and support. Diabetes Spectr. 2022;35(3):284–94.
15. DEEP™ Program Overview | Office of Technology Management | University of Illinois Chicago. https://otm.uic.edu/deep-program-2/deep-program-overview-2. Accessed 15 Mar 2024.
16. Olson AW, Burns AL. From patient centered to person centered: the pharmacist's role and value in community-integrated care transformation. J Am Pharm Assoc. 2023;63(3):736–41.
17. Rathert C, Wyrwich MD, Boren SA. Patient-centered care and outcomes: a systematic review of the literature. Med Care Res Rev. 2013;70(4):351–79.
18. Choi N, Kim J, Kim H. The influence of patient-centeredness on patient safety perception among inpatients. PLoS One. 2021;16(2):e0246928.
19. Kim EJ, Nam IC, Koo YR. Reframing patient experience approaches and methods to achieve patient-centeredness in healthcare: scoping review. Int J Environ Res Public Health. 2022;19(15):9163.
20. Sakthong P, Sangthonganotai T. A randomized controlled trial of the impact of pharmacist-led patient-centered pharmaceutical care on patients' medicine therapy-related quality of life. Res Soc Adm Pharm. 2018;14(4):332–9.
21. Basger BJ, Moles RJ, Chen TF. Uptake of pharmacist recommendations by patients after discharge: implementation study of a patient-centered medicines review service. BMC Geriatr. 2023;23(1):183.
22. Daly CJ, Quinn B, Mak A, Jacobs DM. Community pharmacists' perceptions of patient care services within an enhanced service network. Pharm J Pharm Educ Pract. 2020;8(3):172.
23. Rosenbaum S. The patient protection and affordable care act: implications for public health policy and practice. Public Health Rep. 2011;126(1):130–5.
24. About PCORI. About PCORI | PCORI; 2021. https://www.pcori.org/about/about-pcori. Accessed 12 Sep 2022
25. Narayanaswami P, Sanders DB, Thomas L, et al. Comparative effectiveness of azathioprine and mycophenolate mofetil for myasthenia gravis (PROMISE-MG): a prospective cohort study. Lancet Neurol. 2024;23(3):267–76.
26. Rawl SM, Perkins SM, Tong Y, et al. Patient navigation plus tailored digital video disc increases colorectal cancer screening among low-income and minority patients who did not attend a scheduled screening colonoscopy: a randomized trial. Ann Behav Med. 2024;58(5):314–27.

27. Seda V, Moles RJ, Carter SR, Schneider CR. Assessing the comparative effectiveness of implementation strategies for professional services to community pharmacy: a systematic review. Res Soc Adm Pharm. 2022;18(9):3469–83.
28. Pinnock H, Barwick M, Carpenter C, et al. Standards for Reporting Implementation Studies (StaRI): explanation and elaboration document. BMJ Open. 2017;7:e013318.
29. PCORI. The PCORI Strategic Plan: Engagement | PCORI; 2022. https://www.pcori.org/about/about-pcori/pcori-strategic-plan/pcori-strategic-plan-engagement. Accessed 4 Apr 2024
30. Edwards HA, Huang J, Jansky L, Mullins C. What works when: mapping patient and stakeholder engagement methods along the ten-step continuum framework. J Comp Eff Res. 2021;10(12):999–1017.
31. Bird M, Ouellette C, Whitmore C, et al. Preparing for patient partnership: a scoping review of patient partner engagement and evaluation in research. Health Expect. 2020;23(3):523–39.
32. Crumby AS, Holmes ER, Rosenthal M. Patient centered research to improve community involvement (PaRTICIpate) in diabetes self-management: a conference series for developing collaborations between researchers, stakeholders, and patients. J Patient-Rep Outcomes. 2018;2(1):47.
33. Hsieh HF, Shannon SE. Three approaches to qualitative content analysis. Qual Health Res. 2005;15(9):1277–88.
34. PCORI. How to Write a Practical & Useful Research Question. How to Write a Practical & Useful Research Question | PCORI; 2014. https://www.pcori.org/engagement/engage-us/suggest-patient-centered-research-question/how-write-practical-useful-research-question. Accessed 14 Sep 2023.
35. Monika S, Meagen R, Tanvee T, Austin A. Patient centered studies focusing on diabetes self-management: a scoping review. Curr Diabetes Rev. 2020;16(6):557–69.
36. Arnold A, Rosenthal M, Salkar M, et al. Patient centered studies focused on type 2 diabetes management, education, and family support: a scoping review. Curr Diabetes Rev. 2022;18(7):e171121197989.
37. Levac D, Colquhoun HL, O'Brian KK, al. et. Scoping reviews: time for clarity in definition, methods, and reporting. J Clin Epidemiol. 2014;67(12):1291–4.
38. Bauer MS, Damschroder L, Hagedorn H, Smith J, Kilbourne AM. An introduction to implementation science for the non-specialist. BMC Psychol. 2015;3(1):32.
39. Munro CL, Savel RH. Narrowing the 17-Year research to practice gap. Am J Crit Care. 2016;25(3):194–6.
40. Ratnani I, Fatima S, Abid MM, Surani Z, Surani S. Evidence-based medicine: history, review, criticisms, and pitfalls. Cureus. 2023;15(2):e35266.

41. Bauer UE, Briss PA, Goodman RA, Bowman BA. Prevention of chronic disease in the 21st century: elimination of the leading preventable causes of premature death and disability in the USA. Lancet. 2014;384(9937):45–52.
42. Braganza MZ, Kilbourne AM. The Quality Enhancement Research Initiative (QUERI) impact framework: measuring the real-world impact of implementation science. J Gen Intern Med. 2021;36(2):396–403.
43. Alaa Eddine N, Schreiber J, El-Yazbi AF, Shmaytilli H, Amin MEK. A pharmacist-led medication review service with a deprescribing focus guided by implementation science. Front Pharmacol. 2023;14:14.
44. Carpenter DM, Kiser S, Smith M, et al. An implementation science focused practice-based research network for rural community pharmacies: RURAL-CP. Clin Transl Sci. 2024;17(2):e13725.
45. Houle SKD, Charrois TL, Chowdury FF, Tsuyuki RT, Rosenthal M. A randomized controlled study of practice facilitation to improve the provision of medication management services in Alberta community pharmacies. Res Soc Adm Pharm. 2017;13(2):339–48.
46. Brandt J, Lê ML, Jantscher S, et al. Medication review service implementation in community pharmacy settings: scoping review with focus on implementation studies. Res Soc Adm Pharm. 2020;16(7):875–85.
47. Theories, Models, & Frameworks. Implementation science at UW; 2024. https://impsciuw.org/implementation-science/research/frameworks. Accessed 19 June 2024

Index

© The Editor(s) (if applicable) and The Author(s), under exclusive license to Springer Nature Switzerland AG 2025

J. Clements (ed.), *The Pharmacist's Pocket Guide for Diabetes and Obesity*, https://doi.org/10.1007/978-3-031-88835-9